Crib Death - Sudden Infant Death Syndrome (SIDS)

Giulia Ottaviani

Crib Death - Sudden Infant Death Syndrome (SIDS)

Sudden Infant and Perinatal Unexplained Death: The Pathologist's Viewpoint

Second Edition

Springer

Giulia Ottaviani, MD, PhD
Università degli Studi di Milano
Milano
Italy

The University of Texas Health Science Center at Houston
Houston, TX
USA

ISBN 978-3-319-08346-9 ISBN 978-3-319-08347-6 (eBook)
DOI 10.1007/978-3-319-08347-6
Springer Cham Heidelberg Dordrecht London New York

Library of Congress Control Number: 2014946575

Printed on acid-free paper

Springer is part of Springer Science+Business Media (www.springer.com)

A voice is heard in Ramah, lamentation and bitter weeping. Rachel is weeping for her children and refuses to be comforted for her children are no more. (Jeremiah 31:15) [1]

To the memory of my beloved mother, Angela, my first inspiration, and to all parents whose lives are touched by the tragedy of a child's illness or loss.

Reference

1. Holy Bible: New revised standard version catholic edition (NRSV-CE), Catholic Biblical Association (1989) Bible Gateway. http://www.biblegateway.com/. Accessed July 26, 2014.

Foreword to the Second Edition

The second edition of Dr. Giulia Ottaviani's monograph on crib death comes seven years after the first edition of this important work. Some key features of the second edition are reflected in the title and subtitle. The focus has been expanded based on convincing evidence for a continuum involving sudden infant death syndrome (SIDS), sudden perinatal unexpected death (SPUD), and sudden intrauterine death (SIUD). Together these entities continue to constitute a major public health problem with emotionally charged and tragic overtones for the involved parents. SIDS affects one infant in every 1,700–2,000 live births, and represents the most frequent form of demise within the first year of life. SIUD or unexplained stillbirth happens up to ten times more frequently than SIDS. It continues to occur in about half of perinatal deaths in spite of advances in maternal and fetal care. The other key feature of this work is the perspective provided by the viewpoint of a pathologist. Specifically, Dr. Giulia Ottaviani brings to this work very impressive scholarship and a wealth of personal experience in studying and researching this field for many years.

The comprehensive nature of the work is reflected by its organization into five chapters, each of which contains text followed by an extensive list of references and review questions. Chapter 1, Introduction, provides key definitions and also introduces a major focus of the work which is the evolving understanding of the pathogenesis of SIDS and related conditions, based on cardio-respiratory and respiratory-reflexogenic mechanisms, related to minute lesions of the central nervous system, particularly of the brain stem, together with involvement of the cardiac nervous and conduction system. Chapter 2, Techniques and Criteria in Anatomic and Forensic Pathology of SIDS and SIUD, documents in detail a comprehensive approach to documenting the anatomic changes at autopsy. This is an important contribution since these lesions are typically overlooked in routine autopsies. This and other chapters of the book are beautifully illustrated with figures which document gross and histologic features. Chapter 3, Pathological and Related Epidemiological Findings, presents the spectrum of clinical, epidemiological and autopsy findings that may be identified in perinatal and infant deaths, and it provides an expert perspective as to how these findings might explain recognized causes of death in order to distinguish them from SIDS and SIUD. Chapter 4, Moving Forward the Discussion on Sudden Infant and Perinatal Unexplained Death, provides further interpretation and analysis of key findings, weighing the strength of the evidence for their roles in these conditions. The genetics of SIDS and SPUD is discussed here.

Recent developments in genetic testing also are presented. Chapter 5, Concluding Remarks, brings the wealth of information in this work into an integrated perspective.

Dr. Giulia Ottaviani has made the quest for unraveling the pathogenesis of the tragic entity of crib death the major focus of her professional career. Her combination of dedication, passion, experience, scholarship and skill as a writer are clearly manifest in this second edition of her seminal work. Dr. Ottaviani amply makes her case that the initial definition of SIDS as "unexpected death after thorough postmortem examination" should be revised. Rather SIDS, SPUD and SIUD should be considered a spectrum of syndromes in which key anatomic alterations of the central nervous system and cardiac conduction system interact with clinical risk factors to produce the fatal outcome.

In summary, Dr. Giulia Ottaviani has produced an excellent, comprehensive and insightful analysis of crib death based on the unique perspective of a scholarly pathologist. I have been pleased to have her as a colleague at my institution as she has completed the writing of this second edition. I have great admiration for her accomplishment. I think it is mandatory for anyone interested or involved with evaluation of crib deaths to obtain this excellent monograph and to consult it regularly for the insights and perspectives it provides.

March 28, 2014

L. Maximilian Buja, MD
Professor of Pathology and Laboratory Medicine
Distinguished Teaching Professor
Medical School, The University of Texas Health
Science Center at Houston

Chief, Cardiovascular Pathology Research
Texas Heart Institute
Executive Director
The Texas Medical Center Library

Foreword to the First Edition

This new book written by Dr. Giulia Ottaviani is beautifully organized and so well written that it is a genuine pleasure to read. It is enjoyable from both an intellectual and a scientific standpoint. I believe it to be a major contribution, not only to "pathology" as she modestly indicates in the title, but to almost every field of medicine, or to anyone with an intellectual curiosity. But for any special medical discipline it could be a virtual necessity. It should be readily available at locations where medical emergency treatment is necessary, especially in hospital emergency rooms and for ambulance medical services.

Pediatricians, obstetricians, and emergency room nurses will find it enormously valuable. It will also be indispensable in numerous other specialties, particularly cardiology, neurology, and even cardiac surgery. For some particular diseases (such as the long QT syndrome) this book will become essential reading, in part because infants, children, and adults can progress to sudden death with this disease. Very few could have written this book from the standpoint of cardiology and neurology to explain crib death, but I believe that Dr. Ottaviani is uniquely qualified for this mission.

February 4, 2007

Thomas N. James, MD, MACP
Former Chairman of Medicine and Physician in Chief
at the University of Alabama Medical School in Birmingham

Later, President University
of Texas Medical Branch (1987–1997)
Currently Distinguished Professor Emeritus
University of Alabama in Birmingham

Foreword to the First Edition

Infant and perinatal mortality is the most accurate index for evaluating the quality of health in most developed countries. In particular, the fetal mortality rate represents the main indicator of the effectiveness of mother–infant support.

Crib death, also called sudden infant death syndrome (SIDS), strikes an apparently healthy baby every 750–1,000 live births and it is the most frequent natural cause of death in the first year of life. The unexpected death of the near-term fetus and of the newborn in the first week of life is unexplained in 60–80% of cases, even after performing a routine *post mortem* examination. Data from the World Health Organization indicate that fetal death has an incidence of one in every 100–200 pregnancies in developed countries. Its frequency is therefore six to seven times greater than that of SIDS, and has not significantly decreased during recent years, mainly because of limited research activity.

The results of in-depth investigations performed at the Institute of Pathology of the University of Milan have contributed to the identification of the nature and location of the alterations, common to both SIDS and fetal death, underlying the onset of lethal nervous reflexes. They are mostly congenital anomalies of the vegetative nervous system and/or of the cardiac conduction system, i.e. of the electric switchboard of the heart, which is also under the control of the autonomic nervous system.

Italian Law n° 31 of February 2, 2006 "Regulations for diagnostic *post mortem* investigation in victims of sudden infant death syndrome (SIDS) and unexpected fetal death" represents a milestone in health politics. It has been new and revolutionary and states fundamental rules to significantly reduce the toll in human life: the promotion of anatomo-clinical, genetic and epidemiological research, and awareness and information campaigns, and the implementation of programs and projects for the psychological support of victims' families.

The need to submit these small victims to *post mortem* examination and to accurate histological investigations is unanimously recognized. Prevention is mainly based on the recognition of lesions detectable in various organs, particularly of the autonomic nervous system regulating the vital activities (respiratory, cardiac, digestive and arousal) and of the pathogenic role of the major risk factors (cigarette smoking and maternal alcoholism, air pollution, sedatives, etc.).

Being a problem of high scientific complexity, the law enacts rules for the post-mortem procedures, with the necessary parents' consent, and it establishes criteria to identify local reference centers, with recognized professional and scientific competences, according to the diagnostic guidelines devised by the Institute of Pathology of the University of Milan.

In the present book a systematic study is presented of the autonomic nervous system and cardiac conduction system in a large number of infants and fetuses dying suddenly and unexpectedly, as well as in age-matched control cases. The purpose of this book is to describe the nervous and cardiac histopathological findings and to describe an investigated standardized *post mortem* protocol to apply to all cases of sudden unexpected infant and perinatal death.

I wish this monograph all the success it deserves. The book is aimed at pathologists, neonatologists, pediatricians and researchers with a university degree in medicine or biology, laboratory histotechnicians, pediatric nurses, as well as medical students and general practitioners. I am sure that the readers will be able to learn from it useful tools and hints to apply in their research and practice.

January 30, 2007

Luigi Matturri, MD
Full Professor of Pathology
Chairman, Institute of Pathology
University of Milan

Preface to Second Edition

It is a great pleasure for me to accept Springer's invitation for a second edition of my monograph *Crib Death. Sudden Unexplained Death of Infants: The Pathologist's Viewpoint*. This book has been re-written in 2014 with the new title *Crib Death – Sudden Infant Death Syndrome (SIDS). Sudden Infant and Perinatal Unexplained Death: The Pathologist's Viewpoint*". I hope it continues to promulgate the importance of anatomo-pathological studies and findings in the expanding field of SIDS and sudden unexplained perinatal death.

The first edition of this monograph, published in 2007, was in part based on my Ph.D. dissertation defended at the University of Milan in 2004, which was judged to be "suitable for publication" by the board committee. This book has had forewords written by two eminent pathologists, the international experts Prof. Luigi Matturri and Prof. Thomas N. James, both my greatly appreciated teachers, who, together with Prof. Lino Rossi, have been pioneers in the field of the cardiac conduction and the autonomic nervous systems investigation. The reviews of Profs. Syed A. Hoda and Brian D. Robinson on *JAMA* [1], Charles I. Berul on *Circulation* [2], Cristina Basso on *Cardiovascular Pathology* [3] and Gaetano Thiene on *Journal of Cardiovascular Medicine* [4] emphasized the international relevance of the monograph and its importance to specialized teaching and learning histopathological methods in the field of SIDS.

In the seven years since I published the first edition of this book its relevance has continued to grow. The studies on SIDS have been changing and evolving and now encompass sudden perinatal unexplained/unexpected death (SPUD). This revised edition intends to present an updated and expanded text that derives from my experience of over ten years in postmortem investigations, research, and teaching the methods, criteria, and pathological findings of sudden unexplained infant and perinatal death to medical students, residents, fellows, and PhD candidates at the University of Milan, Italy.

The unexpected death of infants has become over the centuries commonly known as crib death in the United States or cot death in the United Kingdom, terms which are still widely used, practically synonymously with SIDS. I wish to underline that SIDS and sudden perinatal unexplained death are considered diagnoses by exclusion as no cause of death is found and the death has been considered *sine materia* and *sine causa*, i.e., without pathological findings and without any evident cause.

Understanding SIDS and sudden perinatal unexplained death is one of the most important challenges for parents, caregivers and physicians worldwide. The sudden unexpected death of a baby in the crib and, even worse, in a mother's womb is surely one of the most heartbreaking tragedies for the family and for society. From the happy event or anticipation of the baby's birth, often a "planned" birth, the parents and even the physicians suddenly have to face the overwhelming grief related to this "unplanned", unexpected death. The sudden and unexpected loss of a child goes beyond any ordinary life and death succession. The tragedy of such loss was expressed by Euripides, who wrote: "*What greater pain can mortals bear than this, to see their children die before their eyes*?".

Everyone who reads this book has always to keep in mind that the sudden unexplained perinatal and infant death is the leading form of death in otherwise healthy babies *in utero* and within the first year of postnatal life.

Most of the people and even physicians underestimate the frequency of this problem and do not know how devastating its consequences are. The sudden unexpected death of a baby is so out of order with the sequence of life, birth, and death that there has been no preparation. The parents' terrible loss is then compounded by feelings of guilt; they blame themselves for overlooking baby's possible symptoms or signs. Poignantly and most sadly, the death occurs too often when no one is around, with the dead infant or fetus only being discovered later. After an unexpected sudden infant or fetal death, a *post mortem* examination has to be performed. This involves examination of the body, organs, and tissues by a pathologist who should always analyze the cardiac conduction system and the brainstem on serial sections.

The continued investigations on SIDS and unexplained stillbirth have been moving forward at an accelerated rate. In this monograph, a systematic study of SIDS and sudden unexplained/unexpected perinatal death pathology is provided along with examination-type multiple-choice questions related to each chapter for independent study and self-assessment. In particular, a systematic study of the cardiac conduction system and of the autonomic nervous system is carried out in a large number of cases.

The first edition has been selling well and it continues to sell year after year. I am pleased and proud to know that hundreds of readers have been helped by it in their studies and research. This second edition is intended to help many more. Comments and suggestions of readers have helped to write this revised edition and will help to improve future editions of this work.

I wish to transmit the current and expanding state of knowledge of SIDS and sudden perinatal death pathology to all readers. This book is designed to keep everyone aware of, involved in, and updated to the current state of the science of SIDS. I hope that this, as the previous edition, continues to fulfill and expand its goals.

Houston, TX Giulia Ottaviani, MD, PhD

References

1. Hoda SA, Robinson BD (2008) Crib death: sudden unexplained death of infants – the pathologist's viewpoint. JAMA 209:1073–1074. http://users.unimi.it/giuliaottaviani/pdf/jama_08.pdf. Accessed July 26, 2014.
2. Berul CI (2008) Crib death: sudden unexplained death of infants – the pathologist's viewpoint. Circulation 117:e173. http://circ.ahajournals.org/content/117/9/e173.full. Accessed July 26, 2014.
3. Basso C (2008) Crib death. Sudden unexplained death of infants: the pathologist's viewpoint. Cardiovasc Pathol 17:256–257. doi:10.1016/j.carpath.2008.04.002.
4. Thiene G (2008) Crib death. Sudden unexplained death of infants: the pathologist's viewpoint. J Cardiovasc Med 9:978. doi:10.2459/JCM.0b013e3282ffd765. http://journals.lww.com/jcardiovascularmedicine/Citation/2008/09000/Crib_death__Sudden_unexplained_death_of_infants_.27.aspx. Accessed July 26, 2014.

Acknowledgments

I am always very grateful to Prof. Luigi Matturri, MD, President of the "Lino Rossi" Research Center for the study and prevention of the unexpected perinatal death and of the sudden infant death syndrome (SIDS), University of Milan, for heartily encouraging me to pursue academic research on the pathology of sudden unexpected infant and perinatal death, from the early years of my medical studies, throughout my residency and PhD program, up to my work as an Assistant Professor of Pathology with tenure at the University of Milan. His valuable support, teaching and mentoring throughout the years made this book possible since its first edition.

I pay respectful tributes to the memory of my valued and much appreciated teachers, Prof. Lino Rossi, MD, University of Milan, Honorary Fellow of the American Heart Association Council on Clinical Cardiology, and to Prof. Thomas N. James, MD, MACP, University of Texas Medical Branch at Galveston, for their everlasting teachings, guidance, support and encouragements.

I wish to thank Prof. Pier Alberto Bertazzi, MD, MPH, Director of the Department of Clinical Sciences and Community Health, University of Milan, for supporting me during this research work, for granting me the official leave in my position as a researcher that allowed me the freedom in my research and allowed me to enhance my academic credentials in the USA. A special thanks go to the histotechnicians who have worked in the "Lino Rossi" laboratories during my tenure at the University of Milan. This research work has been supported by the FIRST and PUR Funding, University of Milan, for the years 2006–2013.

Finally, I offer my heartly thanks and regards to Prof. L. Maximilian Buja, MD, for the privilege of appointing me as a Visiting Professor at the Department of Pathology and Laboratory Medicine, University of Texas Health Science Center at Houston, TX, during the completion of this book's revised edition, and for sharing with me his knowledge of anatomic and cardiovascular pathology, and serving as a role model for excellence in academics.

Contents

Introduction to Sudden Infant and Perinatal Unexplained Death

1

Sudden and unexpected death of a young baby in the crib is surely one of the most emotional tragedies that any parent can experience. An understandable continued and growing concern has led to a search for an explanation with the goal of being able to quickly diagnose or predict infant and perinatal sudden unexpected death.

Sudden infant death syndrome (SIDS) or crib death is defined as "the sudden death of an infant under one year of age which remains unexplained after a thorough case investigation, including performance of a complete autopsy, examination of the death scene, and review of the clinical history" [246]. Crib death is the most frequent form of death in infants between one month and one year of age, accounting for 0.47 death per 1,000 births in the USA, striking one infant every 1,700–2,000 [31]. The emotional consequences among families are devastating, and the social cost is high, especially considering the early loss of many potentially productive individuals. Poignantly and perhaps most sadly, the death occurs too often when no-one is around, with the dead baby only being discovered later. SIDS represents a great enigma as one of the main open issues in the social–medical and scientific setting of modern medicine. Despite a wide spectrum of proposed theories, its etiology remains uncertain.

The most important pathogenetic theories in SIDS are the respiratory (apnea), the cardiac (arrhythmogenic), and the visceral dyskinetic (glottic spasm and/or esophagogastric reflux) theories [70, 71, 205]. It has been stressed that neurogenic factors play a role in all these theories, but particularly in the cardiac arrhythmogenic one since the cardiac conduction system and the accessory pathways are strictly controlled by the respiratory, cardiovascular, and upper digestive autonomic nervous system [49, 67, 103, 113, 136, 138].

There is an association between SIDS and sleep, and there are data indicating impaired autonomic function in infants who subsequently die of SIDS, or suffer from Apparent Life Threatening Events (ALTE) [67, 70, 184].

G. Ottaviani, *Crib Death - Sudden Infant Death Syndrome (SIDS): Sudden Infant and Perinatal Unexplained Death: The Pathologist's Viewpoint*,
DOI 10.1007/978-3-319-08347-6_1

Sudden intrauterine unexplained death (SIUD) is the late fetal death before complete expulsion or removal of the fetus from the mother ≥22 weeks of gestation or ≥500 gm body mass which is unexpected by history and is unexplained after a thorough pathological exam of the fetus and the fetal adnexa [40, 56, 99, 177]. Advances in maternal and fetal care have produced a significant reduction in perinatal mortality [125], but have not significantly changed the prevalence of SIUD. About one-half of perinatal mortalities are unexpected.

The definition of SIDS and sudden unexplained perinatal death as "unexplained" should be revised as studies performed on a large number of cases [136–138, 140, 142–146] indicate that a cardio-respiratory and respiratory–reflexogenic pathology, due to minute lesions of the central nervous system (particularly of the brainstem, the site of confluence of the vagosympathetic reflexes), should be considered significant, together with the involvement of the cardiac nervous and conduction system, lamentably routinely overlooked in necroscopy studies.

Pathologically, SIDS can be included in the extended domain of perinatal-infant pathology, as a continuity of cardiac conduction system and autonomic nervous system findings have been detected without a clear separation between unexplained perinatal and infant death [153, 185, 186]. The in-depth *post mortem* examination is equally mandatory in every case of sudden unexpected infant and perinatal death, i.e., SIUD and sudden neonatal unexplained death (SNUD).

It should be underlined that the primary risk factors for the sudden unexplained perinatal-infant death include exposure to cigarette smoke that, starting *in utero*, acts as a causative agent and triggering factor in vulnerable infants with developmental abnormalities in the cardiac conduction system and/or autonomic nervous system detected at necropsy examinations after the unexpected demise, not definitely separable from the unifying concept of the syndrome.

Sudden infant and perinatal unexplained death (SIDS/SIUD/SNUD) "grey zone" or borderline is a new category in which the sudden death is concomitant with other pathologies, such as a broncho-pneumonic infection or a chorionamnionitis. These concurrent pathologies act as a triggering phenomenon in particularly vulnerable infants or fetuses [152, 171, 179]. Under this model, sudden death would not occur in a baby with pre-existing neuroautonomic or cardiac alterations unless a new pathological event takes place. Therefore, the accurate clinical examination is also essential, since any possible symptom or sign cannot be neglected.

In this book it is reviewed the systematic study of the autonomic nervous system and cardiac conduction system performed in a large number of infants and fetuses dying suddenly and unexpectedly, as well as in age-matched controls. The cardiac and neuropathological findings are described. The relationships between SNUD and SIUD – together collected as sudden perinatal unexplained death (SPUD) – and SIDS are discussed. The purpose of this book is to review all the possible morphological bases of SIDS and to discuss standardized investigational studies to be performed in an autopsy protocol to apply to all cases of sudden unexplained infant and perinatal death.

1.1 Sudden Infant Death Syndrome (SIDS)

1.1.1 History and Definition

The unexpected and sudden death of an apparently healthy infant has been for thousands of years the most devastating event that any parent could experience.

Historically, the aim of investigations into the cause of SIDS was to seek out a potential single cause that could then be held responsible for all cases that occurred [23]. Nevertheless, in the literature of all times, the sudden unexpected infant death has been attributed to multiple causes, and even nowadays cannot be characterized by a unifying etiological concept, so that the term "syndrome" has been adopted.

The earliest report of sudden unexpected infant death, is in the Holy Bible, dating to 950 B.C.E., that describes an infant brought to King Solomon dead as a result of being "overlaid": "*Later, two women who were prostitutes came to the king and stood before him. The one woman said, "Please, my lord, this woman and I live in the same house; and I gave birth while she was in the house. Then on the third day after I gave birth, this woman also gave birth. We were together; there was no one else with us in the house, only the two of us were in the house. Then this woman's son died in the night, because she lay on him*" (*1 Kings 3:16–19*). After finding a baby dead, both women claimed to be the mother of the living son and were brought to king Solomon for a judgment as both said that the dead boy belonged to the other one. Solomon said that there was only one fair solution: the live son must be split in two by a sword, each woman receiving half of the child. But the woman whose son was alive said to the king — because compassion for her son burned within her — "*Please, my lord, give her the living boy; certainly do not kill him!*". The other said, "*It shall be neither mine nor yours; divide it*". Then the king responded: "*Give the first woman the living boy; do not kill him. She is his mother*" (*1 Kings 3:26–27*) [77]. To this day, a judgment of Solomon is synonymous with a wise decision in a difficult dispute.

In Babylonia the cause of sudden infant death was attributed to Larbatu, a demon god.

In the fourth century B.C.E., a record of sudden unexpected infant death was from Euripides, a Greek tragedian of classical Athens: "*What greater pain can mortals bear than this; to see their children die before their eyes?*".

In the first century B.C.E., the Latin literature has many references to sudden infant death as for instance in the sixth book of Virgil's Aeneid [212].

In early history, overlying was considered to be the cause of sudden infant death. Infants dying suddenly and unexpectedly were thought to be suffocated by mothers or bed clothes. A mother whose child died of overlaying was punished. According to the historian Diodorus Siculus, who wrote history between 60 and 30 B.C.E., in Egypt, about the time of King Solomon, mothers judged responsible for overlaying were condemned to hug the infant for 3 days and nights as punishment for their neglect [212].

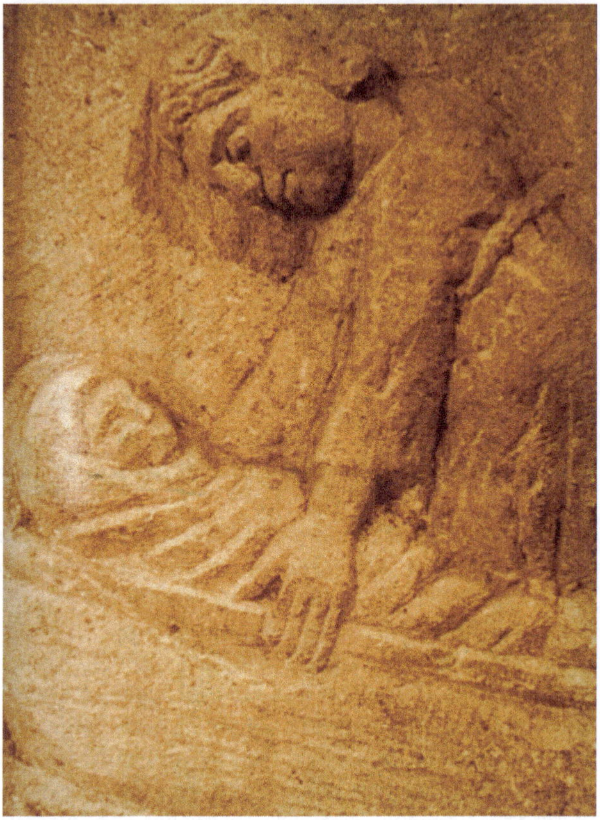

Fig. 1.1 Early representation of crib death in this sculpture dating to 250 A.D. which can be seen at the Cologne museum. The *nutrix Severina* is looking at an infant dead in the crib. This image is adopted as the symbol of the "Lino Rossi" Research Center for the study and prevention of the unexpected perinatal death and SIDS, University of Milan, Italy

An early representation of sudden infant unexpected death is a sculpture dating to 250 A.D. showing the *nutrix Severina* looking at an infant dead in the crib (Cologne museum, Germany) (Fig. 1.1).

In the second century, the first medical report on the danger of overlaying causing soffucation was in a gynecology book by Soranus of Ephesus [225], stating that the infant should be placed in a cradle.

Overlying was considered a common form of infanticide. The early Catholic church did not punish infanticide until the eighth century and even then it was considered only a venial sin [67].

In the twelfth century, a Medieval book by the Welsh priest Giraldus Cambrensis, reported a mother that overlaid her baby that "with more affection than prudence she had brought into her own bed". The Britain's *Children and Young Person's Act* criminally punished adults who in a drunken state slept in a bed with an infant who was later found dead.

In the thirteenth century, a German placard stated that mothers were forbidden to take infants under 3 years into their beds at night [212].

In the fifteenth century, Platter [189], a Swiss physician, was the first to describe infant death due to a large thymus, as translated in 1925 by Ruhrah [211]. However, the translation by Ruharah [211] was faulty, as the original Latin [189] refers to goiter, which was endemic in the Alps.

In the seventeenth century in Sweden, a mother whose child had died was judged by the church. If the church found the mother guilty of overlaying, she was placed in a pillory in front of the church and lost her standing in the church and community. After a public confession, she could be reinstated into the church and community.

In the seventeenth century, the first preventive measure was introduced in Italy, the *arcuccio*, a wood and iron device with arches, resembling a covered wagon, to prevent the mother to roll over the infant and subsequently prevent infant's suffocation. The infant death occurring in absence of the use of this device was punished by the church with excommunication. The punishment was more severe for unmarried mothers who were considered more suspects for infanticide [67].

In the eighteenth century, as described by St. John [228], the *arcuccio* invention reached England, and references of its use are found in Italy up to 1890.

In 1889, Yeats [250], in his poem "Ballad of Moll Magee", described a baby found dead due to overlay: "*…I lay upon my baby. Ye little childer dear, I looked on my cold baby…*".

In the nineteenth century it was found upon autopsy that victims of crib death had an enlarged thymus gland when compared to infants that had died of a chronic disease. At the time, it was thought an enlarged thymus could impinge upon the trachea during sleep resulting in death. In 1830, Kopp [110] reported the first observation of "thymic asthma" in which the thymus impinges directly on the trachea. This quickly gained international acceptance and "Kopp's asthma" [82] is still found in current medical diagnostic codes.

In 1834, Fearn [48] reported on *Lancet* the "Sudden and unexplained death in children", describing two infants aged 5 and 6 months with the same postmortem findings of healthy appearance and concluding that the death may have occurred from a "sudden and violent action of the heart", excluding overlaying. In 1855, Wakely [242] published on *Lancet* an Editorial that dismissed the idea of overlaying.

In 1842, Lee [119] described the removal of thymus to treat thymic asthma as "decisive, because after its performance the infant would not likely be troubled with this or any other complaint!" In 1858, Friedleben [55] published a monograph rejecting the thymic asthma. In 1889, Paltauf [187], while rejecting the theory that thymus exerted lethal pressure on trachea, observed enlarged thymuses compressing the aorta in infants dying unexpectedly, invoking a constitutional illness due to hyperplasia of the entire lymphatic system. In 1896, Escherich [45] named this disease as "Status thymico-lymphaticus". In 1927, Lucas [123] gave advice on preventing the status thymico-lymphaticus with throat irradiation. In the same year, Boyd [19] showed that a stressor, i.e., malnutrition, caused thymic shrinking and suggested that the status thymico-lymphaticus of children who died suddenly might be an artifact. Only in 1945, Nelson [163] concluded that the status thymico-lymphaticus was an artifact and that its treatment was a disaster.

In 1892, Templeman [234] reported the potential role of excessive alcohol consumption and overlaying. He studied postmortem 258 infants dying suddenly and unexpectedly attributing them to suffocation, more than half of deaths occurring

Saturday night. He postulated that alcohol intoxication impaired arousal responses of parents sleeping with infants, thus increasing the risk of accidental suffocation. Templeman [234] also reported an increased incidence of overlaying and sudden infant death in winter time due to huddling of a family in a single bed.

Until the twentieth century, infants were placed to sleep in the family bed, except in the upper class families [108], so that when a sudden infant death occurred in the maternal bed, it was natural for everyone to assume that the baby had been suffocated by being overlaid [212]. Later after cribs and cradles had been invented, the idea of accidental overlaying was gradually abandoned. The diagnosis of overlaying could not be applied to an infant that had died in a separate bed from the mother [195]. The unexpected death of infants has become over the centuries commonly known as crib death in the USA or cot death in the UK, terms which are still widely used, practically synonymously with SIDS.

In 1923, Still [230] first suggested sleep apnea as a cause of crib death, describing in five infants an abrupt cessation of sleep, followed by cyanosis. Between the apnea episodes the infants were unremarkable to observation, though only one survived after receiving artificial respiration, i.e., representing the first near-SIDS case by today's standards. An apnea monitor was recommended to detect and prevent crib death. At the time, an apnea monitor consisted of round-the-clock observation by a trained medical professional [67, 230].

In 1938, Goldbloom and Wigglesworth [62] reported a *post mortem* evidence of respiratory infection in 63% of sudden infant deaths, without specific bacteria found. In 1945, Woolley [249] diagnosed the unexpected infant deaths as suffocation by bed linen or posture. The diagnosis of suffocation was based on the assumption that petechiae noted in the thoracic cavity upon *post mortem* examination could only have resulted from the act of suffocation. This idea received criticism as it did not explain why a weaker infant less than 28 days old had a lower incidence of crib death than a larger infant aged 28 days to 6 months. It was supposed by critics that an older infant was more mobile and less likely to be trapped in bedding than a smaller weaker infant and, therefore, was less likely to be suffocated while sleeping. Additionally, petechiae were not present in all SIDS infants [38, 195].

In 1956, Adelson and Kinney [1] published the first systematic epidemiological report on crib death. The report stated that certain groups of infants were more likely to be victims of crib death. These included male infants, black infants, premature infants, and infants with a history of upper respiratory infection within the 10 days prior to death. Additionally, this report ruled out low levels of gamma globulins as a predisposing factor for infant infection.

In 1963, the first international conference on sudden infant death syndrome was held in Seattle, WA [2]. Detailed gross and histopathological photographs were presented at the conference and published. Statistics were presented showing that sudden infant death syndrome also occurs in higher socioeconomic groups, in any sleeping position and while awake, and that 31% of victims were born premature and many were underweight. It was also concluded that any relationship of SIDS to a virus was nonspecific, as viral isolation had been done successfully in only one-quarter of all case.

In 1968, James [84] published the first evidence of a morphologically definable substrates for cardiac arrhythmias in crib death, analyzing in details the cardiac conduction system.

In 1969, the term Sudden Infant Death Syndrome (SIDS) was first proposed at the second international conference held in Seattle, WA [12], for a distinctive subgroup of unexpected infant deaths that occur during the postneonatal period with consistent clinical, epidemiological, and pathological features. At this conference an updated definition of SIDS was agreed upon. Since then, the term SIDS rapidly achieved a wide international use and acceptance up to now, as evident from the ensuing thousands of articles on SIDS. The 1969 definition of SIDS is as follows: "The sudden death of any infant or young child, which is unexpected by history, and in which a thorough *post mortem* examination fails to demonstrate an adequate cause for death" [12]. This definition contains no limiting criteria, such as a specific age, lists none of the features common to most cases, and suggests that this syndrome is only one of exclusion. Clinical data and death scene investigation are not mentioned, leading to subsequent critics [14]. Sleep apnea was put to the conference as a possible cause of SIDS, and apnea monitoring was suggested to prevent these deaths. Also presented at the conference was the idea that SIDS was the result of a general vulnerability and combined immaturity interacting with coincidental additional less-common events. This idea of interacting events as a cause of SIDS was termed the "multifactorial theory" [195].

In 1970, a symposium was held on sudden and unexpected deaths in infancy in Cambridge, UK [26]. At this conference emerged the idea that somewhere there should be a "near miss" form of SIDS.

In 1974, a conference on SIDS was held in Toronto [229]. At this conference it was agreed that the retention of brown fat in the periadrenal area is the result of hypoxia. This retention in some cases was considered possibly due to exposure of the infant to cigarette smoke. It was further determined that the primary problem in SIDS is the failure of the infant to rouse after an apnea event. It was thought that an infant less than one month old has enough remaining anaerobic metabolism after birth to survive an apnea event. It was also thought at this time that an older infant has a decrease in anaerobic metabolism resulting in a decreased ability to survive an apnea event. Additionally, failure to keep the initial follow-up appointment after hospital discharge was associated with a higher rate of SIDS.

In 1976, Naeye [162] introduced the brainstem hypothesis of SIDS.

In 1991, Willinger et al. [246] published the following new definition of SIDS as redefined by the National Institute of Child Health and Human Development (NICHD) panel convened in 1989: "The sudden death of an infant under one year of age, which remains unexplained after a thorough case investigation, including performance of a complete autopsy, examination of the death scene, and review of the clinical history". Only four of the twelve invited participants and neither of the co-chairs were pathologists, so that most of them had little knowledge of the issues involved in defining cause of death from autopsy examinations. SIDS is a diagnosis made by pathologists, based primarily on autopsy findings and death investigation. It therefore seems appropriate that pathologists should play the leading role in establishing definitional criteria, with other disciplines providing advice and consultation [14]. For over 20 years this definition has been largely adopted all over the world.

In 1992, the American Academy of Pediatrics [4] recommended that infants be laid down for sleep in a nonprone position as a strategy to reduce the risk of SIDS.

In 1993, at the Second SIDS International Conference [13], SIDS was subsequently divided into Category I "typical", Category II "atypical", and Category III where autopsies were not performed, but this further classification failed to gain wide acceptance.

In 1994, the official federal "Back to Sleep" campaign [159, 247] was launched in the USA, by the NICHD jointly sponsored by the AAP, advising caregivers to place infants to sleep on their back or side. Later, also the side position in the crib has been recommended to be avoided [231]. The AAP safe sleep recommendations [231], revised over the years, have the purpose of reducing the risk of infant death from SIDS as well as death from known sleep-related causes. A significant reduction of SIDS incidence has been associated with the "back to sleep" campaign over the last 20 years. According to the NICHD, since that campaign started, the percentage of infants placed on their backs to sleep has increased dramatically, and the overall SIDS rates have declined by more than 50% [5, 159]. The SIDS rate subsequently plateaued [236]. The "Safe to Sleep" campaign, formerly known as the "Back to Sleep" campaign, is the registered trademark of the U.S. Department of Health and Human Services as public education campaign [159] to spread the safe sleep messages to millions of people in communities throughout the world.

In 1994, Filiano and Kinney [50] introduced the triple risk model. This states that SIDS results from the interaction of three overlapping factors: (1) vulnerable infant with an underlying susceptibility, (2) critical developmental time period in homeostatic control with a peak at 2–4 postnatal months, and (3) exogenous stressor/s at the time of death. Current SIDS research [231] supports this theory that intrinsic and extrinsic risk factors provides unification into the underlying triple-risk model.

In 2001, in Italy, the honorable Dr. R. Calderoli [24], presented to the House of Representatives the bill ° 396 of 07-05-2001 "*Post mortem* regulation on SIDS and unexpected fetal death victims", later approved by the Senate of the Italian Republic.

In 2004, Krous et al. [111] defined SIDS as "the sudden unexpected death of an infant less than one year of age, with onset of the fatal episode apparently occurring during sleep, that remains unexplained after a thorough investigation, including performance of a complete autopsy and review of the circumstances of death and the clinical history".

In 2006, the Italian Law n° 31 [36], "Regulations for diagnostic *post mortem* investigation in victims of sudden infant death syndrome and unexpected fetal death" was introduced, imposing rules for postmortem procedures and cases referral, according to standardized diagnostic guidelines [143, 145, 153].

In 2008, then US Senator Barack Obama [191] introduced the Preventing Stillbirth and Sudden Unexpected Infant Death Act, which will enhance public health activities related to understanding and preventing stillbirth and sudden unexpected infant deaths.

Recently, the Centers for Disease Control and Prevention (CDC) [33] has described the SIDS as a subset of "sudden unexpected infant deaths" (SUID). SUID is defined as "sudden unexpected infant deaths are defined as deaths in infants less than one year of age that occur suddenly and unexpectedly, and whose cause of death are not immediately obvious prior to investigation". SIDS represents 50% of SUID deaths.

Currently, the SIDS is attributed to multiple causes, and therefore cannot be characterized by a unifying etiological concept, and this is why the term "syndrome", i.e. the simultaneous manifestation of preliminary and/or terminal symptoms, is still adopted to describe this common form of death in infancy.

The current definition of SIDS as "unexplained after thorough postmortem examination" [246] is hereby under review as the cardiac conduction and brainstem findings described in SIDS cases are indeed the morphological substrates for the sudden unexpected infant and perinatal death. According to Matturri et al. [137], "the sudden death of an infant under one year of age which remains unexplained after a thorough case investigation, including performance of a complete autopsy, examination of the death scene, and review of the clinical history" [246] should be modified by the addition of "complete autopsy examination with an in-depth histopathological analysis of the autonomic nervous system and of the cardiac conduction system that can only be entrusted to experienced reliable pathologists".

1.1.2 Epidemiology and Risk Factors

In the industrialized countries, SIDS is the most frequent form of death in apparently healthy infants between one month and one year of age, striking one every 1,700–2,000 otherwise healthy infants. According to Centers for Disease Control and Prevention (CDC) [31], from 2009 to 2010 the SIDS rate has dropped from 0.54 to 0.47 per 1,000 births.

SIDS occurs within the first year of life, with a maximum incidence in the first 6 months of life and a peak incidence from the second to the fourth month [78, 149]. Death generally occurs during sleep, in prone sleep position [247], almost always at night between 10 p.m. and 7 a.m. [73]. SIDS is more frequent in males [149, 157], in twins [98], in premature infants [73, 129], in infants with a low weight at birth [18], during the winter months [67, 149], in urban areas [109], in children exposed to thermal stress [72, 190, 215], bed sharing [27, 75], and in families with a low economic level [9]. The mothers of SIDS infants more frequently are young and unmarried [9] and have more children [9, 73] with a short interval between pregnancies [226], and are more frequently smokers [107, 149, 222], drug addicts [47] or alcoholics [164, 222]. SIDS infants are more frequently the sibling of an infant that previously died of SIDS [73]. Most SIDS victims suffered from infection of the upper respiratory pathways [51, 131, 243]. Over the years, numerous investigations [5, 21, 96, 156, 233] have been carried out to identify the possible risk represented by the type of mattress, bedding, and pillows.

The parents of a SIDS infant, besides suffering the obvious emotional consequences of the loss of a child [20, 240], also face problems of a juridical nature, as they are immediately questioned to determine whether they provoked the death of their own child [6, 15]. Besides the psychological trauma from the loss of a child [240], the judicial investigation and forensic autopsy is often the cause of additional suffering.

Table 1.1 Risk factors for SIDS

Risk factors	Preventive interventions
Amenable to interventions	
Cigarette smoking by parents/ caregivers	Stop smoking
Substance-abusing mother	Diagnosis and treatment
Formula feeding (disputed)	Breast feeding except if mother smokes
Hypoxia in premature infants	Oxygen supplementation at home
Infections, particularly respiratory	Infant isolation, hygiene, maternal education
Short interpregnancy interval	Pregnancy interval >6 months
No pacifier	Use pacifier during sleep, particularly if bottle fed
No prenatal care	Early prenatal care
Prolonged apnea, ALTE, near-miss	Work-up, home monitoring
Poverty, uneducated mothers	Better housing, education
Sleep-related	
Bed sharing	Avoid
Loose bedding, toys in bed	Avoid
Prone or side sleep position	Supine sleep position
Sleeping in separate rooms	Crib in parents/ caregivers' bedroom
Soft sleep surfaces, loose bedding	Firm mattress, avoid loose bedding
Thermal stress-related	
Head covered	Avoid duvets
Room heated	Avoid excessive heating
Non-Amenable to interventions	
Gender (male)	
Ethnicity (American Indians, Alaskan Natives, and African Americans)	
Age (infant)	
Season (winter)	
Prematurity	
Sleep time	

None of the risk factors identified can be considered a specific cause of SIDS. They can be arbitrarily subdivided into amenable and non-amenable to prevention

Many cases previously recorded as crib death have been proven to be infanticide [188]. On the other hand, cases of repeated sudden infant death within a family punished as murder were instead proven to be SIDS [43]. The prevalence of non-natural causes of death in babies recorded as SIDS [44] has led to the view that every unexpected infant death should be considered as homicide until proven otherwise.

Many risk factors for SIDS have been described over the years. None of the risk factors identified can be considered a specific cause of SIDS. According to Guntheroth [68], they can be arbitrarily subdivided into amenable and non-amenable to interventions and thus prevention (Table 1.1).

Risk factors associated with a higher risk of SIDS mortality are not claimed to have a causal relationship with SIDS, but have shown a positive statistical relationship. Such factors include the following:

- **Prone sleeping position**. Over the years, much attention [21, 69, 95, 166, 213, 247] has been given to the position of the infant in the crib as prone sleep position is an important and well known risk factor for SIDS and increases risk for SIDS two fold or more. Thus the "Safe to sleep" campaign, formerly known as "Back to Sleep" campaign [159, 166, 231], has been conducted to encourage mothers and caregivers to place babies to sleep on their back. According to the Task Force on SIDS [231], side sleeping is considered to be unsafe and is currently not advised.

Supine sleeping position has been shown in studies [21, 95, 231] to significantly reduce the risk for SIDS in healthy full-term infants. Thanks to the "Back to Sleep" campaign launched in 1994 [159, 247], a consistent decrease by over 50% has been registering in the SIDS rate over the last 20 years [5, 159] and then subsequently plateaued [236].

- **Cigarette smoke**. A high incidence of SIDS has been associated with exposure to cigarette smoke [10, 149, 161, 178, 182]. Exposure to cigarette smoke *in utero* has been shown to adversely affect the infant's neural and cardiovascular development [116, 149, 151, 185]. If the parent stops smoking, the risk is decreased [161]. Cigarette smoke is also associated with initial atherosclerotic lesions detected in victims of sudden unexpected perinatal and infant death [147].
- **Drugs and alcohol abuse**. Maternal drug and alcohol abuse affect the fetal development and expose the infant to a higher risk for SIDS [47, 164, 222].
- **Overheating of the infant**. The increased risk of SIDS associated with overheating has been attributed to sleep position, room temperature, excess bedding and infection. A strong association between thermal regulation and ventilatory control has been demonstrated in infants and is thought to play a role in certain cases. Infants that are loosely covered without restricting evaporation do not appear to have as high a risk of SIDS [72, 190, 215].
- **Bed sharing**. Bed sharing with parents or other children has been associated with an increased risk of SIDS. Placing the infant in a crib or bassinet will reduce this risk [21, 27, 29].
- **Soft sleep surfaces and loose bedding**. Epidemiological studies [5, 21] have shown that SIDS is associated with a higher incidence of soft and loose bedding, such as pillows, quilts, comforters, sheepskins, and porous mattresses. Sleep surfaces designed for adults should be avoided as they often have loose bedding, in addition to the risk of entrapment between the mattress and the structure of the bed, i.e., the headboard, footboard, side rails, and frame, the wall, the adjacent furniture, or railings in the headboard or footboard. According to the recommendations of the Task Force on SIDS [231], infants should be placed to sleep on firm mattresses that maintain their shape, without gaps between the mattress and the side of the crib, bassinet, portable crib, or play yard. Soft materials or objects such as pillows, quilts, comforters, or sheepskins. A mattress cover to protect against wetness can be used only if it is tightly fitting.
- **Preterm birth and low birth weight**. Research studies [18, 53, 54, 129] have shown a higher risk of SIDS in preterm and low birth weight infants. No specific mechanism has been proposed for this relationship. The risk is decreased when preterm and low birth weight infants are placed on their back to sleep.
- **Marginal nutrition** *in utero* or after birth. Thiamine and magnesium abnormalities have been reported in SIDS victims. It has been proposed that a deficiency in nutritional intake or an abnormality of metabolism may contribute to these abnormalities [122].

- **Winter season**. SIDS is more frequent in the winter months [67, 149].
- **Infection**. A history of a recent upper respiratory infection has been associated with a higher incidence of SIDS mortality [51, 131]. In particular, Weber et al. [243], performed a 10-year systematic retrospective case review of autopsies of over 500 infants who died suddenly and unexpectedly, reporting evidence of *Staphylococcus Aureus* and *Escherichia Coli*, in SIDS cases. Concurrent pathogens would act as a triggering phenomenon in particularly vulnerable infants. Under this model, sudden death would not occur in a baby with pre-existing neuroautonomic or cardiac alterations unless a new pathological event, i.e., a concurrent infection, takes place [171, 179].
- **Lower socioeconomic status**. A higher incidence of SIDS has been associated with a lower socioeconomic status. Overall this group tends to have a higher rate of multiple risk factors [9, 23, 67].
- **Other maternal factors**. Maternal factors associated with a higher rate of SIDS include: mother's age less than 20 years, short intervals between pregnancies, little or no prenatal care, placental abnormalities, and urinary tract infection during pregnancy [23, 60, 67, 226].
- **Pacifier lack**. Pacifier use during sleep decreases SIDS risk. The association between adverse environmental factors and SIDS risk is modified favorably by pacifier use [158, 231]. Pacifier should be offered to infants at naptime and bedtime during the first year. It does not need to be reinserted once the infant falls asleep. If the infant refuses the pacifier, he/she should not be forced to take it. The protective effect of pacifier persists throughout the sleep period, even if it falls out of the infant's mouth. Pacifiers should not be hung around the infant's neck, in order to avoid the risk of strangulation. Pacifiers attached to infant clothing should not be used during infant's sleep. In order to avoid the risk of suffocation, objects such as toys should not be attached to pacifiers. For breastfed infants, the introduction of pacifier should be delayed until breastfeeding has been firmly established, usually by 3–4 weeks of age. There is insufficient evidence that finger-sucking is also protective against SIDS [231].
- **Drenching night sweats**. The increased incidence of night sweats in SIDS infants may be related to an abnormality of brainstem function [72].
- **Atmospheric pressure changes**. An increase rate of SIDS mortality following a drop in barometric pressure from high to low has been reported [25].
- **Ethnicity**. Nearly one-third of all SIDS deaths in the USA occur in American Indians, Alaskan Natives, and African Americans. The much lower incidence of SIDS in Caucasians may be determined by genetic, cultural, and socioeconomic influences [32, 53, 126].
- **Vaccination**. Vaccines are not considered to be associated with an increased risk of SIDS [241] and the concern that vaccinations might have a causal relationship with SIDS was raised by the fact that the peak age for SIDS is 2–4 months is coincidental with the age for vaccinations. A possible role of hexavalent vaccine in triggering a lethal outcome in a vulnerable infant presenting with hypoplasia of the arcuate nucleus (ARCn) and/or cardiac conduction system abnormalities has been suggested [173].

The current recommendations described in the policy statement of the Task Force on SIDS [231] include supine positioning, use of a firm sleep surface, breastfeeding, room-sharing without bed-sharing, routine immunizations, consideration of using a pacifier, and avoidance of soft bedding, overheating, and exposure to tobacco smoke, alcohol, and illicit drugs.

1.1.3 Etiopathogenesis

The etiopathogenesis of SIDS is still an unsolved medical problem. SIDS seems to be a "lethal multifactorial dysfunction" due to something not sufficiently developed or to something working in an anomalous way. In the few cases where it has been possible to observe this catastrophic event, a child in apparently good health mysteriously and suddenly stops breathing without crying and without being excited.

Most of the babies before the fatal event show only a mild infection of the upper respiratory pathways [51, 131] and mild acute inflammatory infiltrate in the lungs are classically reported in SIDS [239].

According to Berry [16], the multifactorial problems in the pathophysiology and clinical presentation of SIDS are the result of a controversial and multifaceted pathology. In order to explain SIDS, several theories have been proposed:

1. The cardiac theory, based on myocardial dysfunction altering the diffusion stimulus. Based on this theory, SIDS is considered as a cardiac arrhythmogenic death – QT long syndrome and/or preexcitation with malignant tachycardia, atrioventricular (AV) blocks, accessory pathways [84, 89, 170, 203, 210, 220, 237].
2. The respiratory theory, based on respiratory alterations, with episodes of sudden and prolonged apnea [70, 131].
3. The visceral dyskinetic theory, based on alterations in upper digestive pathways (motility abnormalities of the glottis and/or gastroesophageal reflux) [67, 94, 245].

It has been stressed that the autonomic nervous reflexes play a role in all such mechanisms. Thus, the anatomo-pathological study must include examination of the autonomic nervous system structures involved in the activities of the respiratory, cardiovascular, upper digestive, and cardiac conduction systems [113, 136, 138, 204].

From the anatomo-pathological plane, different findings have been reported as possible causes of SIDS: brainstem abnormalities [93, 105, 106, 142], cardiac conduction system developmental defects [135, 170, 237, 238], immaturity of the paraganglia or of the carotid bodies [192–194, 204]. In particular, much importance has been placed on the autonomic innervation of the heart and respiratory apparatus [103, 132, 140, 181].

1.1.3.1 Reflexogenic SIDS

Overall, the abnormalities detected in the autonomic nervous and cardiac conduction systems represent a plausible basis for SIDS being reflexogenic in nature.

The dive reflex, feigned death, auditory, oculo-cardiac, trigemino-cardiac, vagal cardio-respiratory, and Ondine's curse reflexes, if pathological, could all lead to SIDS as a final common pathway.

Dive Reflex

The reflex mechanism more frequently considered in the etiopathogenesis of SIDS is the dive reflex, which seems to persist in humans as an inheritance from diver birds and amphibians. It has been reported that washing the face with cold water or plunging into cold water provokes in humans a cardiac deceleration through the ambiguous and the dorsal vagal nuclei. In individuals with an increased sensitivity, bathing the face with cold water can provoke a cardiac arrest. Some people die of cardiac and respiratory arrest while diving, without evidence of drowning. It seems that some newborns with a developmental defect of these reflexogenic centers, i.e. interacting through the glossopharyngeal or trigeminal nerves, die of apnea following absence of breath [121, 144, 204]. Diving reflex in humans is characterized by breath-holding, slowing of the heart rate, reduction of limb blood flow and a gradual rise in the arterial blood pressure [58, 63]. Diving reflex can terminate supraventricular paroxysmal tachycardia [11, 63, 102].

Feigned Death/Fear Paralysis Reflex

Another reflex that seems to play a role in SIDS is the tonic immobility, known as feigned death reflex or fear paralysis reflex. Small mammals develop a reflex by which they stop breathing or drastically decrease their heart rate when exposed to the danger of a large carnivore. They instinctively realize that the carnivore does not usually devour carrion. The carotid glomus and sinus in the adult mainly regulate cardiac pulsation. In Los Angeles, the police sought to restrain a suspected criminal by pressing the carotid glomus and the sinus provoking death, and this led to the suspension of the police chief because he had encouraged the maneuver [97, 154, 204].

Auditory Reflex

A violent sudden auditory stimulus has been reported to be able to trigger SIDS. This is termed the auditory reflex. About 10% of patients with long QT syndrome fall into syncope as a result of the acoustic reflex which is carried by the vestibular nerve along the lateral lemniscus down to the brainstem centers [204, 235].

Oculo-Cardiac Reflex

Cardiac arrest can also occur as a result of the inhibitory oculocardiac reflex, possibly elicited by a prone sleep position [205].

Trigemino-Cardiac Reflex (TCR)

The TCR has been described as a reflexive response of bradycardia, hypotension and gastric hypermotility as a result of mechanical, electrical or chemical stimulation of the trigeminal nerve at the level of the cerebellopontine angle. The TCR, consisting of autonomic changes such as bradycardia or even asystolia along with arterial hypotension. TCR is characterized by a drop in the mean arterial blood pressure and the heart rate of more than 20%, compared with the baseline values before the stimulation and coinciding with the manipulation of the trigeminal nerve [216–219].

Vagal Cardio-Respiratory Reflexes

Vagal cardio-respiratory reflexes, if pathological, could lead to SIDS [204]. They represent common instinctive conditionings and are physiologically programmed to maintain life under conditions of danger; for example, the dive reflex is vital in diving birds and in amphibians. It is most likely that even minimal alterations along the neural pathways of the reflex arc could interfere with the triggering and/or the reflexogenic response and thus could transform a paraphysiological action into a lethal event. Cardiac or cardio-respiratory arrest could happen whenever such lesions are located in the centers and in the most delicate and complex brainstem neuronal circuitry [200, 204].

Ondine's Curse Reflex

Another reflex considered in SIDS is the so-called "Ondine's curse" reflex. In German mythology, and in a play by J. Giraudoux, Ondine was a water nymph who placed a curse on her unfaithful human lover which took from him all automatic vital functions. He therefore had to remember to breathe and thus would stop breathing when he fell asleep. The Ondine's curse reflex seems to play a pathological role in SIDS as the infants while sleeping "forgets" to breathe due to agenesis of the arcuate nucleus [204].

Ondine's syndrome is a rare autosomal dominant disorder of the autonomic nervous system, also called Congenital Central Hypoventilation Syndrome (CCHS), characterized by alveolar hypoventilation during sleep from a lack of physiological response to hypercarbia and hypoxemia. The paired-like homeobox 2B (PHOX2B) has been identified as the major gene causing CCHS, resulting from polyalanine repeat expansion mutations. CCHS typically presents in newborns, but some cases have been described in adults as late onset CCHS, reflecting the variable penetrance of PHOX2B mutations [244].

1.1.3.2 SIDS due to Metabolic Impairment

In some rare cases of SIDS a hereditary metabolic defect has been detected. The hypothesis that there is a subgroup of SIDS in which death is due to congenital metabolic defects originated from the autopsy findings, in some SIDS victims, of a massive fatty degeneration of the liver similar to that seen in Reye syndrome [22, 59, 65, 124]. Several studies reported in the literature, particularly from the second half of the 1980s, confirm the validity of this hypothesis, but they are discordant as to what percentage of sudden deaths can be attributed to this metabolic factor. Elevated values, ranging from 5 to 27% reported by some authors, are not in agreement with the findings of other studies, which have shown that fewer than 3% of SIDS deaths have a metabolic etiology [66, 124].

Although many metabolic diseases can potentially lead to sudden death, only enzymatic defects associated with serious hypoglycemia (often triggered by a subclinical infection), i.e. defects in gluconeogenesis, glycogen metabolism (glycogenosis type I) and beta-oxidation of fatty acids, seem to play a role [22]. In most cases the symptoms suddenly appear following fasting during infection (usually viral in nature) that seems to increase tissue dependence on fatty acid beta-oxidation as an energy source [22, 59, 124].

Among the enzymatic mitochondrial defects involved in the fatty acid beta-oxidation cycle, deficiency in medium-chain acyl-CoA-dehydrogenase (MCAD) has the richest documentation as a cause of SIDS [59, 124]. In fasting, the metabolic block leads to an insufficient formation of ketone bodies with a reduction in the availability of alternative energy substrates for the brain and the muscles, including the cardiac muscle. This also leads to accumulation of esterified acyl-CoA-dehydrogenase and consequent hypoketonic hypoglycemia [22, 59, 124].

In gluconeogenesis defects one of the key enzymes for the process is missing and it is impossible to build glucose from nonglucidic sources (pyruvic acid, lactic acid, amino acids, etc.). Therefore, following fasting, intermediate glycolysis products accumulate with consequent lactic acidemia and hypoglycemia accompanied by a rapid deterioration in the vital functions. In the case of glucogenosis, SIDS has been reported in association with types Ia, Ib and Ic, that imply a deficit in intrahepatic microsomal glucose-6-phosphatase. The activity of this enzyme also seems to remain absent for a prolonged period in most preterm newborns, a group commonly at higher risk of SIDS. The diagnosis is based on the activity of the hepatic enzyme [22, 124].

Likewise, metabolic alterations, acidosis or alkalosis, unbalanced electrolytic state, hypoglycemia, or enzymatic defects could eventually provoke lethal cardiac arrhythmias [184].

1.1.4 Near-SIDS and ALTE Episodes

The SIDS baby is generally found dead in the crib without prodromic signs. If the infant is seen in the agonic phase, it could be saved with cardio-respiratory resuscitation maneuvers. The terms "near SIDS" and "near miss" have been used to indicate babies nearly lost, near to death and "resuscitated" after such an episode. Unfortunately, in most cases the dying baby is discovered when the hypoxia and ischemia have already caused irreversible damage to the central nervous system and the myocardium, and every therapeutic measure is too late [223, 224].

In 1923, Still [230] first described the modern near-SIDS as an abrupt cessation of sleep, followed by cyanosis, in five infants. Between the apnea episodes the infants were unremarkable to observation, though only one survived after receiving artificial respiration, i.e., representing the first near-SIDS case by today's standards. At the time, an apnea monitor was recommended; it consisted of round-the-clock observation by a trained medical professional.

Babies with Apparent Life-Threatening Event (ALTE), which is characterized by apnea and/or alterations in muscular tone or cutaneous color, are at increased risk of SIDS. ALTE, according the definition of the National Institutes of Health Consensus Development Conference on Infantile Apnea and Home Monitoring [160], is "an episode that is frightening to the observer and that is characterized by some combination of apnea (central or occasionally obstructive) color change (usually cyanotic or pallid but occasionally erythematous or plethoric), marked change in muscle tone (usually marked limpness), choking, or gagging". ALTE is not a diagnosis, but rather a constellation of symptoms and anything that causes an infant to appear in danger of dying can be interpreted as ALTE, i.e., metabolic disorders, neurological diseases, cardiac arrhythmias and child abuse [28]. An ALTE event is considered an abortive SIDS, and infants experiencing an ALTE could possibly be saved by continuous cardio-respiratory monitoring [3, 28, 39, 52].

On one hand, an infant dying of SIDS can be saved with very prompt cardio-respiratory resuscitation maneuvers, resulting in a near-SIDS event. On the other hand, it should be underlined that these maneuvers, if not properly performed, can cause damage to the cardiac conduction system due to the intense force exerted on the interventricular septum [139, 141, 172, 202].

1.1.5 SIDS Prevention

Prevention of SIDS and stillbirth is the object of the bill S. 3142 introduced in 2008 in the Senate of the USA [191], which enhances public health activities in order to understand and prevent sudden unexpected infant and perinatal deaths. The aim of the bill is to significantly reduce the toll in human life, to promote the anatomo-clinical, genetic and epidemiological research, as well as information campaigns, programs and projects to support of victims' families.

Since the etiopathogenetic factors in SIDS are still largely unknown, it is not possible to adopt a therapeutic strategy. The incidence of SIDS can be reduced only through preventive approaches. Cigarette smoking is the most preventable risk factor, and should mandatorily be avoided [116, 149, 178].

Once the drama of the loss of a child to SIDS has passed [240], and the trauma of the consequent judicial investigations has been overcome, the parents ask the family practitioner, the gynecologist, the pediatrician or the pathologist: "Can we have another child? Will he/she have any abnormalities? Will he/she be predisposed to SIDS?" The need to give all necessary information to the parents is self-evident [37, 38]. Although cases of SIDS from congenital metabolic dysfunction are rare [124], genetic and metabolic investigations are necessary in families with a SIDS victim in the following circumstances:

- The sudden infant death was preceded by prodromic signs suggestive of metabolic disease;
- There is a history of sudden death;
- There is a history of Reye syndrome;

- The autopsy of the young victim disclosed fatty degeneration of the liver or of other tissues;
- There has been more than one case of SIDS in the same family [79, 124].

Using the polymerase chain reaction (PCR) method, it is possible to carry out a prenatal diagnosis of a deficit in M-CAD on the chorial villus [66].

In order to recognize babies with long QT syndrome at increased risk of SIDS, it has been suggested performing screening electrocardiography in all newborns to evaluate cardiac function [220]. A fundamental way to prevent SIDS is by placing newborns and infants to sleep in the crib on their back (supine position) [166]. The incidence of SIDS has decreased after the health authorities have encouraged families to avoid the prone sleeping position for their babies [159, 160, 213]. Because children of mothers who smoke [107, 222], who are alcoholic [222] or drug addicts [47] are at higher risk of SIDS, avoiding the parents' smoke, and abuse of alcohol and drugs helps prevent SIDS. Since infants exposed to thermal stress are at greater risk of SIDS [190, 215], it is also necessary to avoid covering the baby excessively. The children of mothers with a short interval between one pregnancy and the next are also at a higher risk of SIDS [226], so it would seem that the probability of SIDS could also be reduced by informing mothers on this issue.

The domiciliary use of cardio-respiratory monitoring, largely based on the hypothesis that sleep apnea plays a fundamental role in the etiopathogenesis of SIDS, and that the terminal event in SIDS is considered to be reversible with prompt intervention and appropriate resuscitative maneuvers. Generally, babies with a birth weight lower than 1,500 gm, those born of drug addict mothers, and those who have presented with idiopathic ALTE episodes are considered at risk of SIDS [39, 224]. Before monitoring it is necessary to perform all relevant tests to exclude any underlying disease as in ill infants, targeted etiological therapeutic strategies are instituted, and to personalize the monitoring program to follow at home. "Home monitors" allow respiratory and cardiac parameters to be controlled. The monitors have alarm ranges set on a case-by-case basis and have a memory that allows cardio-respiratory activity to be evaluated. The monitor is generally used during the night and while the baby sleeps, mainly during the first 7–8 months of life. If a crisis occurs, the parents are alerted by the monitor when the crisis starts, and generally the infant needs simple "stimulations" administered by the parents. The parents are trained in the appropriate resuscitative maneuvers [3, 39, 52, 80, 160].

The current recommendations from the AAP described in the policy statement of the Task Force on SIDS for a safe infant sleeping environment [231] are divided into three different levels:

Level A Recommendations are based on good and consistent scientific evidence:

Back to sleep for every sleep; Use a firm sleep surface; Room-sharing without bed-sharing is recommended; Keep soft objects and loose bedding out of the crib; Pregnant women should receive regular prenatal care; Avoid smoke exposure during pregnancy and after birth; Avoid alcohol and illicit drug use during pregnancy and after birth, Breastfeeding is recommended; Consider offering a pacifier at nap time and bedtime; Avoid overheating; Do not use home cardiorespiratory monitors as a strategy for reducing the risk of SIDS; Expand the national campaign to reduce the risks of SIDS to include a major focus on the safe sleep environment and ways to reduce the risks of all sleep related infant deaths, including SIDS, suffocation, and other accidental deaths; pediatricians, family physicians, and other primary care providers should actively participate in this campaign.

Level B Recommendations are based on limited or inconsistent scientific evidence: Infants should be immunized in accordance with recommendations of the AAP and Centers for Disease Control and Prevention; Avoid commercial devices marketed to reduce the risk of SIDS; Supervised, awake tummy time is recommended to facilitate development and to minimize development of positional plagiocephaly.

Level C Recommendations are based primarily on consensus and expert opinion: Health care professionals, staff in newborn nurseries and NICUs, and child care providers should endorse the SIDS risk-reduction recommendations from birth; Media and manufacturers should follow safe-sleep guidelines in their messaging and advertising; Continue research and surveillance on the risk factors, causes, and pathophysiological mechanisms of SIDS and other sleep-related infant deaths, with the ultimate goal of eliminating these deaths entirely.

1.2 Sudden Intrauterine Unexplained Death (SIUD)

There is a continuity between SIDS and sudden perinatal unexplained death (SPUD) – sudden intrauterine unexplained death (SIUD) and sudden neonatal unexplained death (SNUD) – as common developmental abnormalities have been detected.

SIUD is the late unexplained fetal death before the complete expulsion or removal of the fetus from the mother ≥20–22 weeks of gestation or ≥500 gm body mass which is unexpected by history and is unexplained after a thorough pathological exam of the fetus and the fetal adnexa [40, 56, 99]. Unexplained stillbirth represent about one-half of perinatal deaths, with a prevalence of 5–12 per 1,000 births [41, 81]. Advances in maternal and fetal care have produced a significant reduction in perinatal mortality [125], but have not significantly changed the prevalence of SIUD or unexplained stillbirth.

SIUD and SIDS have similar epidemiology, risk factors [56], pathological and genetic findings [113, 150, 177], though SIUD is up to 10 times more frequent than SIDS [31, 41, 81]. In both SIUD and SIDS victims, despite they are defined as "unexplained", frequent developmental abnormalities in the brainstem, particularly in the arcuate nucleus [113, 116, 142, 143] and in the cardiac conduction system [177] have been observed. Pulmonary immaturity [140, 181] and fibromuscolar hyperplasia of the pulmonary artery have also been detected [180].

In the cardiac conduction system of unexpected perinatal death several abnormalities have been identified, i.e., accessory atrioventricular pathways, mostly Mahaim fibers, cartilaginous hypermetaplasia, abnormal resorptive degeneration, junctional islands, fetal dispersion, hypoplasia of the cardiac conduction system or of the central fibrous body, splitting of the atrioventricular node or of the His bundle, similar to those detected in SIDS cases [175–177, 184].

The arcuate nucleus (ARCn) is an important cardio-respiratory center of the ventral medullary surface, characterized by great morphological variability [104, 136, 138]. ARCn hypoplasia, detected in over 50% of SIDS and SIUD victims [136, 138, 142], is of great interest, particularly because of its frequency and pathogenetic implications. Sometimes the ARCn hypoplasia or immaturity is associated with alterations in other centers regulating the vital functions, i.e., the respiratory reticular formation, the solitary tract nucleus, the hypoglossus nucleus, the ambiguus nucleus, the locus coeruleus; and the parabrachial Kölliker-Fuse complex and the cerebellum [115, 117, 118, 138, 146, 155, 174]. It is remarkable, particularly because of the functional consequences, that ARCn hypoplasia may be unilateral and when bilateral may involve only part of the nucleus [138, 142].

All these findings in SIUD need further study in larger series which should include the examination of the brainstem and the cardiac conduction system in serial sections in a complete and standardized way.

1.3 Cardiac Conduction System (CCS)

The heart is regulated by involuntary rhythmic contractions not produced by nervous impulses. The only role of the cardiac innervation, which is primarily sympathetic in nature, is to modify the cardiac rhythm, accelerating or decelerating it. In the common or working myocardium there is a system of particular muscle fibers, called the specialized myocardium or cardiac conduction system (CCS), which produces the impulses for contraction which is propagated to the atrial musculature functionally connecting it to the ventricle. The CCS is composed of myocardial fibers modified in structure as well as function in comparison to common fibers. Myocardial fibers have scarce myofibrils, abundant glycogen and are slender or star-shaped. They show an elevated spontaneous frequency of contraction and a high speed of impulse conduction. However, these specific or specialized myocells are morphologically not uniform [30].

The cytological components of the CCS have several differences. Such morphological heterogeneity reflects the different physiological characteristics of the specialized conduction myocardium in its various centers, in relation to both its autonomic nature and its conductive role.

In the human heart, the system of conduction and formation of the stimulus (Fig. 1.2) is considered to comprise:

- The sinoatrial node (SAN) or Keith-Flack node;
- Internodal pathways (superior, middle, posterior);
- The atrio-ventricular node (AVN) or Aschoff-Tawara node;

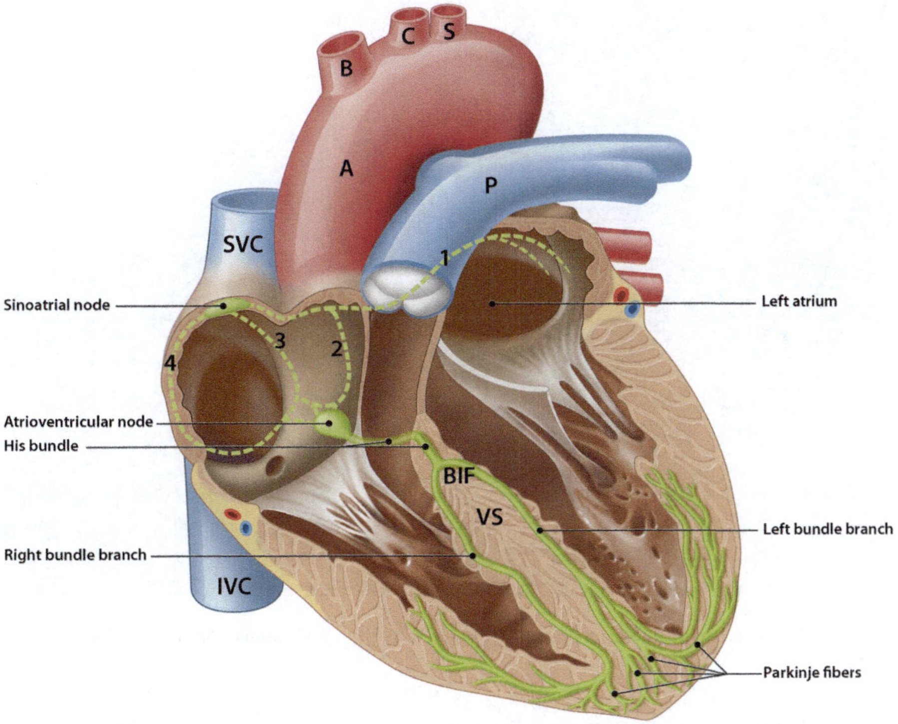

Fig. 1.2 Diagram of the human heart showing schematically the location of the cardiac conduction system (*A* aorta, *B* brachiocephalic artery, *C* left common carotid artery, *L* left subclavian artery, *BIF* Bifurcating His bundle/Bifurcation, *IVC* inferior vena cava, *P* pulmonary trunk, *SVC* superior vena cava, *VS* ventricular septum, *1* interatrial pathway, *2* anterior internodal Bachmann-James pathway, *3* middle internodal Wenckeback tract, *4* posterior internodal Thorel pathway corresponding to the *crista terminalis*)

- The atrio-ventricular (AV) node, His bundle (HB) or common trunk;
- The bifurcation or bifurcating His bundle;
- The right bundle branch (RBB) and LBB.

However, first, it is to be underlined that the anatomo-histological junctions between the common trunk and the bifurcation, and between the bifurcation and bundle branches are not well delimited. Second, it should be underlined that in many cases there is longitudinal partition of the CCS destined to become each of the two bundle branches in the background of the common trunk, much above the actual bifurcation; therefore the position of the AV junction–subjunction is uncertain [196, 203, 206, 209].

1.3.1 Sinoatrial Node (SAN)

The SAN, also known as sinuatrial node, sinus node or Keith-Flack node [100], is an oval formation measuring about 0.5 × 1.5 cm in adults, comprising specialized

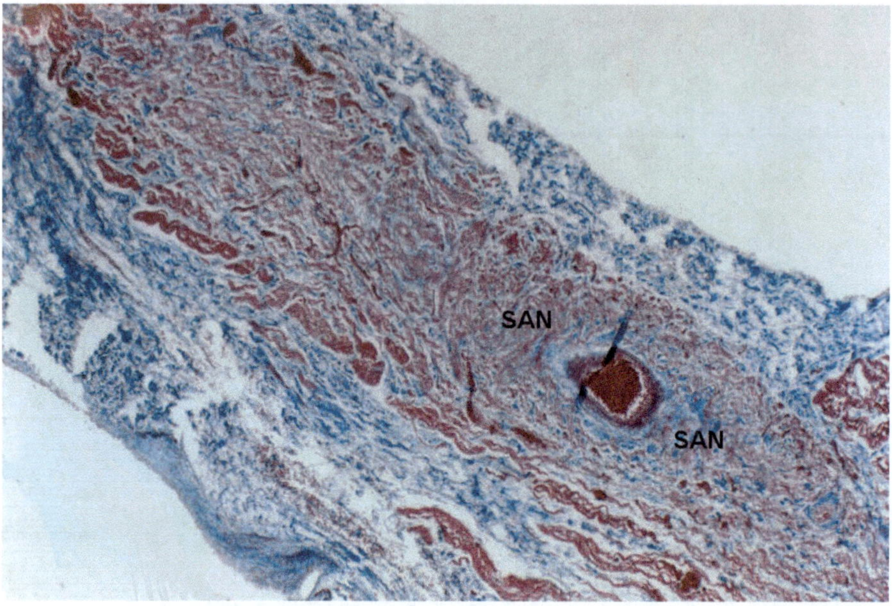

Fig. 1.3 Normal human sinoatrial node (*SAN*) centered by the SAN artery (Trichromic Heidenhain, ×25)

myocardial fibers with abundant interposition of connective tissue. The node is located in the subepicardium, in the superior third of the *crista terminalis*, directed along its greater axis, in the back wall of the right atrium. Its cranial part reaches the outlet of the caval vein. The superficial part of the SAN is generally in contact with the subepicardial adipose tissue, while the inner layers variably anastomose with the common atrial myocardium. The SAN artery crosses longitudinally at the center of the SAN (Fig. 1.3). The specialized myocardial cells of the SAN are small, measuring 3.0–4.5 μm, clear, with a little evident striation. In the central part of the node the cells weave forming a pluridirectional anastomosis while at the periphery they tend to be parallel and show morphological transitional characteristics towards the adjacent common myocardium. The connective stroma is rich in elastic and reticular fibers close to collagen fibers that, around the SAN artery, tend to have a circular aspect.

1.3.1.1 Histology

According to James [88], four types of specialized myocardial cells of the SAN can be distinguished:

1. Pacemaker (P) cells, primarily located at the center of the node, rather small and round, assembled in groups with a common basal membrane, characterized by a shortage of myofibrils, sarcosomes and cytoplasmic granules, and by apparent absence of intercalary disks, since the cell–cell contacts are simple juxtaposition of the plasma membranes. In the general organization of the SAN around its artery, the P cells tend to be located centrally [85].

2. Slender cells, rather short and thin, often in relationship with P cells. They are distributed along the whole SAN, but mainly in its external half. Some of these cells extend from the periphery of the SAN for some millimeters into the right atrial myocardium [88]. The slender cells may contain a small or a great number of myofibrils, longitudinally directed (rather than directed randomly as in P cells) with interposition of mitochondria, as in ordinary myocardium. Transitional cells, unlike P cells, contain much glycogen. P cells connect only with each another and with transitional cells, while transitional cells exclusively contact the SAN, as well as the internodal and interatrial tracts. The junctions of slender cells with P cells are simple, consisting of apposition of the plasma membranes with many desmosomes, while the junctions among the transitional cells or between these and the cells of the internodal tracts are complex, resembling the ordinary intercalary disks. The framework of these thin fibers is one of the more readily recognizable characteristics of the SAN [85].
3. Common myocardial fibers at the periphery.
4. Purkinje fibers (shorter and wider than the common myocardial cells) with few filaments, with a frayed appearance, clear perinuclear halo, indentations of the sarcolemma in correspondence with the Z stripes. Peculiar to the Purkinje cells is, according to James [88], a "specialized" intercellular junction, an oblique course, constituted by juxtaposition of the plasma membranes, with basal membrane interposition.

Also particular to these cells is their rapid myocardial conduction capability, and the lack or paucity of the T-tubular system. Many nerve fibers are intercalated with and adjacent to the nodal cells [61, 133].

Among these specialized types of cells, it is important to recognize the two principal types of cells of the SAN, and it is equally important to understand that the SAN works as a non-elementary biological unit together with three other important anatomic systems: the central artery, the collagen framework, and the innervations [85].

1.3.1.2 Vascular Supply

The vascular supply of the SAN is represented by the main atrial artery that lies longitudinally in the SAN. This may originate from the right sinusal nodal artery deriving from the right coronary artery in most cases, from the left sinusal nodal artery or from the posterior sinusal nodal artery, deriving from the left coronary artery. Histologically, the SAN artery shows marked development of the longitudinal layer of the tunica media [196, 203, 206]. The normal human SAN is disposed coherently around its homonymous central artery (Fig. 1.3). The SAN has been described as being an enormous adventitia of its artery. The blood introduced into the SAN artery with every cardiac cycle seems to have a modulatory effect. It seems to synchronize the basically random P cell activity stabilizing it from the extranodal influence. Experimental modifications of the pressure of the SAN artery have been shown to have a significant effect on the sinusal pacemaker. This has been further supported by the presence of arrhythmias and sudden death in individuals with anomalous thickness and narrowing of the SAN artery which decrease or eliminate its pulsatility [85, 92].

1.3.1.3 Collagen Framework

After birth, the collagen content of the SAN increases progressively up to adulthood. The growth rate and the final total amount of collagen vary greatly from one human heart to another. The volume of collagen in the adult SAN is so great as to represent the predominant staining feature in histological slides. SAN collagen is a mixture of P cells and slender cells which form a periarterial framework. Furthermore, the collagen separates into small groups of cells, so limiting the extension of cellular contacts. Collagen is an inherent component of both the SAN artery and the basal membrane of the nodal cells. Whatever the exact mechanism by which the central artery influences the pacemaker rate of the SAN, without doubt the normal framework of dense collagen contributes significantly to this functional relationship. Any disease damaging the collagen framework is associated with arrhythmias partly due to the loss of this functional relationship and to the consequent instability of the SAN [42]. This suggests that adult individuals with decreased collagen in the SAN could have an intrinsically less stable cardiac pacemaker. If this is the case, then the postnatal development of the fibrous framework of the SAN would play a key role in optimizing the stability of the cardiac pacemaker [85, 92, 203].

1.3.1.4 Innervation

The innervation of the SAN is extremely rich. Numerous and conspicuous nerve trunks reach the SAN, particularly its external surface, through the subepicardial adipose layer where many ganglia, the ganglionar plexus, are located. Nerve cells, isolated or in small groups, are sometimes observed in the superficial layers of the SAN. From the perinodal ganglionar plexus, nervous ramifications penetrate the SAN. They seem to form a network with small trunks parallel to the greater nodal axis, gathered by oblique transverse tracts. From this nervous network fascicles or isolated fibers, amyelinated or poorly myelinated, originate with regular swellings or with small variations of caliber to form the preterminal and terminal plexuses. The autonomic innervation influences the SAN and is the principal bond between the normal cardiac pacemaker and the extracardiac regulatory centers, i.e. brain and carotid sinus [30, 85, 203, 209].

In the human heart, both the SAN and the AVN are the two most efficient pacemaker units, the SAN normally being predominant. This predominance is partly due to the more elevated speed and partly to its pacemaker signal distribution pathway to the atria and ventricles, to its abundant adrenergic and cholinergic innervation, and to its disproportionately wide central artery around which the SAN is located in a background of dense collagen [85, 92].

1.3.2 Internodal and Interatrial Pathways

Myocardial fascicles in the right atrium connecting the SAN with the AVN have been described by several researchers. They are: the anterior internodal Bachmann-James tract, also including the principal interatrial connection; the middle internodal Wenckeback tract; and the posterior internodal Thorel tract corresponding to the *crista terminalis* [91, 196, 203, 206, 209]. The anterior and posterior internodal pathways are more developed and more readily detectable than the middle internodal pathway [88]. The area crossed by the three internodal pathways corresponds to the residual primitive sinus venosus [85, 92]. Experience suggests that the presence of these specific internodal pathways is uncertain. This is mainly due to the long posterior extension of the SAN that, adjacent to the *crista terminalis*, is rich in "slender cells" of nodal type [61, 203]. James emphasized the existence and functional importance of the internodal pathways, and has reported their histological features, both at the light and electron microscopic levels, as characterized by the presence of Purkinje cells, but also by nodal P cells and slender cells, which are seen predominantly in the conduction system [91, 92]. Of interest, James described two electrical pathways, which are named for him the James fibers, one physiologic anterior internodal and one pathologic atriofascicular that originate in the atrial internodal tracts and pass to the ventriculum bypassing the atrioventricular node [91, 183].

Such pathways are not covered or otherwise separated from the adjacent tissue. They are anatomically distinguished, being a continuum of myocardial cells in an area otherwise largely consisting of adipose tissue and collagen. The speed of the internodal pathways is significantly higher than in the common myocardium, although it is lower than in the bundle of His and the bundle branches. Moreover, in the normal human heart there is an internodal pathway connecting the SAN with the left atrium [85, 92].

1.3.3 Atrioventricular Node (AVN)

The AVN, or Aschoff-Tawara node [232], is an oval structure measuring about 1×3×5 mm, located in the subendocardium of the right atrium, adherent to the central fibrous body, above the septal surface of the tricuspid valve and anterior to the coronary sinus ostium. The proximal border of the AVN is a region where a network of slender nodal fibers contacts the bigger cells and fibers of the internodal pathways [88, 92]. Its supraanterior, lateral and posteroinferior surfaces receive fibers from the adjacent atrial myocardium. In the adult they are fascicles crossing the adipose tissue and partially embracing the AVN before penetrating it (Fig. 1.4). In humans, the dimensions of the AVN and the number and type of the atrionodal connections show a certain variability [88, 196].

1.3.3.1 Histology

The AVN is composed of specialized myocardial cells similar to the cells of the SAN but with a rather smaller volume. Their color is weaker than that of the common atrial fibers and they anastomose through short pluridirectional ramifications to form a three-dimensional net, mixed with a collagen and elastic network. Ultrastructurally, James [88, 92] distinguishes four AVN cell types:

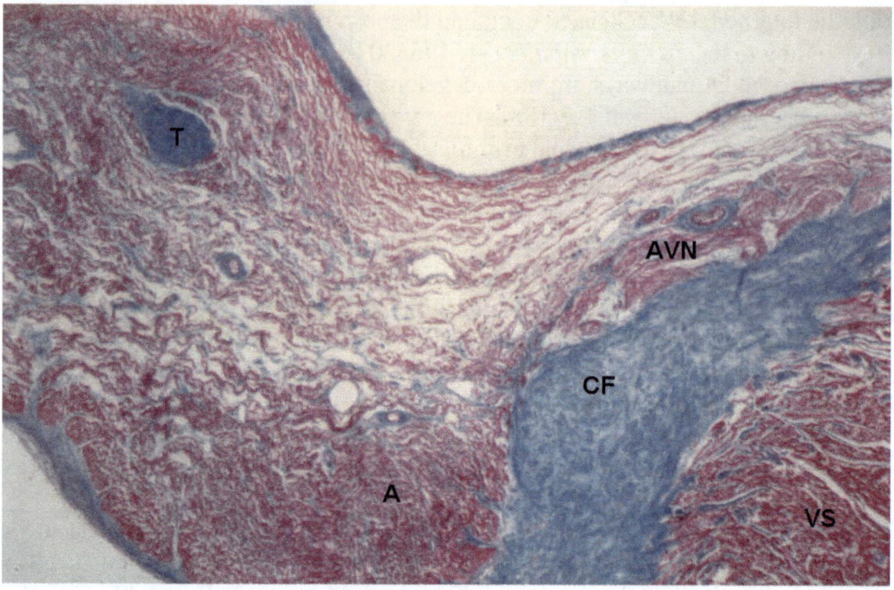

Fig. 1.4 Normal human atrioventricular node (*AVN*). It adheres to the central fibrous body (*CF*), a dense structure of collagen. The AVN node artery is located eccentrically. The tendon of Todaro (*T*) is separated from the AVN and located in the right atrium (*A*), but its location varies greatly in the human heart (*VS* interventricular septum) (Trichromic Heidenhain, ×25)

1. P cells (see Sect. 1.3.1). These are located mainly in the deepest portion of the AVN. They are fewer numbers in the AVN than in the SAN.
2. Star cells. These are the predominant cell type in the AVN. They anastomose through short pluridirectional ramifications to form a three-dimensional net, mixed with a collagen and elastic network. In the distal portion of the AVN the specialized fibers tend to become parallel [196]. Some star cells are located in the atrial septum with direct contact with the cells of the internodal pathways [85, 92].

   Also detected rarely are the following cells:

3. Common myocardial cells [196].
4. Purkinje cells, particularly in the periphery of the AVN and in the area between the AVN and the right atrial endocardium.

In the AVN there is much less collagen than in the SAN. It has been suggested that the abundant collagen in the SAN interferes with its pacemaker activity. Therefore, the relatively scanty collagen in the AVN would explain its accessory rather than primary pacemaker role [85, 92].

1.3.3.2 Vascular Supply

The blood to the AVN is assured, in more than 80% of cases, by the branch of the fibrous septum, that is the first perforant septal branch (posterior) of the right coronary artery. The AVN artery, sometimes double or triple, penetrates the node in the inferior posterior portion and crosses it near the center [196]. Unlike in the SAN, in the AVN the homonymous artery is not normally located centrally. The AVN artery is usually eccentric and is often detected out from the node, but almost always it is partly included in the central fibrous body [85, 92]. The AVN artery differs in caliber and in richness of internodal ramifications. It should not be considered a terminal artery, as was previously thought in normal and pathological anatomy. The venous outflow is assured by big channels and sinusoids in the superior part of the node; the veins drain into the coronary sinus or directly into the right atrium [196].

1.3.3.3 Lymphatic Drainage

The lymphatic drainage of the AVN is assured by a conspicuous system of lymphatic channels originating from the superior portion of the interventricular septum. They reach the cardiac center near the AVN [209].

1.3.3.4 Innervation

Innervation is less relevant in the AVN than in the SAN. However, nerve trunks cross the adipose perinodal tissue and penetrate the node though thin ramifications. Nerve cells have been noted rarely in the human AVN, while some ganglia are readily detected around it [30, 61, 88, 203, 209].

1.3.4 Morphological Concept of the Atrioventricular Junction (AVJ)

According to the classical description of Tawara [232], which has been little modified over the years, the AVN, the His bundle, and the two bundle branches represent a myocardial conduction pathway known as the "atrioventricular system" or Tawarian system that is normally the only connection between the atrial and the ventricular myocardium [30, 203, 209].

Electrophysiological studies tended to designate the undivided part of the AVN with its atrial junctions and the His bundle, up to the bifurcation, by the term of AV junction (AVJ), tissue, or area. This definition which primarily reflects the functional significance, does not offer, from the anatomic point of view, particular advantages in comparison to the traditional nomenclature of the conduction system. Rather, such a definition could lead to a misunderstanding by inferring an incomplete anatomo-physiological continuity of the system itself whose proximal part (undivided) and distal part (divided into two branches) are generally considered to constitute unique entities [30, 196, 203, 206, 209]. The AVJ contains not only the AVN and the bundle of His with its proximal branches, but also the AVN artery (terminal divisions of the septal branches of the anterior descending left coronary artery), the central fibrous body, the tendon of Todaro, the *pars membranacea septi*, some nerves and ganglia, and the septal surface of both the mitral and tricuspid valves. The origins of both the aorta and the principal pulmonary arteries do not belong to the AVJ, but are adjacent to the AVJ. Being near these mitral and tricuspid valvular surfaces, cardiac contractile movements produce marked stress on the AVJ. The central fibrous body and the tendon of Todaro are two important functional structures for the mechanical strength of the AVJ [88, 92, 209].

1.3.4.1 Central Fibrous Body

The central fibrous body of the adult human heart is a dense structure of collagen, while in the fetus and in the newborn it is almost entirely a gelatinous substance (Fig. 1.4). Based on its mechanical function, the central fibrous body can be described as a septal anchor for the mitral valve, extending directly from the valvular edge to the crest of the interventricular septum where it also provides an attachment for the septal edges of the tricuspid valve. Since both the AVN and the His bundle lie directly on the central fibrous body, due to their proximity, they are considered at risk in case of alteration to the central fibrous body, for example, in calcification of the mitral ring [88]. The mitral valve, facing the maximal systolic pressure normally produced by the left ventricle, has a strong influence on the central fibrous body. Therefore, it is also clear why the central fibrous body insertion in the crest of the interventricular septum is rich in fibrous tissue. It is a mistake to think that this fibrous tissue in the crest of the interventricular septum represents a pathological process. Such fibrous tissue is not only normal, but is even necessary to ensure local mechanical strength. The dynamic role played by fibroblasts in the central fibrous body during postnatal morphogenesis of the AVN and the His bundle has been a matter of controversy [8, 42, 237].

1.3.4.2 Tendon of Todaro

The tendon of Todaro is more prominent in the heart of the dog than in the human heart, in which it is rudimentary. In its typical form (Fig. 1.4), the tendon of Todaro originates in the tissue of the atrial septum, anterior to the coronary sinus and well above of the central fibrous body. Rarely it is attached to the wall of the coronary sinus or to the pons of Eustachio. From its origin, it becomes adjacent to the AVN but usually above or separate from it. Then it goes directly to the central fibrous body or, more rarely, to the origin of the aorta [88]. According to its site, which varies greatly in the human heart, it can join the central fibrous body posteriorly adjacent to the coronary sinus or more anteriorly adjacent to the aorta. At both these sites, it can also influence the morphogenesis of the AVN [88, 209].

1.3.5 His Bundle (HB)

The His bundle (HB) or bundle of His is also known as common trunk. Without any clear histocytological borders with the AVN, it enters the central fibrous body (Fig. 1.5). The direction followed by the bundle of His in the central fibrous body is not constant; generally it follows the basis of the central fibrous body on the right side, toward the crest of the interventricular myocardial septum. However, a central location or a location toward the left within the fibrous septum are not rare [196].

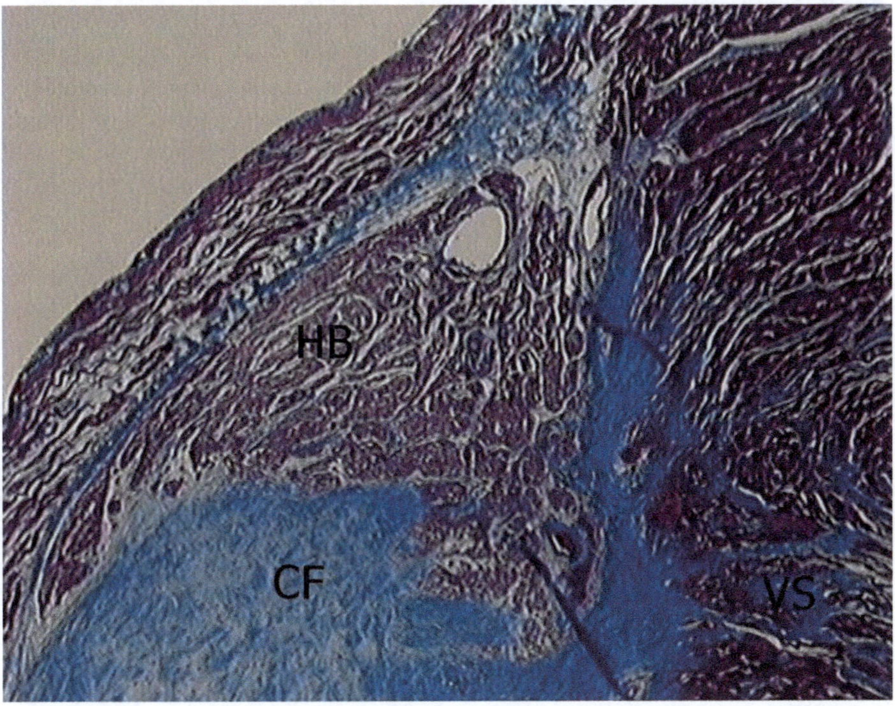

Fig. 1.5 Normal human bundle of His (*HB*) located in the central fibrous body (*CF*) (*VS* interventricular septum) (Trichromic Heidenhain, ×25)

The proximal portion of the bundle of His is sometimes distinguished by the penetrating portion entering the fibrous septum. The section of the bundle of His generally has an oval shape, but can vary notably case-by-case if examined at different levels. The best criteria to establish where the AVN ends and the bundle of His begins and what the AVN includes are still unclear [238]. The origin of the bundle of His can be defined in two different ways. According to the first definition, the bundle of His begins where the AVN becomes separate, through the fibrous body surrounding it, from the atrial septal fibers. According to the second definition, the bundle of His begins where the network of slender cells is connected to the parallel Purkinje fibers oriented longitudinally [88]. From the histological point of view, the fibers appear longer and more regularly located than in the AVN. Their caliber is basically uniform, except in the area close to the bifurcation where tortuous and irregular fibers appear. The transverse striation is more evident; the nuclei are smaller. The color remains in general less evident than in the common myocardium. The subdivision of the bundle of His into fibers directed to the two branches, as described by Sciacca et al. [221] several years ago, has been confirmed in the modern physio-pathological concept of the functional dualism in the longitudinal dissociation of the AV pathway, as well as in the "junctional" pathogenesis of the AV blocks [30, 196, 203, 209].

1.3.5.1 Histology

The bundle of His is composed, from its origin, of small nodal fibers of mean cross section 7×5 μm. The fibers gradually increase in diameter and become oriented parallel. James [85, 92] states that the common trunk is mainly composed of Purkinje cells oriented longitudinally and separated by basically continuous collagen, with few transverse anastomoses [88].

1.3.5.2 Vascular Supply

Usually the common trunk and the bifurcation are vascularized by arterioles originating from the *ramus septi fibrosi* (right coronary artery). However, some anatomo-clinical cases have shown that damage to the common trunk has been caused by alterations to the anterior descendant of the left coronary artery [30, 196, 203, 206, 209].

1.3.5.3 Innervation

Small nerves run down along the vessels of the common trunk; they are also observed in the fibrous septum [203, 209].

1.3.6 Bifurcating His Bundle or Bifurcation

The common trunk bifurcates after having assumed, in frontal section, a markedly more prismatic shape (Fig. 1.6). The division is at the level of the interventricular myocardial crest; it is almost never symmetrical and therefore it is observed with difficulty in single histological sections. Usually the bifurcation is located on the right side, the right bundle branch (RBB) being the continuation of the common trunk. However, in some cases it has been observed on the left side. In single sections, the appearance is characterized by the scarcity of bundles directed to the left compared to those of the RBB. This is not so much due to a great quantity of fibers in the RBB, but due to the fact that the fibers of the left bundle branch (LBB) radiate precociously, departing from the common trunk at the single levels as isolated ramifications. The fibers of the RBB represent instead a compact bundle. An interesting but generally neglected aspect of the Tawarian bifurcation is its variability, in both site and direction. This variability is not a purely anatomic issue, but also seems to play a role in the field of anatomo-pathological "vulnerability", with the well-known consequences on atrial and intraventricular conduction. In fact, the bifurcation sometimes does not appear to be located as a "rider" of the ventricular myocardial septal crest, according to the classical description, but on the contrary is located on a side, usually the right side, of the ventricular myocardium. So, as mentioned above, the bifurcation is displaced to the left side and the LBB runs down directly in the left subendocardium, while instead the RBB originates as a bundle included in the septal myocardium. Then the RBB runs an "intramural" course before reaching a subendocardial location. In rare cases the bifurcation is totally intramyocardial. It is located in the ventricular septum, so that both the branches have an intramural origin, and then go towards the respective endocardium [30, 203].

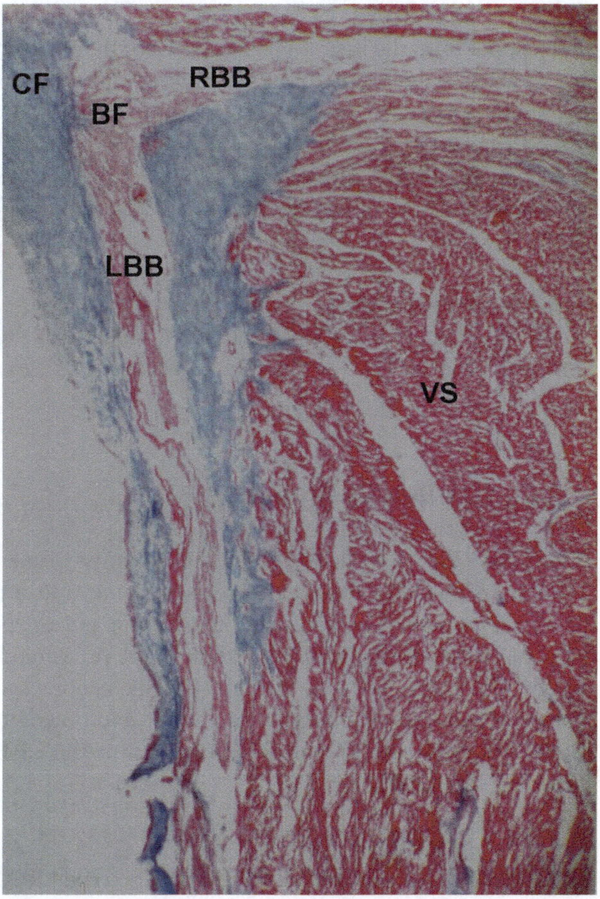

Fig. 1.6 Normal human bifurcating bundle of His (*BF*). The left bundle branch (*LBB*) runs directly down in the left subendocardium, while the right bundle branch (*RBB*) originates in the septal myocardium and has an intramural course before reaching a subendocardial location (*VS* interventricular septum, *CF* central fibrous body) (Trichromic Heidenhain, ×25)

1.3.7 Right Bundle Branch (RBB)

The RBB (Fig. 1.6) appears as the continuation of the common trunk, from which it continues first in a horizontal direction, and after passing under the confluence of the anterior and middle cuspides, passes under the right septal endocardium for about 0.5 cm. It then turns to the lower part and penetrates the muscular septum staying separate from it by a connective fold. After 1 cm it becomes subendocardial again and frays out near the base of the anterior papillary tricuspid muscle. Not rare in humans is the anatomic variant connected to that described as bifurcation where the root of the RBB directly penetrates the interstitium of the septal myocardium, so underlining a first intramural rather than a subendocardial portion. Such a variant may have anatomo-pathological significance if it causes an alteration in the branch with regional myocardial infarctions leading to direct or indirect compromise through a perifocal inflammatory reaction [30, 196, 203, 206, 209].

1.3.7.1 Histology

In its upper third the histological features of the RBB are the same as those observed at the level of the bifurcation. In the middle third it does not show any remarkable difference compared with the myocardium [196, 203].

1.3.7.2 Vascular Supply

The RBB is fed by a branch of an anterior septal artery (left coronary artery) [203, 209].

1.3.7.3 Innervation

In the RBB amyelinated fibrils are always detectable close to the myocardial fibers and to the capillaries by electron microscopy [30, 196, 203, 209].

1.3.8 Left Bundle Branch (LBB)

The LBB (Fig. 1.6) arises from the common trunk and is directed toward the homologous side of the ventricular septum as a thin bundle of fibers maintaining along their course a subendocardial location and an appearance similar to Purkinje fibers. A rare intramyocardial variant of the proximal LBB has been recently identified. The LBB, 1–2 cm from its origin, becomes fan-shaped subdividing in a complex and variable manner into richly and precociously anastomosed ramifications. A frankly dichotomous subdivision of the LBB is rare in the human heart [30, 196, 203, 209].

1.3.8.1 Histology

In the LBB there are many cells of Purkinje type [203, 209].

1.3.8.2 Vascular Supply

The anterior and middle ramifications of the LBB, which is broadly located on the left surface of the septum, are vascularized by the anterior perforant arteries (left coronary artery), and the posterior ramifications by the posterior perforant arteries (right coronary artery). Since the anterior perforant arteries are long, they also supply the intermediate area of the LBB. It must be underlined that the LBB, due to its subendocardial location and extension, is also oxygenated trans-endocardially by blood circulating in the ventricle [30, 196, 203, 209].

1.3.8.3 Innervation

The innervation of the LBB is limited, histologically at the light microscopic level, to thin and rare amyelinated subendocardial fibrils. On electronic microscopy, in contrast, the richness of the innervation of the branch is evident [30, 203, 209].

1.3.9 Fetal and Postnatal Development

The cardiac conduction system, proportionally wider in the fetus, is reduced in the newborn and even more in the adult. It seems that this reduction happens mainly by apoptosis. This is genetically programmed cellular death, not a result of illness, but perhaps secondarily caused by illness [35, 89]. In fact, developmental alterations in the cardiac conduction system after birth could lead to arrhythmias responsible for sudden and unexpected infant death [17, 86, 88, 91, 92, 130, 167–169].

1.3.9.1 Sinoatrial Node: Fetal and Postnatal Development

During the 6th to the 8th gestational week, the heart already shows many of its adult features and the SAN is already detectable. The cells of the SAN originate in the venous sinus. At this early stage, the cells of the SAN are all similar and appear as small dark cells. It seems that these cells are specialized since they arise and develop from primordial pacemaker sites. Nearing birth, the P cells and the slender cells quickly also become distinguishable on light microscopy, but they are a site of continuous further differentiation during the first years of life. In the adult SAN there are relatively fewer P cells than in the fetus and the newborn, while the slender cells are more frequent in the adult SAN [85, 92].

SAN Artery

During the early stages of fetal development, the SAN already contains a small artery, but its size increases during childhood and adolescence. During fetal development it appears as part of the arterial ring distributed at the junction of the venous sinus and the atrium. Some cells of the developing SAN are able to produce an electric impulse functionally totally independent of the central artery. The sinusal rhythm in the fetus and the newborn is fast and relatively unstable, unlike in the adult where it is slower and much more stable [85, 92].

Collagen Framework

A concomitant and tightly correlated feature during development is the increasing content of collagen. After birth, the collagen content of the SAN increases progressively up to adulthood, but the growth rate and the final amount of collagen vary greatly from one human heart to another. The volume of collagen in the adult SAN is so high as to represent the most readily distinguishable staining feature in histological slides for light microscopy. The postnatal development of the fibrous stroma of the SAN plays a key role in optimizing the stability of the normal cardiac pacemaker [85, 92].

SAN Innervation

Early during fetal development, there is clear evidence of cardiac cholinergic innervation, while adrenergic innervation develops afterwards and is completed only some months after birth. The scarcity of adrenergic innervation of the fetal and neonatal SAN can be compensated for by an increased sensitivity of the SAN to circulating catecholamines. The variability in autonomic influence through intranodal release of neurotransmitters should be one of the most efficient forms of control. The nervous control of the fetal and infant SAN is mainly cholinergic. The balanced autonomic innervation is developed in the postnatal SAN when the SAN has become intrinsically a generator of more stable impulses [85, 92].

1.3.9.2 Internodal Pathways: Fetal and Postnatal Development

Little is known about the fetal and postnatal development and changes in the internodal pathways, although many markers can be seen in the adult since the fetal heart completes its subdivision in the second month of gestation. Since the anterior and middle internodal pathways merge in the interatrial septum and since normally the oval foramen closes shortly after birth, it is probable that the septal course of the internodal pathways becomes well defined only during postnatal life. In cases of anomalous development of the atrial septum or of the primitive venous valves, it can be anticipated that the internodal conduction pathways will be altered [85, 92].

1.3.9.3 Atrioventricular Node Development

During embryonal development, the primitive AVN migrates inside the heart from its original epicardial center when the dorsal endocardial pillow invaginates during formation of the AV valves. The artery supplying the AVN originates from a large vessel that penetrates directly into the interventricular posterior vein near the junction with the coronary sinus. This suggests that the dorsal endocardial pillow migrates to the inside transporting with it the AVN and its artery [85]. Additional evidence for this migration of the AVN to the inside is the onset of mesotheliomas which certainly originate from primitive residual cells incorporated in the primitive heart by the adjacent epithelial tissue during embryonal development. The primitive AVN is thought to originate at the level of the junction of the superior cardinal vein and the venous sinus. Then, with the development of the left atrium and the incorporation of the venous sinus into the atrium, the AVN may move towards its adult location or may remain in the same location while the atria develop around it. The terminal portion of the left superior cardinal vein becomes the coronary sinus, while the proximal portion usually atrophies. In the human embryonic heart, immediately after the first month of gestation, the AVN can already be detected on histological examination. At this stage, it is vaguely organized, but is already in its characteristic location in relation to the central fibrous body that is still gelatinous in consistency. Both the AVN and the bundle of His are modified little or not at all during the remaining fetal life, but within one or two weeks of birth they undergo dramatic transformation [85, 88]. In the infant heart, there are fragments of nodal AV tissue dispersed along all the borders of the central fibrous body (including the ventricular septal crest). They are gradually reabsorbed during postnatal development, so that they are rarely seen in the adult heart [85]. Postnatal morphogenesis of the AVN and bundle of His is an important part of the normal development of the cardiac conduction system. The term "resorptive degeneration" was originally suggested by James in 1968 [84] to indicate the normal process of postnatal cardiac molding, consisting of degeneration, cell death and replacement in an orderly programmed way [35, 85, 88, 89]. The nature of the changes in the conduction system during the postnatal period and their relationship to sudden death in infancy has been a subject of debate [85, 167, 170].

1.3.9.4 Bundle of His and Bundle Branches Development

It seems that the bundle of His and bundle branches originate in a different way from the AVN. Some factors suggest that the bundle of His and its branches originate separately from the ventricular crest [85]:

1. Mesotheliomas rarely extend beyond the proximal border of the bundle of His, with a predominant location around and inside the AVN:
2. The action potential of the membranes of the cells of the AVN and bundle of His are very different;
3. All cases of congenital AV block studied histologically have basically shown the same lesion: an interruption between the AVN and the bundle of His, despite the presence of both structures;
4. In a clinical–pathological study of the absence of SAN activity and AV block in a dog, the cells of the SAN and of the AVN appeared not to be differentiated in their adult configuration, while the cells of the bundle of His and its proximal branches were normal;
5. The area of the junction between the AVN and the bundle of His appears to be a *locus minoris resistentiae* from the electrophysiological point of view, and because of its tendency to undergo focal ischemic degeneration.

None of these factors prove in themselves the separate origin of the AVN and the bundle of His, but taken together they strongly suggest this [85].

In the human embryonic heart, soon after the first gestational month, the bundle of His, similarly to the AVN, can be easily distinguished on histological examination. At this stage it is vaguely organized, but it is already in its characteristic site in relation to the central fibrous body that is still gelatinous in consistency [88]. The bundle of His in fetal life differs from its adult configuration in at least two important aspects: it is disproportionately large and wide, and it is widely attached to or in direct continuity with the myocytes of the interventricular septal crest. The AVN and the bundle of His do not change or change little during the remaining fetal life, but within one or two weeks of birth they undergo some "dramatic" transformations [85, 88].

1.3.9.5 AVN and Bundle of His Postnatal Molding

It has been shown that the human AVN and the bundle of His undergo extensive postnatal molding before reaching their adult configuration [84]. This should not be surprising, there being already many well-known examples of cardiac and great vessel molding after birth, for example, the closure of the oval foramen and the ductus arteriosus [85].

When the central fibrous body starts to change from a large gelatinous mass to a thin but strong fibrous mass in the adult heart, the AVN and the bundle of His undergo what Grant [64] in 1962 initially defined as a formation and remodeling process. Grant [64] described many postnatal events of the heart, such as the closure of the oval foramen and of the ductus arteriosus, and the thinning of the right ventricle wall. Similarly, the AVN and the bundle of His also undergo a remarkable postnatal transformation [64, 88]. In general terms, this postnatal molding of the AVN and the bundle of His can be considered as a molding and shaping process through which the surplus tissue is gradually reabsorbed so that these two electrically important structures are refined into their adult configuration. Many strands of surplus AVN tissue protruding into the central fibrous body of the fetal heart, the abundant conductive tissue connecting the fetal bundle of His with the ventricular septum, and most of the surplus volume of the bundle of His are reabsorbed [84, 87, 88]. It is interesting that this postnatal reabsorption of the bundle of His in humans takes place exclusively on its left side and never on the right.

The postnatal molding of the AVN and the bundle of His is ubiquitous in all normal hearts. This represents their transformation from a rough configuration, that may be electrically dangerous in the fetus and newborn, into their more smooth, and safe adult configuration. During the molding, the gradual reabsorption of the AVN and bundle of His cells seems to be a genetically programmed process. What begins and finishes the process within the first or second year of life in normal infants is unknown [88]. Inevitably, this process of postnatal morphogenesis is correlated with cellular death [84, 88], but this should be considered normal as many other examples of cellular death are associated with human morphogenesis [214].

The molding of young fibroblasts of the central fibrous body and of young growing cells of the AVN and bundle of His includes cellular death and focal cellular degeneration that can have dangerous consequences [84]. It has been proposed that congenital AV block represents an excessive growth of collagen along the bundle of His, jeopardizing its connection with the AVN. However, since homeostasis between the AVN/bundle of His and the central fibrous body cells is reached only some months or years after birth, the hypothesis of "over development" to explain congenital AV block would require that the block appears initially in the postnatal period, while it is already detectable prenatally. This strongly suggests, but it does not prove, that congenital AV block is due to incomplete development of the junction between the AVN and the bundle of His, rather than to a postjunctional overdevelopment of collagen [88].

Since AVN/bundle of His molding normally does not begin before birth, it can be suggested that postnatal events trigger the process. Hemodynamic cardiac and great vessel modifications at birth could be responsible for this process. If so, then the great physical stress normally involving the central fibrous cardiac body could induce modification of the functional relationship between young fibroblasts located therein and the adjacent AVN/bundle of His cells. There is also the possibility that the AVN/bundle of His cells are subject to genetic control leading to degeneration at a particular time or under particular conditions, as for instance during the postnatal hemodynamic changes. It is uncertain what factors control AVN/bundle of His molding in the postnatal period, but it is certain that the process takes place as one of the most important developmental changes of the cardiac conduction system [85].

1.3.10 Accessory Cardiac Conduction Pathways

Tawara [232], in his original description of the AVN, considered it as the beginning of the bundle of His and therefore the tract through which all the electrical activity of the atria is transmitted to the ventricles. This is true only in normal circumstances [88]. The impulse goes down from the SAN towards the ventricle, stops in the AVN where its speed is 2 cm/s. The point where the impulse passes from the bundle of His to the two bundle branches can be compared to a highway crossroads. In the SAN and in the AVN the impulse slows down, while in the bundle of His it speeds up [203, 209].

At the level of the AVJ there are transmission pathways, both normal and abnormal, in which the AVN can be partially or completely bypassed. A complete bypass of the AVN represents both an anatomic and a physiological abnormality, and it can be both near to or far from the AVN and the bundle of His [88]. When a complete bypass is next to the AVN, the fibers pass from the atrial septum through the central fibrous body independently of the AVN but directly connecting with the bundle of His [88, 198]. In some cases a defective reabsorption of the fetal tissue, perinatal or postnatal, as well as the same "highway", there are also accessory pathways directed toward the ventricles. Such malformations, under a neurovegetative influence, can induce cardiac activity dysfunction leading to cardiac arrhythmias and sudden death [90, 198].

When there is a working accessory AV connection, the whole AV system or its junctional tract can become part of the classic circuit of a tachycardic macroloop. It is well known that preexcitation depends on the presence of AV accessory pathways where the impulse can diffuse in an antegrade direction [197, 205].

The AV accessory connections are divided in three principal categories:

1. Direct accessory pathways, completely connecting the atrium to the ventricle through the conduction system: Kent fibers. They are subdivided into right, left, and medial.
2. Indirect accessory pathways, connecting the atrium to the ventricle through an anatomo-functional interposition of junctional tissue. They are subdivided into:
   - Mediate pathways for distal "input" within the cardiac conduction system, known as atriofascicular James fibers. They come down from the atrium and enter the junctional area beyond the nodal AV site of impulse deceleration.
   - Mediate pathways for "output", known as Mahaim fibers. They originate from the AVN, from the bundle of His and/or from the bifurcation and anastomose early with the septal ventricular myocardium. These mediate emission bundles of the Mahaim type, and are subdivided into superior (nodoventricular), middle (fascicular-ventricular), and inferior (ventricular-bifurcation).
3. Mixed accessory pathways, direct and indirect. They are represented by Kent medial and Mahaim superior pathways [128, 197, 198, 205].

The Kent-type direct bundles can be found anywhere on the contour of the AV rings, mostly on the subepicardial area and in the region of the trigonum (defective in such cases). Differently, James and Mahaim fibers are always located in the junctional area. The presence of AV accessory pathways is the necessary, but not sufficient, condition to determine preexcitation and/or reciprocating tachyarrhythmias. Such arrhythmias can start or stop depending on their uni- or bidirectional conductive activity under neurovegetative control [197, 198]. Embryology suggests that such anomalous connections represent the vestiges of the incomplete separation of the cardiac conduction system from the adjacent myocardium, and/or of the primordial mixture of atrial and ventricular myocardium in the fetal, newborn or infant heart. In fact, anomalous AV pathways are not rare. The malformations of accessory and/or double AV pathways have two possible causes. First, there may be defective reabsorption and shaping of the junctional tissue in the pre- and postnatal period, when the so-called "archipelago" of specific myocardial islands constituting the AVN/bundle of His axis should partly degenerate at the periphery and reunite in the mature AVJ. Second, there may be defective development of the AV fibrous rings and of the central fibrous body. This frequently seems to occur concomitantly with a low insertion of the medial tricuspid leaflet, so configuring a cardiac malformation microscopically similar to Ebstein disease called "micro-Ebstein" malformation. This micro-Ebstein malformation is characterized by a narrow muscular septum–septal connection composed of a direct mediate Kent bundle, mediate Mahaim fibers, or both the accessory AV pathway types [197, 198, 203].

1.3.10.1 Mahaim Fibers

The Mahaim fibers were first described in 1938 by Mahaim and Benatt [127]. In 1981, Gallagher et al. [57] pointed that the role of Mahaim fibers in the genesis of cardiac arrhythmias in man has been controversial since they were first described.

The Mahaim fibers are accessory pathways consisting of bundles of conducting tissue directly connecting the AVN, bundle of His or bifurcation directly to the ventricular myocardium. The Mahaim fibers are subdivided into superior (nodo-ventricular), middle (fascicular-ventricular) and inferior (ventricular-bifurcation), depending if the accessory pathway connects to the ventricle the AVN, bundle of His or bifurcation respectively. They are associated with forms of pre-excitation syndrome [7, 198, 203, 206] and are of great interest as morphological substrates for lethal arrythmias in fetuses and infants dying suddenly and unexpectedly [135, 176, 177].

1.3.10.2 James Fibers

The James fibers have been first described by James in 1961 [83]. They are atrio-fascicular accessory pathways connecting the atrium with the AVN or the bundle of His. The pathogenetic significance of the mediate bundles of James and Mahaim types is unclear, both in relation to the Lown-Ganong-Levine (LGL) syndrome [206, 208].

1.3.10.3 Kent Fibers

In 1893, Kent [101], while studying the AV muscular connections, proposed that there are multiple muscular links which crossed the AV groove, in particular a muscular connection between the right auricle and right ventricle at the lateral right border of the heart. In 1925, Lewis [120], not finding adequate anatomo-physiological evidence, questioned the role of "Kent's bundle" in the AV conduction. In 1930, Wolff, Parkinson, and White [248] reported 11 patients with the pre-excitation syndrome. In 1932, Holzmann and Scherf [74] suggested bypass tracts as the most likely mechanism of preexcitation syndrome that was called Wolff-Parkinson-White (WPW) syndrome. In 1947, Mahaim [128] stated that if Kent's fibres existed, they should be regarded as an accessory form of conduction: a para-specific conduction.

Kent fiber are considered to be accessory direct arrhythmogenic pathways that connect the atrium with the ventricle bypassing the classical conduction system. This anatomic defect results in double conductive pathways, with an accessory conduction pathway that does not slow down in the AVN. This represents the anatomic substrate for the ventricular preexcitation syndrome or WPW syndrome. The Kent bundle allows the passage of a faster impulse than the normal pathway because the deceleration in the AVN is skipped. Kent fibers may cause a tachycardic preexcitation of the ventricle, and the possibility of retrograde excitation of the atrium through the Kent fibers themselves. The impulse through the Kent bundle enters directly into the ventricle and can reenter along the septum crossing the conduction system in a retrograde way. The anomalous flow of reentry can cause a sudden ventricular fibrillation [203, 209].

Direct Kent fibers have been described in over 60% of patients with WPW syndrome who show a short P–Q time and delta wave. The pathogenetic role of the Kent bundle is confirmed by remission of preexcitation malignant arrhythmias after resection of the anomalous bundle [197, 207].

1.4 Central, Peripheral and Autonomic Nervous Systems

The regulation of cardiac rhythm is hardly distinguishable from that of vessel motility and respiratory activity, both from the anatomic and the physiological points of view. The neurovegetative innervation, cardiovascular and respiratory, comprises the central structures, i.e., nuclei of the brainstem and of the spinal cord, and the peripheral receptors, together with the nerves and ganglia. They are part of the mechano- or baroreceptor reflex arc that, with particular superior psycho-emotional integrations, seem to condition dysfunctions of varied intensity and sudden reflex death. The nervous control of the heart is due to the antagonism between sympathetic and vagal innervation. The central parasympathetic nuclei are situated in the brainstem while those of the sympathetic nervous system are located in the thoracic spinal cord [30, 134, 200].

1.4.1 Brainstem

There is a continuity between SIDS and unexpected perinatal death as common developmental abnormalities have been detected in the brainstem, in particular in the hypoplasia and neuronal immaturity of the arcuate nucleus and the other centers of regulation of the vital functions, i.e., hypoglossus nucleus, vagal dorsal motor nucleus, nucleus of the solitary tract, ambiguous nucleus, reticular ventrolateral formation in the medulla oblongata, the locus coeruleus, and the parabrachial Kölliker-Fuse complex in the junction between pons and midbrain; the red nucleus and the substantia nigra in the midbrain [153, 165, 184].

1.4.1.1 Arcuate Nucleus (ARCn)

The arcuate nucleus (ARCn) is located in the ventral surface of the medulla, close to the pyramidal bundles, and it extends longitudinally from the caudal border of the pons to the inferior pole of the olivary body. The neurons, which are polygonal or oval in shape, have average dimensions. The ARCn plays an important role in chemoreception, modifying blood gas exchange of oxygen and carbon dioxide, and acidity. The neuronal circuits of this vital area of the brainstem elaborate afferent and efferent stimuli, integrating both with impulses of the sympathetic thoracocervical chain, and with corticomesencephalic psychosensorial descending impulses. The reflexogenic reply is carried particularly along the motor fibers of the dorsal vagal nucleus. It is well known that barochemoreptorial reflexogenesis changes the cardiovascular vagal-sympathetic equilibrium in favor of the first (bradycardia, vasodilatation). However, in pathological cases with neurovegetative impairment, an altered vagal response may predispose to a violent sympathetic predominance (tachycardia, hypertension), lowering the threshold of ventricular fibrillation, leading to a high risk of sudden death. Moreover, the receptors are activated by circulating catecholamines [134, 200].

1.4.1.2 Parabrachial/Kölliker-Fuse Complex

The parabrachial/Kölliker-Fuse (PB/KF) complex is located in the junction between the pons and midbrain and plays an important role in modulating respiratory function. Morphologically, the PB/KF complex has been described as a group of neurons that surrounds the superior cerebellar peduncle, subdivided into three well-defined regions:

1. The medial parabrachial nucleus, localized ventromedially to the superior cerebellar peduncle.
2. The lateral parabrachial nucleus, located dorsally to the superior cerebellar peduncle.
3. The Kölliker-Fuse (KF) nucleus, located ventrally to the lateral parabrachial nucleus.

The complex has inhibitory activity, during fetal life, acting on chemoreceptor function and particularly on the pulmonary motor responses to blood changes in pO2, pCO2, and pH. After birth, the structures of the PB/KF complex participate in modulation of respiratory activity [34, 76, 114, 165].

1.4.1.3 Dorsal Motor Vagal Nucleus

The two principal vagal visceromotor nuclei are located in the brainstem above the ependymal and they are the dorsal vagal nucleus and the ambiguous nucleus.

The dorsal motor vagal nucleus consists of neurons of average size. It contains different neurochemical subpopulations with distinct physiological roles. It has been well established that the caudal region of this nucleus is involved in vagal reflexes controlling gastric motility, while the motoneurons with respiration-related activity are located at the rostral-intermediate levels [30, 165, 200].

1.4.1.4 Ambiguous Nucleus

The ambiguous nucleus has a major glossopharyngeal component; it has large neurons. Indeed, it is considered one of the magnocellular nuclei of the respiratory ventrolateral reticular formation, a respiratory center [165].

1.4.1.5 Solitary Tract Nucleus

The solitary tract nucleus consists of neurons of rather small size and is located lateral to the dorsal vagal nucleus. Like the ambiguous nucleus, it is glossopharyngeal, but has small neurons. Viscerosensitive fibers of the glossopharyngeus, coming from the intercarotid and mediastinal baroreceptors are carried along the solitary tract to the solitary tract nucleus. The nucleus has close anatomic relationships with the adjacent vagal nuclei (dorsal vagal nucleus and ambiguous nucleus), with the reticular formation and with the superior centers, particularly the locus coeruleus, and is involved in control of baroreflexogenesis [165].

1.4.1.6 Locus Coeruleus

The locus coeruleus is a complex of catecholaminergic neurons located in the rostral dorsolateral pons, and has been extensively studied in numerous animal species. Projections from this nucleus are responsible for more than half of the noradrenergic connections throughout the brain, including the neocortex, thalamus, amygdala, hippocampus, hypothalamus, cerebellum, medulla oblongata and spinal cord. The locus coeruleus is known to be the major producer of noradrenaline, and subserves several important physiological functions including the sleep-waking cycle and control of the cardiovascular and respiratory systems [117].

1.4.1.7 Hypoglossal Nucleus

The hypoglossal nucleus is the motor nucleus innervating the intrinsic and four of the five extrinsic muscles of the tongue. It is located in the medulla oblongata near the midline, immediately beneath the floor of the inferior recess of the rhomboid fossa. Impairment of deglutition due to hypoplasia and/or neuronal immaturity of the hypoglossal nucleus seems to play a role in SIDS [174].

1.4.2 Spinal Cord

The sympathetic neurons gathered in the lateral horns of levels T1–T5 of the spinal cord send their axons through communicating branches to the ganglia T1–T5 of the sympathetic chain from which the cardiac branches originate. From the first thoracic ganglion the sympathetic trunk extends toward the neck together with the stellate ganglion (cervical inferior, sometimes fused with the first thoracic ganglion), the middle ganglion (small) and the superior cervical ganglion (great), which contribute to the cardiac innervation. The nervous ramifications coming from these ganglionar structures anastomose with those of the vagus nerve [30, 200].

1.4.3 Extrinsic Cardiac Innervation

1.4.3.1 Right Side of the Heart

The nerves of the right side of the human heart, belonging to the right thoracic sympathetic chain, converge in the right stellate ganglion from which originates a thin right stellate cardiac nerve that is directed medially toward the superior vena cava and the aortic sulcus. From the middle cervical ganglion a right dorsolateral cardiac thoracic nerve also originates. The inferior laryngeal recurrent vagus nerve gives off a recurrent cardiac branch and cardiac cranio- and caudovagal nerves [209].

1.4.3.2 Left Side of the Heart

The cardiac innervation of the left portion consists of a prominent sympathetic left stellate ganglion that gives origin to a left stellate cardiac nerve that reaches the left auricula. Most of the left vagal cardiac left branches, in contrast to those of the right, interconnect with the sympathetic branches [209].

All these cardiac nerves, of right and of left, tend to converge in an undefined, varying, but conspicuous extrinsic cardiac plexus (including the intertruncal and/or aorticocoronary plexuses) where there is a rich neuroreceptor paraganglial component. The usual indication of a connection between the aortic and pulmonary glomera is purely conventional.

The first branch of the left coronary artery, sometimes called the intertruncal artery, connects with the system of the paraganglia of the left coronary artery. In the nerve of the extrinsic cardiac plexus there are numerous united cells similar to paraganglial cells (rich in granules containing aminic neurotransmitter) mixed with neurons [206, 209].

1.4.4 Intrinsic Cardiac Innervation

The intrinsic innervation of the heart is represented by a diffused vagal-sympathetic plexus. The plexuses are differentiated into intracardiac, ganglionar, subepicardial, intramyocardial diffused particularly along the coronary ramifications, and terminal to the receptor and afferent structures. The sympathetic neuroreceptors are mostly located in the anterior wall, while the vagal neuroreceptors are in the post-inferior wall. It is almost impossible to distinguish anatomically the sympathetic from the parasympathetic structures, and the afferent from the efferent functions [203].

The vagal and sympathetic nerves, arising or not from the extrinsic cardiac plexus, reach the subepicardium where they form the ganglionar plexus at the level of the sinoatrial inlet of the superior vena cava, around the SAN and along the *crista terminalis*. Numerous ganglia are gathered around the AV sulcus, but these are rare in the ventricles. The ganglionar sinoatrial plexus is mainly vagal in nature, and seems to decrease from the AV sulcus toward the lower part. From the ganglionar plexus, the so-called "coarse plexus" is branched and divided within the myocardium into a thinner plexus and a terminal or preterminal one. Recently a diagram of the intrinsic cardiac innervation, in which the sympathetic ventricular fibers from the AV sulcus continue into a subepicardial position, from the base toward the apex, becoming intramural and subendocardial, has been proposed. The vagal fibers, instead, cross proximally toward the epicardium and send fibers to the wall and distally to the epicardium near the apex. Regarding the terminal axonal branches, electron microscopy reveals axonal swelling with synaptic vesicles, granular or agranular and rich in neurotransmitters while the cardiac receptor structures are very difficult to visualize morphologically. Vagal and sympathetic receptors might have different spatial densities in the inferior and anterior ventricular walls [206].

1.4.5 Nervous Structures Regulating Cardiac Activity

In relation to the reflexogenic stimuli of mechano- and chemoreceptor type, i.e., variations in cardiac activity in relation to arterial pressure, pO2 and pCO2, nervous structures regulating cardiac activity include sympathetic ganglia, carotid cardioinhibitory receptors, and juxtacardiac and mediastinal ganglia and paraganglia.

The sympathetic ganglia comprise the stellate ganglion and the cervicosuperior ganglion. The carotid cardioinhibitory receptors comprise the carotid body or glomus and the carotid sinus.

The carotid body is a classical chemoreceptor paraganglion, formed principally by cells of neuronal origin whose cytoplasm is rich in argyrophilic granules containing catecholamine neurotransmitter. These cellular elements, gathered in glomeruli (Zellballen), are surrounded by sustentacular cells of schwannian type. The organelles connect with the adventitia of carotid-derived arterioles and with mixed glossopharyngeal nervous plexuses of vagal and, less frequently, sympathetic origin [134, 205] (Fig. 1.7).

The carotid sinus, unlike the carotid body, is a paraganglial organelle. The carotid sinus comprises mechanoreceptor glossopharyngeal and in small measure vagal nerve terminations called Krause's club-like, partially anastomosed along the external portion of the middle tunica of the initial tract of the internal carotid artery. The carotid sinus configures an anatomic area inside the arterial tunica media (outer layer), in which many nerve endings lie that are also called Krause's club-like. The clear structural difference between the carotid body and the carotid sinus does not correspond to a substantial distinction between, respectively, chemo- and baroreception. In fact, a small paraganglion can sometimes be found in the inside portion of the adventitia of the carotid sinus adjacent to Krause bodies which are likewise innervated. Moreover, paraganglial cells are sometimes present in the trunk of the vagus nerve at the level of the carotid bifurcation.

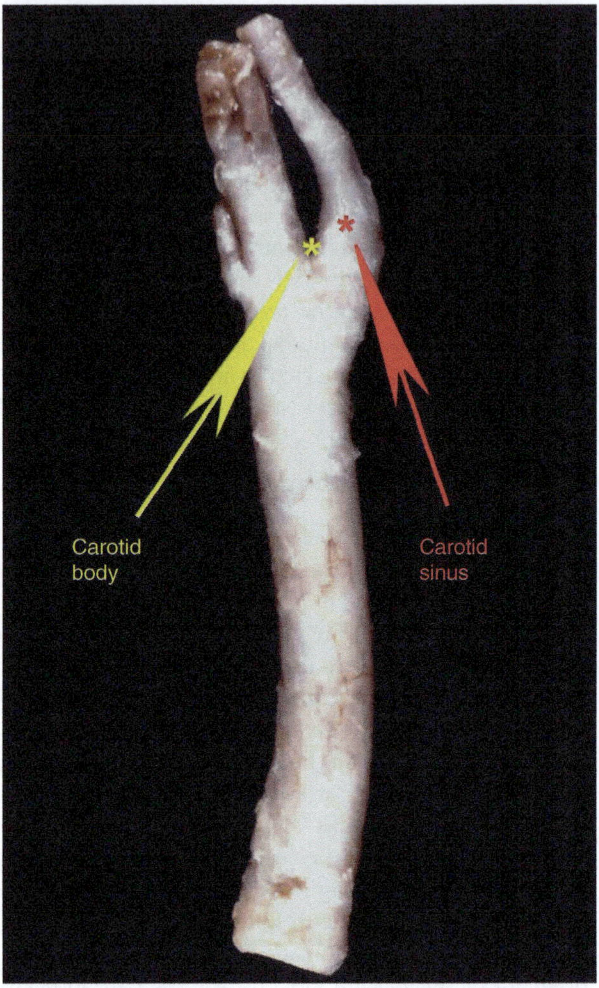

Fig. 1.7 The carotid body or glomus is located between the two carotid branches; it is found in the area of the carotid bifurcation, on the internal carotid artery side, close to the "swelling" of the carotid sinus. A little above the bifurcation, the carotid sinus is located just at the root of the internal carotid artery

This complex histological structure reflects the difficulty in distinguishing baro and chemoreflexogenesis in the neuronal glossopharyngeal-vagal circuits of the brainstem [134, 205, 209]. The baroreflexogenic function of the carotid sinus correlates with the chemoreflexogenic function of the inherent glomeruli so forming a unique anatomic complex. Performing a stimulating maneuver, so-called "massage of the carotid sinus" in this region, produces abnormal reflexes provoked not only by the stimulation of the carotid sinus, but also of the local glomerula (carotid body, glomus of the carotid sinus and/or sometimes intravagal paraganglia). Moreover, argyrophilic cells have been observed in the cervical sympathetic ganglia. They are considered interneurons that control the general level of afferent and efferent activity. Experimental evidence suggests that modifications of the cardiac rhythm are due only to the action of the low neuroreceptors rather than to that of the carotid sinus [209] (Fig. 1.7).

1.4.5.1 Juxtacardiac and Mediastinal Ganglia and Paraganglia

These are situated in the fibroadipose tissue between the ascending aorta, the aortic arch and the bifurcation of the pulmonary artery. They are neuroreceptors, microscopic structures whose fundamental function is to modulate cardiac activity [205]. In the modern literature, different paraganglial structures corresponding to embryonal branchiomeric levels I–IV are distinguished. Beyond the carotid sinuses the mediastinal glomera and the coronary glomus are included. However, the histological picture appears to be more complex: rather than glomera distinguished as "aortic", "pulmonary" and "coronary", minute disseminated receptors are observed, present also in nervous ramifications sometimes with the principal cells mixed with neurons, with no relationship to vascular structures. These ganglial-paraganglial intraneural and extravascular units within the cardiac plexus participate in the regulation, and to the possible disorder, of reflexogenic activity. The juxtacardiac ganglia paraganglia, as well as the intracardiac receptors, influence the arterial pressure and the cardiac rhythm for vagal and/or sympathetic stimulation [192–194].

Although there is glomus tissue in a variety of sites throughout the body, the most important are the carotid bodies and the aortic bodies, also known as aorticopulmonary paraganglia (APP), which are a more diffuse group of small glomera primarily situated in the aortic arch [112, 148]. Little is known about the pathology of the APP. Although they are a critical component of respiratory control, their neuroanatomic complexity has been investigated to only a limited extent in human disease [199, 201, 204]. Histologically they consist of small groups of lobules of glomic tissue separated by a well-vascularized connective tissue with a prolific supply of nerve bundles and ganglion cells [112]. Each lobule contains several distinct cell clusters consisting of central cores of chief (glomus type I) cells surrounded by thin rims of elongated sustentacular (glomus type II) cells [112]. Most investigators [46] consider the chief cells, containing a dense core of neurosecretory granules, to be the chemosensitive element or transducer within the APP with a presumed chemoreceptor function. Only a few investigators [148, 192] have studied the possible role of the APP in pathological processes involving cardiorespiratory disturbances.

Stephan-Blanchard et al. [227] reported the current knowledge on peripheral chemoreceptor function in preterm neonates, measuring the peripheral chemoreceptor activity at thermoneutrality in neonates born to nonsmoking and smoking mothers, performing a 30 s hyperoxic test during active and quiet sleep. They reported that prenatal smoking exposure in neonates have a negative impact on peripheral chemoreceptor tonic activity, hypothesizing the presence of preexisting damage in the brainstem and cardiac conduction. The common physiopathology of sudden unexplained infant and perinatal death is attributed to impaired developmental processes in the peripheral chemoreceptors, i.e., in the carotid and aortic bodies and the aorticopulmonary paraganglia. At the functional level, a sudden death implies a defective resetting, slow or incomplete, of the sensitivity to hypoxia and hypercapnia and/or a defective processing of signals in the brainstem cardio-respiratory centers. A normal infant's nervous system receives prompt information on a progressive hypercapnia and hypoxia event, and triggers respiration or arousal. In infants with peripheral or central chemoreception defects, these protective reflexes are not released, and prolonged apnea can develop which may be fatal and lead to sudden death. Smoke exposure *in utero* acts as a triggering phenomenon in fetuses and infants with developmental abnormalities located the in brainstem centers regulating vital functions or in the cardiac conduction system [182].

1.5 Review Questions

This test, composed of 10 multiple-choice questions, is designed to measure knowledge about the contents of this chapter on Introduction to Sudden Infant and Perinatal Unexplained Death. Questions have only one correct answer and cover the major content areas of this chapter. Check the correct responses and score your test using the answer keys on page 48.

1. Which of the following statements about SIDS is correct?
   - □ A. SIDS is completely preventable.
   - □ B. SIDS is the leading cause of death of infants aged one month to one year.
   - □ C. Most infants were not considered to be healthy before they were found dead from SIDS.
   - □ D. SIDS is caused by aspiration or choking.
   - □ E. SIDS is caused by immunization.
2. How often does SIDS occur in the USA?
   - □ A. SIDS strikes one infant in every 500–750 live births.
   - □ B. SIDS strikes one infant in every 750–1,000 live births.
   - □ C. SIDS strikes one infant in every 1,750–2,000 live births.
   - □ D. SIDS strikes one infant in every 2,500–3,000 live births.
   - □ E. SIDS strikes one infant in every 3,000–5,000 live births.
3. Current SIDS research supports the theory that intrinsic and extrinsic risk factors provides unification into the underlying triple-risk model called:
   - □ A. Triple risk model
   - □ B. Vulnerable infant model
   - □ C. Critical development theory
   - □ D. Double risk theory
   - □ E. Exogenous stressors model
4. Since 1994, when the NICHD launched the official federal "Back to Sleep" campaign, advising caregivers to place infants to sleep on their back, the SIDS rate in the USA has decreased by:
   - □ A. 15%
   - □ B. 30%
   - □ C. 50%
   - □ D. 70%
   - □ E. 75%

5. The SIDS incidence is disproportionately higher in which of the following ethnic groups:
   □ A. American Indians, Alaskan Natives, and African Americans
   □ B. Hispanics
   □ C. Caucasians
   □ D. American Indians
   □ E. African Americans
6. Which of the following does not belong to the cardiac conduction system?
   □ A. His bundle
   □ B. Aortic valve
   □ C. Atrio-ventricular node
   □ D. Sino-atrial node
   □ E. Purkinje cells
7. Where is the arcuate nucleus, often hypoplastic in SIDS, located?
   □ A. Pons
   □ B. Midbrain
   □ C. Medulla oblongata
   □ D. Spinal cord
   □ E. Cerebellum
8. Which of the following is a safe sleeping environment for infants?
   □ A. Soft sleeping surfaces free of loose bedding and free of stuffed toys surrounding the infant
   □ B. A firm mattress with loose bedding
   □ C. Loose bedding, such as quilts and comforters
   □ D. A firm mattress, free of loose bedding and free of stuffed toys surrounding the infant
   □ E. A soft mattress with loose bedding
9. Which of the following statements on the current recommendations from the American Academy of Pediatrics described in the policy statement of the Task Force on SIDS is correct?
   □ A. Recommendations are divided into three levels based respectively on good and consistent scientific evidence (Level A), limited or inconsistent scientific evidence (Level B), consensus and expert opinion (Level C).
   □ B. Level A Recommendations are based on limited or inconsistent scientific evidence, such as, infants should be immunized in accordance with recommendations of the AAP and Centers for Disease Control and Prevention.
   □ C. Level B Recommendations are based primarily on consensus and expert opinion, such as Health care professionals, staff in newborn nurseries and NICUs, and child care providers should endorse the SIDS risk-reduction recommendations from birth.
   □ D. Level C Recommendations are based on good and consistent scientific evidence, such as Back to sleep for every sleep.
   □ E. Level B Recommendations are based on good and consistent scientific evidence, such as room-sharing without bed-sharing.

10. Which of the following is not a SIDS risk reduction recommendation?
    - □ A. Place infants to sleep in a firm sleep surface.
    - □ B. Do not use fluffy bedding or stuffed toys in the crib.
    - □ C. Do not smoke around infants.
    - □ D. Keep infants warm by wrapping tightly with blankets.
    - □ E. Place infants on their backs to sleep for every sleep.

1.6 Answer Keys

Block 1 (Questions 1–10)

1. B
2. C
3. A
4. C
5. A
6. B
7. C
8. D
9. A
10. D

References

1. Adelson L, Kinney ER (1956) Sudden and unexpected death in infancy and childhood. Pediatrics 17:663–697.
2. Adelson L (1963) Specific studies of infant victims of sudden death, Sudden Death in Infants. In: Wedgewood RJ, Benditt EP (eds) Proceedings of the Conference on Causes of Sudden Death in Infants. September 1963, Seattle, WA. GPO PHS Publ. 1412, Washington, DC, pp 1–40.
3. Al-Kindy HA, Gélinas JF, Hatzakis G, Côté A (2009) Risk Factors for extreme events in infants hospitalized for apparent life-threatening events. J Pediatr 154:332–337.
4. American Academy of Pediatrics AAP Task Force on Infant Positioning and SIDS (1992) Positioning and SIDS. Pediatrics 89:1120–1126.
5. American Academy of Pediatrics Task Force on Sudden Infant Death Syndrome (2005) The changing concept of sudden infant death syndrome: diagnostic coding shifts, controversies regarding the sleeping environment, and new variables to consider in reducing risk. Pediatrics 116:1245–1255.
6. American Academy of Pediatrics, Hymel KP, Committee on Child Abuse and Neglect, National Association of Medical Examiners (2006) Distinguishing sudden infant death syndrome from child abuse fatalities. Pediatrics 118:421–427.
7. Anderson RH, Becker AE, Brechenmacher C, Davies MJ, Rossi L (1975) Ventricular preexcitation. A proposed nomenclature for its substrates. Eur J Cardiol 3:27–36.
8. Anderson RH (2000) Sudden and unexpected death in infancy and the conduction system of the heart. Cardiovasc Pathol 9:147–148.
9. Arntzen A, Moum T, Magnum P, Bakketeig LS (1995) Is the higher postneonatal mortality in lower social status due to SIDS? Acta Paediatr 84:188–192.

10. Balk SJ, Bearer CF, Etzel RA, Falk H, Hendrick JG, Miller MD, Miller RW, Rogan W, She KM, Simon PR (1997) Environmental tobacco smoke: a hazard to children (RE9716). Pediatrics 99:639–642.
11. Bamford OW, Jones DR (1976) Respiratory and cardiovascular interaction in ducks: the effect of lung degeneration on the initiation of and recovery from some cardiovascular responses to submergence. J Physiol 259:575–596.
12. Beckwith JB (1970) Discussion of terminology and definition of the sudden infant death syndrome. In: Bergman AB, Beckwith JB, Ray CG (eds) Sudden infant death syndrome: proceedings of the second international conference on the causes of sudden death in infants. University of Washington Press, Seattle, pp 14–22.
13. Beckwith JB (1993) A proposed new definition of sudden infant death syndrome. In: Walker AM, McMillen C (eds) Second SIDS international conference. Perinatology Press, Ithaca, pp 431–434.
14. Beckwith JB (2003) Defining the sudden infant death syndrome. Arch Pediatr Adolesc Med 157:286–290.
15. Benedetti G (1994) Risvolti giuridico-pratici della morte improvvisa cardiaca che attengono alla Procura della Repubblica. Pathologica 86:430–433.
16. Berry PJ (1992) Pathological findings in SIDS. J Clin Pathol 45(11 Suppl):11–16.
17. Bharati S, Krongrad E, Lev M (1985) Study of the conduction system in a population of patients with sudden infant death syndrome. Pediatr Cardiol 6:29–40.
18. Bigger HR, Silvestri JM, Shott S, Weese Mayer DE (1998) Influence of increased survival in very low birth weight, low weight, and normal birth weight infants on the incidence of sudden infant death syndrome in the United States: 1985–1991. J Pediatr 133:73–78.
19. Boyd E (1927) Growth of the thymus, its relation to status thymicolymphaticus and thymic symptoms. Am J Dis Child 33:867–879.
20. Boyle FM, Vance JC, Najman JM, Thearle MJ (1996) The mental health impact of stillbirth, neonatal death or SIDS: prevalence and patterns of distress among mothers. Soc Sci Med 43:1273–1282.
21. Brooks JG, Kattwinkel J, Keenan ME, Malloy M, Scheers NJ, Willinger M (2000) Changing concepts of sudden infant death syndrome: implications for infant sleeping environment and sleep position. Pediatrics 105:650–656.
22. Burchell A, Lyall H, Busuttil A, Bell E, Hume R (1992) Glucose metabolism and hypoglycemia in SIDS. J Clin Pathol 45(11 Suppl):39–45.
23. Byard RW, Krous HF (eds) (2001) Sudden infant death syndrome. Problems, progress & possibilities. Arnold, Hodder Headline Group, London.
24. Calderoli R, Martini F, Galli S, Matturri L (2002) Post mortem discipline on the sudden infant death syndrome (SIDS) and of unexpected late fetal stillbirth victims. In: Proceedings of the 7th SIDS International Conference, Florence, p 135.
25. Campbel MJ, Julious SA, Peterson CK, Tobias A (2001) Atmospheric pressure and sudden infant death syndrome in Cook County, Chicago. Paediatr Perinatal Epidemiol 3:287–289.
26. Camps FE, Carpenter RG (1970) Sudden and unexpected deaths in infancy (cot deaths): report of the proceedings of the Sir Samuel Bedson Symposium. April 17–18th. Addenbrook's Hospital, Cambridge, UK.
27. Carpenter R, McGarvey C, Mitchell EA, Tappin DM, Vennemann MM, Smuk M, Carpenter JR (2013) Bed sharing when parents do not smoke: is there a risk of SIDS? An individual level analysis of five major case-control studies. BMJ Open 3:e002299.
28. Carroll J (2004) Apparent life threatening events (ALTE) assessment. Pediatr Pulmonol 26(Suppl):108–109.
29. Carroll-Pankhurst C, Mortimer EA (2001) Sudden infant death syndrome, bedsharing, parental weight, and age at death. Pediatrics 107:530–536.
30. Castano P, Cocco L, De Barbieri A, D'Este L, Floriani F, Gheri G, Mondello MR, Papa S, Petriglieri P, Pizzini G, Ridola C, Sirigu P, Spinella S (1986) Anatomia Umana. Edi-Ermes, Milan, pp 434–440.
31. Centers for Disease Control and Prevention (CDC) (2014) Linked birth/infant death records, 2007–2010 results. http://wonder.cdc.gov/lbd-current.html. Accessed July 26, 2014.

32. Centers for Disease Control and Prevention (CDC) (2012) Postneonatal mortality among Alaska Native infants – Alaska, 1989–2009. MMWR Morb Mortal Wkly Rep 61:1–5.
33. Centers for Disease Control and Prevention (2014) Sudden unexpected infant death and sudden infant death syndrome. http://www.cdc.gov/sids/. Accessed July 26, 2014.
34. Chamberlin NL, Saper CB (1994) Topographic organization of respiratory responses to glutamate microstimulation of the parabrachial nucleus in the rat. J Neurosci 414:6500–6510.
35. Colombo B, Ottaviani G, Ramos SG, Matturri L (1998) Apoptosis in cardiac conduction system in sudden infant death syndrome (SIDS): preliminary results. In: Proceedings of the 5th SIDS International Conference, Rouen, p 157.
36. Constitution of the Italian Republic, February 2, 2006, Law n° 31 (2006) Regulations for diagnostic post mortem investigation in victims of sudden infant death syndrome and unexpected fetal death. Official Gazette of the Italian Republic General Series 34:4. http://users.unimi.it/giuliaottaviani/pdf/legge.pdf. Accessed July 26, 2014.
37. Cooper RM, Lumley J (1996) Mother's knowledge of the risk factors and anxiety about SIDS. J Paediatr Child Health 32:310–315.
38. Corr CA, Fuller H, Barnickol CA, Corr DM (eds) (1991) Sudden infant death syndrome: who can help and how. Springer, New York.
39. Côtè A, Hum C, Brouillette RT, Themens M (1998) Frequency and timing of recurrent events in infants using home cardio-respiratory monitors. J Pediatr 132:783–789.
40. Cotzias CS, Paterson-Brown S, Fisk NM (1999) Prospective risk of unexplained stillbirth in singleton pregnancies at term: population based analysis. BMJ 319:287–288.
41. Crotti L, Tester DJ, White WM, Bartos DC, Insolia R, Besana A, Kunic JD, Will ML, Velasco EJ, Bair JJ, Ghidoni A, Cetin I, Van Dyke DL, Wick MJ, Brost B, Delisle BP, Facchinetti F, George AL, Schwartz PJ, Ackerman MJ (2013) Long QT syndrome-associated mutations in intrauterine fetal death. JAMA 309:1473–1482.
42. Davies MJ, Anderson RH, Becker AE (1983) The conduction system of the heart. Butterworth, London.
43. Eastman Q (2003) Genetics. Crib death exoneration could usher in new gene tests. Science 300:1858.
44. Emery JL (1993) Child abuse, sudden infant death syndrome, and unexpected infant death. Am J Dis Child 147:1097–1100.
45. Escherich T (1896) Status thymico-lymphaticus. Berlin klin, Woeschesucher, p 29.
46. Eyzaguirre C, Nishi K, Fidone S (1972) Chemoreceptor synapses in the carotid body. Fed Proc 31:1385–1393.
47. Fares T, McCulloch KM, Raju TN (1997) Intrauterine cocaine exposure and the risk for sudden infant death syndrome: a meta-analysis. J Perinatol 17:179–182.
48. Fearn SW (1834) Two cases of sudden and unexplained death of children during sleep. Lancet 1:246–248.
49. Filiano JJ, Kinney HC (1992) Arcuate nucleus hypoplasia in the sudden infant death syndrome. J Neuropathol Exp Neurol 51:394–403.
50. Filiano JJ, Kinney HC (1994) A perspective on neuropathologic findings in victims of sudden infant death syndrome: the triple risk model. Biol Neonate 65:194–197.
51. Fleming KA (1992) Viral respiratory infection and SIDS. J Clin Pathol 45(11 Suppl):29–32.
52. Franco P, Montemitro E, Scaillet S, Groswasser J, Kato I, Lin JS, Villa MP (2011) Fewer spontaneous arousals in infants with apparent life-threatening event. Sleep 34:733–743.
53. Frahna JG, Pollack HA (2001) A competing risk model of sudden infant death syndrome incidents in two US birth cohorts. J Pediatr 138:661–667.
54. Freeman DH, Malloy MH (2000) Birth weight- and gestational age-specific sudden infant death syndrome mortality: United States, 1991 versus 1995. Pediatrics 105:1227–1231.
55. Friedleben A (1858) Die physiologie der thymusdruese. Gesundheit and Krankheit, Frankfurt, p 336.
56. Frøen JF, Arnestad M, Vege A, Irgens LM, Rognum TO, Saugstad OD, Stray-Pedersen B (2002) Comparative epidemiology of sudden infant death syndrome and sudden intrauterine unexplained death. Arch Dis Child Fetal Neonatal Ed 87:F118–F121.

57. Gallagher JJ, Smith WM, Kassell JH, Benson DWJ, Sterba R, Grant AO (1981) Role of Mahaim fibers in cardiac arrhythmias in man. Circulation 64:176–189.
58. Gandevia SC, McCloskey DI, Potter EK (1978) Reflex bradycardia occurring in response to diving, nasopharyngeal stimulation and ocular pressure, and its modification by respiration and swallowing. J Physiol 276:383–394.
59. Gerbitz KD, Jaksch M (1994) Mitochondrial DNA, aging and sudden infant death syndrome. Eur J Clin Chem Clin Biochem 32:487–488.
60. Getahun D, Amre D, Rhoads GG, Demissie K (2004) Maternal and obstetric risk factors for sudden infant death syndrome in the United States. Obstet Gynecol 103:646–652.
61. Ghidoni P, Giudici E, Matturri L, Rossi L (1986) Extranodal specialized sinoatrial cells. Anal Quant Cytol Histol 8:255–258.
62. Goldbloom A, Wigglesworth FW (1938) Sudden death in infancy. Can Med Assoc J 38:119–129.
63. Gooden BA (1994) Mechanism of the human diving response. Integr Physiol Behav Sci 29:6–16.
64. Grant RP (1962) The embryology of ventricular flow pathways in man. Circulation 25:756–779.
65. Green A (1993) Biochemical screening in newborn siblings of cases of SIDS. Arch Dis Child 68:793–796.
66. Gregersen N, Winter V, Jensen PK, Holmskov A, Kolvraa S, Andresen BS, Christensen E, Bross P, Lundemose JB, Gregersen M (1995) Prenatal diagnosis of medium-chain acyl-CoA dehydrogenase (MCAD) deficiency in a family with a previous fatal case of sudden unexpected death in childhood. Prenat Diagn 15:82–86.
67. Guntheroth WG (1995) Crib death: the sudden infant death syndrome, 3rd edn. Futura Publishing Company, Armonk/New York.
68. Guntheroth WG (1999) Risk factors for SIDS. In: Proceedings of the 19th International Symposium on Neonatal Intensive Care, Milan, p 36.
69. Guntheroth WG, Spiers PS (1992) Sleeping prone and the risk of sudden infant death syndrome. JAMA 267:2359–2362.
70. Guntheroth WG, Spiers PS (1996) Are bedding and rebreathing suffocation a cause of SIDS? Pediatr Pulmonol 22:335–341.
71. Guntheroth WG, Spiers PS (1999) Prolongation of the QT interval and the sudden infant death syndrome. Pediatrics 10:813–814.
72. Guntheroth WG, Spiers PS (2001) Thermal stress in sudden infant death: is there an ambiguity with the rebreathing hypothesis? Pediatrics 107:693–698.
73. Haas JE, Taylor JA, Bergman AB, Van Belle G, Felgenhauer JL, Siebert JR, Benjamin DR (1993) Relationship between epidemiologic risk factors and clinicopathologic findings in the sudden infant death syndrome. Pediatrics 91:106–112.
74. Holzmann M, Scherf D (1932) Uber Elektrokardiogramme mit verkurzter Vorhof-Kammerdiztanz und positiven P-Zacken. Z Klin Med 121:404–423.
75. Hawkes N (2013) Sharing a bed with your baby increases the risk of sudden infant death syndrome, UK study shows. BMJ 346:f3296.
76. Hirano T, Simbulan D, Kumayawa T (1994) Effects of kainic acid in the parabrachial region for ongoing respiratory activity and reflexive respiratory suppression. Brain Res 665:54–62.
77. Holy Bible: New revised standard version catholic edition (NRSV-CE), Catholic Biblical Association (1989) Bible Gateway. http://www.biblegateway.com/. Accessed July 26, 2014.
78. Hoffman HJ, Damus K, Hillman L, Kangrad E (1988) Risk factors for SIDS. Results of the National Institute of Child Health and Human Development SIDS cooperation epidemiological study. Ann N Y Acad Sci 533:13–30.
79. Hunt CE (2001) Sudden infant death syndrome and other causes of infant mortality: diagnosis, mechanisms, and risk for recurrence in siblings. Am J Respir Crit Care Med 164:346–357.
80. Hunt CE, Corwin MJ, Lister G, Weese-Mayer DE, Ward SL, Tinsley LR, Neuman MR, Willinger M, Ramanathan R, Rybin D, Collaborative Home Infant Monitoring Evaluation (CHIME) Study Group (2008) Precursors of cardio-respiratory events in infants detected by home memory monitor. Pediatr Pulmonol 43:87–98.

81. Iams JD, Lynch CD (2011) Stillbirth and lessons for pregnancy care. JAMA 306:2506–2507.
82. 2013 ICD-10-CM Diagnosis Code E32.8. http://www.icd10data.com/ICD10CM/Codes/E00-E89/E20-E35/E32-/E32.8. Accessed July 26, 2014.
83. James TN (1961) Morphology of the human atrioventricular node, with remarks pertinent to its electrophysiology. Am Heart J 62:756–777.
84. James TN (1968) Sudden death in babies: new observation in the heart. Am J Cardiol 22:479–506.
85. James TN (1970) Cardiac conduction system: fetal and postnatal development. Am J Cardiol 25:213–226.
86. James TN (1976) Sudden death of babies. Circulation 53:1–2.
87. James TN (1983) Change and sudden death. J Am Coll Cardiol 1:164–183.
88. James TN (1983) The Mikamo lecture. Structure and function of AV junction. Jpn Circ J 47:1–47.
89. James TN (1994) Normal and abnormal consequences of apoptosis in the human heart. From postnatal morphogenesis to paroxysmal arrhythmias. Circulation 90:556–573.
90. James TN (1997) Apoptosis in congenital heart disease. Coron Artery Dis 8:599–616.
91. James TN (2001) The internodal pathways of the human heart. Prog Cardiovasc Dis 43:495–535.
92. James TN (2002) Structure and function of the sinus node, AV node and His bundle of the human heart: Part I – stucture. Prog Cardiovasc Dis 45:235–267.
93. Jaster JH, Ottaviani G, Matturri L, Lavezzi AM, Zamecnik J, Smith TW (2008) Sudden unexpected death related to medullary brain lesions. Am J Forensic Med Pathol 29:371–374.
94. Jeffery HE, Page M, Post EJ, Wood AK (1995) Physiological studies of gastro-oesophageal reflux and airway protective responses in young animal and human infant. Clin Exp Pharmacol Physiol 22:544–549.
95. Jeffery HE, Megevan A, Page M (1999) Why the prone position is a risk factor for sudden infant death syndrome. Pediatrics 104:263–269.
96. Jenkins RO, Craig PJ, Goessler W, Irgolic KJ (1998) Antimony leaching from cot mattresses and sudden infant death syndrome (SIDS). Hum Exp Toxicol 17:138–139.
97. Kaada B (1986) Sudden infant death syndrome: the possible role of "the fear paralysis reflex". Norwegian University Press, Oslo.
98. Kahn A, Blum D, Muller MF, Montauk L, Bochner A, Monod N, Plouin P, Samson-Dollfus D, Delagree EH (1986) Sudden infant death syndrome in twins: a comparison of sibling histories. Pediatrics 78:146–150.
99. Kalousek DK, Gilbert-Barness E (1997) Causes of stillbirth and neonatal death. In: Potter's pathology of the fetus and infant. Mosby-Year book, New York, pp 128–162.
100. Keith A, Flack MW (1906) The auricolo-ventricular bundle of the human heart. Lancet 2:359–364.
101. Kent AFS (1893) Researches on the structure and function of the mammalian heart. J Physiol 14:233–254.
102. Khurana RK, Watabiki S, Hebel JR, Toro R, Nelson E (1980) Cold face test in the assessment of trigeminal-brainstem-vagal function in humans. Ann Neurol 7:144–149.
103. Kinney HC, Filiano JJ, Harper RM (1992) The neuropathology of the sudden infant death syndrome. A review. J Neuropathol Exp Neurol 51:115–126.
104. Kinney HC, Filiano JJ, Panigraphy A, Rava LA, White WF (1995) Anatomic and neurochemical studies of the ventral medulla oblongata in early life. Observation relevant to the sudden infant death syndrome. In: Trouth CO, Millis RH, Kiwull-Schone H, Schlafke ME (eds) Ventral brainstem mechanisms and control respiration and blood pressure. Dekker, New York, pp 589–609.
105. Kinney HC, Filiano JJ, Sleeper LA, Mandell F, Valdes-Dapena M, White WF (1995) Decreased muscarinic receptor binding in the arcuate nucleus in sudden infant death syndrome. Science 269:1446–1450.
106. Kinney HC, Thach BT (2009) The sudden infant death syndrome. N Engl J Med 361:795–805.
107. Klonoff-Cohen HS, Edelstein SL, Lefkowitz ES, Srinivasan IP, Kaegi D, Chang JC, Wiley KJ (1995) The effect of passive smoking and tobacco exposure through breast milk on sudden infant death syndrome. JAMA 273:795–798.

108. Knight B (1983) Sudden death in infancy – the cot death syndrome. Faber and Faber, London.
109. Knobel HH, Chen CJ, Liang KY (1995) Sudden infant death syndrome in relation to weather and optimetrically measured air pollution in Taiwan. Pediatrics 96:1106–1110.
110. Kopp JH (1830) Denkwordigkeiten in der artzlichen praxis. Herman JC. http://archive.org/stream/denkwrdigkeiten02koppgoog#page/n11/mode/2up. Accessed July 26, 2014.
111. Krous HF, Beckwith JB, Byard RW, Rognum TO, Bajanowski T, Corey T, Cutz E, Hanzlick R, Keens TG, Mitchell EA (2004) Sudden infant death syndrome and unclassified sudden infant deaths: a definitional and diagnostic approach. Pediatrics 114:234–238.
112. Lack EE (1994) Pathology of adrenal and extra-adrenal paraganglia. W.B. Saunders, Philadelphia.
113. Lavezzi AM, Ottaviani G, Mauri M, Matturri L (2004) Hypoplasia of the arcuate nucleus and maternal smoking during pregnancy, in perinatal and infant sudden unexpected death. Neuropathology 24:284–289.
114. Lavezzi AM, Ottaviani G, Rossi L, Matturri L (2004) Cytoarchitectural organization of the Parabrachial/Kölliker-Fuse complex in man. Brain Dev 26:316–320.
115. Lavezzi AM, Ottaviani G, Rossi L, Matturri L (2004) Hypoplasia of the parabrachial/Kölliker-Fuse complex in perinatal death. Biol Neonate 86:92–97.
116. Lavezzi AM, Ottaviani G, Matturri L (2005) Adverse effects of prenatal tobacco smoke exposure on biological parameters of the developing brainstem. Neurobiol Dis 20:601–607.
117. Lavezzi AM, Ottaviani G, Mingrone R, Matturri L (2005) Analysis of the human locus coeruleus in perinatal and infant sudden unexplained deaths. Possible role of the cigarette smoking in the development of this nucleus. Brain Res Dev Brain Res 154:71–80.
118. Lavezzi AM, Ottaviani G, Mauri M, Matturri L (2006) Alterations of biological features of the cerebellum in sudden perinatal and infant death. Curr Mol Med 6:429–435.
119. Lee CA (1842) Art XII On the thymus gland: its morbid affections, and the diseases which arise from its abnormal enlargement. Am J Med Sci 3:135–154.
120. Lewis T (1925) The mechanism and graphic registration of the heart beat. Shaw and Sons Ltd, London, p 13.
121. Lobban CD (1995) The oxygen-conserving dive reflex re-examined as the principal contributory factor in the sudden infant death. Med Hypotheses 44:273–277.
122. Lonsdale D (2001) Sudden infant death syndrome requires genetic predisposition, some form of stress and marginal malnutrition. Med Hypotheses 57:382–386.
123. Lucas W (1927) Modem practise of pediatrics. Macmillan, New York.
124. Lundemose JB, Gregerson N, Kolvara S, Pederson BN, Gregersen M, Helweg-Larsen K, Simonsen J (1993) The frequency of a disease-causing point mutation in the gene coding for medium-chain acyl-CoA dehydrogenase in sudden infant death syndrome. Acta Paediatr 82:544–546.
125. MacDorman MF, Kirmeyer SE, Wilson EC (2012) Fetal and perinatal mortality, United States, 2006. Natl Vital Stat Rep 60:1–23. www.cdc.gov/nchs/data/nvsr/nvsr60/nvsr60_08.pdf. Accessed July 26, 2014.
126. MacDorman MF, Mathews TJ (2011) Understanding racial and ethnic disparities in U.S. infant mortality rates. NCHS Data Brief 74:1–8.
127. Mahaim I, Benatt A (1938) Nouvelles recherches sur les connexions superiors de la branche gauche du faisceau de His-Tawara avec cloison interventriculaire. Cardiologia 1:61–120.
128. Mahaim I (1947) Kent's fibers and the A-V paraspecific conduction through the upper connections of the bundle of His-Tawara. Am Heart J 33:651–653.
129. Malloy MH, Hoffman HJ (1995) Prematurity, sudden infant death syndrome, and age at death. Pediatrics 96:464–471.
130. Marino TA, Kane BM (1985) Cardiac atrioventricular junctional tissues in hearts from infants who died suddenly. J Am Coll Cardiol 5:1178–1184.
131. Martinez FD (1991) Sudden infant death syndrome and small airway occlusion: facts and hypothesis. Pediatrics 87:190–198.
132. Matthews TG (1992) The autonomic nervous system: a role in sudden infant death syndrome. Arch Dis Child 67:654–656.

133. Matturri L, Ghidoni P, Rossi L (1986) Miocellule specifiche senoatriali extranodali nella cresta terminale. G Ital Cardiol 16:947–954.
134. Matturri L, Rossi L (1998) Patologie del sistema nervoso legate all'embriogenesi ed allo sviluppo nella SIDS. CIC Edizioni Internazionali, Rome, pp 8–13.
135. Matturri L, Ottaviani G, Ramos SG, Rossi L (2000) Sudden infant death syndrome (SIDS). A study of cardiac conduction system. Cardiovasc Pathol 9:137–145.
136. Matturri L, Biondo B, Suàrez-Mier MP, Rossi L (2002) Brain stem lesions in the sudden infant death syndrome: variability in the hypoplasia of the arcuate nucleus. Acta Neuropathol (Berl) 194:12–20.
137. Matturri L, Lavezzi AM, Rossi L (2002) Proposal to modify the definition of SIDS, with regard to the post-mortem exam. In: Proceedings of the 7th International Conference on SIDS, Florence, p 103.
138. Matturri L, Minoli I, Lavezzi AM, Cappellini A, Ramos S, Rossi L (2002) Hypoplasia of medullary arcuate nucleus in unexpected late fetal death (stillborn infants): a pathological study. Pediatrics 109:E43.
139. Matturri L, Ottaviani G, Rossi L (2002) Should overdone external cardiac massage in infants dying of SIDS be discouraged? In: Proceedings of the 7th International Conference on SIDS, Florence, p 136.
140. Matturri L, Lavezzi AM, Minoli I, Ottaviani G, Cappellini A, Rubino B, Rossi L (2003) Association between pulmonary hypoplasia and hypoplasia of arcuate nucleus in stillbirth. J Perinatol 23:328–332.
141. Matturri L, Ottaviani G, Rossi L (2003) External cardiac massage in infants. Intensive Care Med 29:1199–1200.
142. Matturri L, Ottaviani G, Alfonsi G, Crippa M, Rossi L, Lavezzi AM (2004) Study of the brainstem, particularly the arcuate nucleus, in sudden infant death syndrome (SIDS) and sudden intrauterine unexplained death (SIUD). Am J Forensic Med Pathol 25:44–48.
143. Matturri L, Ottaviani G, Benedetti G, Agosta E, Lavezzi AM (2005) Unexpected perinatal death and sudden infant death syndrome (SIDS): anatomopathologic and legal aspects. Am J Forensic Med Pathol 26:155–160.
144. Matturri L, Ottaviani G, Lavezzi AM (2005) Sudden infant death triggered by dive reflex. J Clin Pathol 58:77–80.
145. Matturri L, Ottaviani G, Lavezzi AM (2005) Techniques and criteria in pathologic and forensic-medical diagnostics in sudden unexpected infant and perinatal death. Am J Clin Pathol 124:259–268.
146. Matturri L, Ottaviani G, Lavezzi AM (2005) Unexpected sudden death related to medullary brain lesions. Acta Neuropathol (Berl) 109:554–555.
147. Matturri L, Ottaviani G, Lavezzi AM, Grana D, Milei J (2005) Madres fumadoras y aterosclerosis prenatal. Rev Argent Cardiol 73:366–369.
148. Matturri L, Ottaviani G, Lavezzi AM, Ramos SG (2005) Peripheral chemoreceptors and sudden infant death syndrome: a wide open problem. Curr Cardiol Rev 1:65–70.
149. Matturri L, Ottaviani G, Lavezzi AM (2006) Maternal smoking and sudden infant death syndrome: epidemiological study related to pathology. Virchows Arch 449:697–706.
150. Matturri L, Ottaviani G, Nonnis Marzano F, Lavezzi AM (2006) Stillbirth versus SIDS. Pathology of the autonomic nervous system and DNA polymorphisms in SIUD and SIDS. In: Proceedings of the 9th SIDS International Conference, Yokohama, pp 105–106.
151. Matturri L, Ottaviani G, Lavezzi AM (2006) Maternal smoking as the most preventable risk factor for sudden infant death syndrome (SIDS): epidemiological and histopathological study. XI Congresso Nazionale della Società Italiana di Medicina Perinatale. June 15–17th, 2006; Parma, Italy. J Perinat Med 34(Suppl):A25–A26.
152. Matturri L, Ottaviani G, Mingrone R, Lavezzi AM, Fulcheri E (2007) Sudden Intrauterine Unexplained Death (SIUD) «Gray Zone» or borderline. 8th World Congress of Perinatal Medicine. Florence, Italy. J Perinat Med 35(Suppl):210.
153. Matturri L, Ottaviani G, Lavezzi AM (2008) Guidelines for neuropathologic diagnostics of perinatal unexpected loss and sudden infant death syndrome (SIDS) – a technical protocol. Virchows Arch 452:19–25.

154. Milner AD (1987) Recent theories on the cause of cot death. Br Med J 295:1366–1368.
155. Mingrone R, Tosi D, Ottaviani G, Matturri L (2007) Possible role of the nucleus ambiguus in sudden infant death syndrome (SIDS). 8th World Congress of Perinatal Medicine. Florence, Italy. J Perinat Med 35(Suppl):210.
156. Mitchell EA, Scragg L, Clements M (1996) Soft cot mattresses and the sudden infant death syndrome. N Z Med J 109:206–207.
157. Mitchell EA, Stewart AW (1997) Gender and the sudden infant death syndrome. New Zealand Cot Death Group. Acta Paediatr 86:854–856.
158. Moon RY, Tanabe KO, Yang DC, Young HA, Hauck FR (2012) Pacifier use and SIDS: evidence for a consistently reduced risk. Matern Child Health J 16:609–614.
159. National Institute of Child Health and Human Development. Safe to Sleep Public Education Campaign. http://www.nichd.nih.gov/SIDS/Pages/sids.aspx. Accessed July 26, 2014.
160. National Institutes of Health Consensus Development Conference on Infantile Apnea and Home Monitoring, Sept 29–Oct 1, 1986 (1987) Pediatrics 79:292–299.
161. Nattie E, Kinney H (2002) Nicotine, serotonine, and sudden infant death syndrome. Am J Respir Crit Care Med 166:1544–1549.
162. Naeye RL (1976) Brain-stem and adrenal abnormalities in the sudden-infant-death syndrome. Am J Clin Pathol 66:526–530.
163. Nelson W (1945) Nelson's texbook of pediatrics, 4th edn. Saunders, Philadelphia.
164. O'Leary CM, Jacoby PJ, Bartu A, D'Antoine H, Bower C (2013) Maternal alcohol use and sudden infant death syndrome and infant mortality excluding SIDS. Pediatrics 131: e770–e778.
165. Olszewski J, Baxter D (1982) Cytoarchitecture of the human brain stem. Karger, Basel.
166. Orenstein SR, Mitchell AA, Ward SD (1993) Concerning the American Academy of Pediatrics recommendation on sleep position for infants. Pediatrics 91:497–499.
167. Ottaviani G, Ramos SG, Matturri L (1997) Defective "resorptive degeneration" of the heart's conduction system and sudden infant death syndrome. Ann Españ Pediatr 92(Suppl):53.
168. Ottaviani G, Matturri L, Ramos SG, Rossi L (1998) Resorptive degeneration of the heart's conduction system and sudden infant death syndrome: preliminary results. In: Proceedings of the 5th SIDS International Conference, Rouen, p 156.
169. Ottaviani G, Rossi L, Varesi C, Ramos SG, Matturri L (1999) Pathology of the cardiac conduction system in sudden infant death syndrome (SIDS): preliminary results. Pediatr Res 45(Suppl):23A.
170. Ottaviani G, Matturri L, Rossi L, James TN (2003) Crib death: further support for the concept of fatal cardiac electrical instability as the final common pathway. Int J Cardiol 92:17–26.
171. Ottaviani G, Matturri L, Bruni B, Lavezzi AM (2005) Sudden infant death syndrome "gray zone" disclosed only by a study of the brain stem on serial sections. J Perinat Med 33:165–169.
172. Ottaviani G, Rossi L, Matturri L (2005) Myocardial injury attributable to external cardiac massage in infants. Cardiology 1:25–29.
173. Ottaviani G, Lavezzi AM, Matturri L (2006) Sudden infant death syndrome (SIDS) shortly after hexavalent vaccination: another pathology in suspected SIDS? Virchows Arch 448:100–104.
174. Ottaviani G, Matturri L, Mingrone R, Lavezzi AM (2006) Hypoplasia and neuronal immaturity of the hypoglossal nucleus in sudden infant death. J Clin Pathol 59:497–500.
175. Ottaviani G, Matturri L (2007) Cardiovascular causes of perinatal loss. In: Conference Handbook of the 3rd annual Conference of the International Stillbirth Alliance ISA 2007. Perinatal loss: improving care and prevention. Birmingham, UK. p 49.
176. Ottaviani G, Matturri L (2007) Cardiovascular pathology of sudden perinatal unexpected death (SPUD) and sudden infant death syndrome (SIDS). 8th World Congress of Perinatal Medicine. Florence, Italy. J Perinat Med 35(Suppl):229–230.
177. Ottaviani G, Matturri L (2008) Histopathology of the cardiac conduction system in sudden intrauterine unexplained death. Cardiovasc Pathol 17:146–155.
178. Ottaviani G, Schaller B (2008) A major modifiable risk factor for sudden infant death syndrome (SIDS). J Community Med 4:1–3.

179. Ottaviani G, Bergui G (2009) Sudden unexpected death in infancy (SUDI): a new anatomo-clinical approach. Europace 11:395.
180. Ottaviani G, Lavezzi AM, Matturri L (2009) Fibromuscular hyperplasia of the pulmonary artery in sudden infant and perinatal unexpected death. Cardiovasc Pathol 18:223–230.
181. Ottaviani G, Mingrone R, Lavezzi AM, Matturri L (2009) Infant and perinatal pulmonary hypoplasia frequently associated with brainstem hypodevelopment. Virchows Arch 454:451–456.
182. Ottaviani G (2010) In utero exposure to smoking and peripheral chemoreceptor function. Pediatrics [E-letter]. http://pediatrics.aappublications.org/content/125/3/e592/reply. Accessed July 26, 2014.
183. Ottaviani G (2011) Dr. Thomas N. James, MD, MACP (1925–2010): in memoriam. Am J Cardiol 108:330.
184. Ottaviani G (2011) Sudden infant and perinatal unexplained death: are we moving forward yet? Cardiovasc Pathol 10:302–306.
185. Ottaviani G (2011) Sudden unexplained neonatal deaths. Arch Dis Child Fetal Neonatal Ed. http://fn.bmj.com/content/96/6/F440/reply. Accessed July 26, 2014.
186. Ottaviani G (2011) Sudden deaths in term infants within 24 hours of birth. Pediatrics. http://pediatrics.aappublications.org/content/127/4/e869/reply. Accessed July 26, 2014.
187. Paltauf A (1889) Uber die Beziehung der Thymus zum plotzlichen Tod. Wien Klin Wochenschr 2:877–881.
188. Pinholster G (1995) Multiple "SIDS" case ruled murder. Science 268:494.
189. Platter F (1614) Observationum Libre Tre. Konig & Bradmylieri, Basel, part IX, p 161.
190. Ponsonby AL, Dwyer T, Gibbson LE, Cochrane JA, Jones ME, McCall MJ (1992) Thermal environment and sudden infant death syndrome: case-control study. BMJ 304:277–282.
191. Preventing Stillbirth and SUID. Act of 2008, Bill introduced in the Senate of the United States, June 17, 2008 by Mr. Reid (for Mr. Obama). S3142 IS. 110th Congress, 2nd Session, S. 3142. Available at: http://www.thomas.gov/cgi-bin/query/z?c110:S.3142. Accessed July 26, 2014.
192. Ramos SG, Matturri L, Biondo B, Ottaviani G, Rossi L (1998) Hyperplasia of the aorticopulmonary paraganglia: a new insight into the pathogenesis of sudden infant death syndrome? Cardiologia 43:953–958.
193. Ramos SG, Matturri L, Ottaviani G, Rossi L (1998) Maternal smoking and aorticopulmonary paraganglia in sudden infant death syndrome. In: Proceedings of the 5th SIDS International Conference, Rouen, p 169.
194. Ramos SG, Ottaviani G, Biondo B, Rossi L, Matturri L (1999) Hyperplasia of the aortico-pulmonary paraganglia in infants dying of SIDS: further supports for the cardio-respiratory hypothesis. In: Proceedings of the International Symposium on SIDS and Lombardy Region project for the reduction of the risk for sudden infant death and unexplained intrauterine death, Milan, pp 117–128.
195. Raring RH (1975) Crib death: scourge of infants–shame of society. Exposition Press, Hicksville/New York.
196. Rossi L (1969) Histopathologic features of cardiac arrhythmias. Casa Editrice Ambrosiana, Milan.
197. Rossi L (1975) A histological survey of pre-excitation syndrome and related arrhythmias. G Ital Cardiol 5:816–828.
198. Rossi L (1983) The pathologic basis of cardiac arrhythmias. Cardiol Clin 1:13–17.
199. Rossi L (1985) Cardioneuropathy and extracardiac neural disease. JACC 5(Suppl):66B–70B.
200. Rossi L (1999) Bulbo-spinal pathology in neurocardiac sudden death of adults: a prognostic approach to a neglected problem. Int J Legal Med 112:83–90.
201. Rossi L, Matturri L (1985) Histopathology of aortocoronary glomera: modern anatomo-clinical approach to the understanding of cardiocirculatory disorders. G Ital Cardiol 15:718–724.
202. Rossi L, Matturri L (1988) His bundle haematoma and external cardiac massage: histopathological findings. Br Heart J 59:586–587.

203. Rossi L, Matturri L (1990) Clinicopathological approach to cardiac arrhythmias. A color atlas. Centro Scientifico Torinese, Turin.
204. Rossi L, Matturri L (1995) Anatomo-histological features of the heart's conduction system and innervation in SIDS. In: Rognum TO (ed) Sudden infant death syndrome: new trends in the nineties. Scandinavian University Press, Oslo, pp 207–212.
205. Rossi L, Matturri L (1995) Cardiac conduction and nervous system in health disease and sudden death: an anatomoclinical overview. Osp Maggiore 89:239–257.
206. Rossi L, Thiene G (1983) Arrhythmologic pathology of sudden cardiac death. Casa Editrice Ambrosiana, Milan.
207. Rossi L, Thiene G, Knippel M (1978) A case of surgically corrected Wolff-Parkinson-White syndrome: clinical and histological data. Br Heart J 40:581–585.
208. Rossi L, Piffer R, Turolla E, Frigerio B, Coumel P, James TN (1985) Multifocal purkinje-like tumor of the heart. Occurrence with other anatomic abnormalities in the atrioventricular junction of an infant with junctional tachycardia, Lown-Ganong-Levine syndrome, and sudden death. Chest 87:340–345.
209. Rossi L, Matturri L, Lotto A (1988) Cardiac conduction blocks and pacemaking. An anatomoclinical color atlas. Clas International, Brescia.
210. Rossi L, Pozzato R, Matturri L (1991) L'anatomia patologica della morte cardiaca oggi. Riv Ital Med Leg 13:93–110.
211. Ruhrah J (1925) Felix platter. In: Pediatrics of the past. Paul B Hoeber, New York, p 239.
212. Russell-Jones DL (1985) Sudden infant death in history and literature. Arch Dis Child 60:278–281.
213. Ruth G (1994) The changing epidemiology of SIDS. Arch Dis Child 70:445–449.
214. Saunders JW (1966) Death in embryonic systems. Science 154:604–612.
215. Sawczenko A, Fleming PJ (1996) Thermal stress, sleeping position, and the sudden infant death syndrome. Sleep 19:267–270.
216. Schaller B, Cornelius JF, Prabhakar H, Koerbel A, Gnanalingham K, Sandu N, Ottaviani G, Filis A, Buchfelder M, Trigemino-Cardiac Reflex Examination Group (TCREG) (2009) The trigemino-cardiac reflex: an update of the current knowledge. J Neurosurg Anesthesiol 21:187–195.
217. Schaller B, Cornelius JF, Sandu N, Ottaviani G, Perez-Pinzon MA (2009) Oxygen-conserving reflexes of the brain: the current molecular knowledge. J Cell Mol Med 13:644–647.
218. Schaller B, Sandu N, Filis A, Ottaviani G, Rasper J, Nöethen C, Buchfelder M, Trigemino-Cardiac-Reflex-Examination-Group (T.C.R.E.G.) (2009) Trigemino-cardiac reflex: the trigeminal depressor responses during skull base surgery. Clin Neurol Neurosurg 111.
219. Schaller B, Sandu N, Ottaviani G, Filis A, Noethen C, Buchfelder M, for the Trigemino-Cardiac Reflex Examination Group (TCREG) (2009) Transient asystole during endoscopic transsphenoidal surgery: an example of trigeminocardiac reflex. Pituitary 12:271–272.
220. Schwartz PJ, Stramba-Badiale M, Segantini A, Austoni P, Bosi G, Giorgetti RR, Grancini F, Marini ED, Perticone F, Rositi D, Salice P (1998) Prolongation of the QT interval and the sudden infant death syndrome. N Engl J Med 338:1709–1714.
221. Sciacca A, Mascagni MT, De Andreis M (1958) Morphological contribution to the knowledge of pathogenesis of branch block; serial histological study and reconstruction of His-Tawara bundle in man. Cuore Circ 42:321–345.
222. Scragg R, Mitchell EA, Taylor BJ, Stewart AW, Ford RPK, Thompson JMD, Allen EM, Becroft DMO (1993) Bed sharing, smoking and alcohol in the sudden infant death syndrome. BMJ 307:1312–1318.
223. Shannon DC, Kelly DH (1982) SIDS and near-SIDS (first of two parts). N Engl J Med 306:959–965.
224. Shannon DC, Kelly DH (1982) SIDS and near-SIDS (second of two parts). N Engl J Med 306:1022–1028.
225. Soranus of Ephesus. Gynecology (trans: O'Temkin) (1956) Johns Hopkin Press, Baltimore, p 90.
226. Spiers PS, Onstad L, Guntheroth WG (1996) Negative effect of a short interpregnancy interval on birth weight following loss of an infant to sudden infant death syndrome. Am J Epidemiol 143:1137–1141.

227. Stéphan-Blanchard E, Chardon K, Léké A, Delanaud S, Djeddi D, Libert JP, Bach V, Telliez F (2010) In utero exposure to smoking and peripheral chemoreceptor function in preterm neonates. Pediatrics 125:e592–e599.
228. St. John O (1732) Letter. Philos Trans R Soc, London.
229. Steinschneider A (1974) The concept of sleep apnea as related to SIDS. In: Robinson RR (ed) SIDS 1974: Proceedings of the Francis E. Camps International Symposium on Sudden and Unexpected Deaths in Infancy. Canadian Foundation for the Study of Infant Death, Toronto, pp 177–190.
230. Still GF (1923) Attacks of arrested respiration in the new-born. Lancet 1:431–432.
231. Task Force on Sudden Infant Death Syndrome, Moon RY (2011) SIDS and other sleep-related infant deaths: expansion of recommendations for a safe infant sleeping environment. Pediatrics 128:1030–1039.
232. Tawara S (1906) Das Reizleitungssystem des Sàugetierherzens. G. Fisher, Jena.
233. Taylor A (1996) Antimony, cot mattresses, and SIDS. Lancet 347:616.
234. Templemann C (1892) Two hundred and fifty-eight cases of suffocation of infants. Edinburgh Med J 38:322–329.
235. Topaz O, Castellanos A, Grobman LR, Myerburg RJ (1988) The role of arrhythmogenic auditory stimuli in sudden cardiac death. Am Heart J 116:222–226.
236. Trachtenberg FL, Haas EA, Kinney HC, Stanley C, Krous HF (2012) Risk factor changes for sudden infant death syndrome after initiation of Back-to-Sleep campaign. Pediatrics 129:630–638.
237. Valdès-Dapena M (1985) Are some crib deaths sudden cardiac deaths? J Am Coll Cardiol 5(6 Suppl):113B–117B.
238. Valdés-Dapena MA, Greene M, Basavanand N, Catherman R, Truex RC (1973) The myocardial conduction system in sudden death in infancy. N Engl J Med 289:1179–1180.
239. Valdès-Dapena M, McFreeley PA, Hoffman HJ, Damus KH, Franciosi RR, Allison DJ, Jones M, Hunter JC (1993) Histopathology atlas for the sudden infant death syndrome. Armed Forces Institute of Pathology, Washington, DC.
240. Vance JC, Boyle FM, Najman JM, Thearle MJ (2002) Couple distress after sudden infant or perinatal death: a 30-month follow up. J Paediatr Child Health 38:368–372.
241. Vennemann MM, Butterfass-Bahloul T, Jorch G, Brinkmann B, Findeisen M, Sauerland C, Bajanowski T, Mitchell EA, GeSID Group (2007) Sudden infant death syndrome: no increased risk after immunisation. Vaccine 25:336–340.
242. Wakely T (1855) Medical jurisprudence: infants found dead in bed. Lancet 1:103.
243. Weber MA, Klein NJ, Hartley JC, Lock PE, Malone M, Sebire NJ (2008) Infection and sudden unexpected death in infancy: a systematic retrospective case review. Lancet 371:1848–1853.
244. Weese-Mayer DE, Berry-Kravis EM, Ceccherini I, Keens TG, Loghmanee DA, Trang H (2010) An official ATS clinical policy statement: congenital central hypoventilation syndrome. Am J Respir Crit Care Med 181:626–644.
245. Widdicombe JG, Tatar M (1988) Upper airway reflex control. Ann N Y Acad Sci 533:252–261.
246. Willinger M, James LS, Catz C (1991) Defining the sudden infant death syndrome (SIDS): deliberations of an expert panel convened by the National Institute of Child Health Development. Pediatr Pathol 11:677–684.
247. Willinger M, Hoffman HJ, Hartford RB (1994) Infant sleep position and risk for sudden infant death syndrome: report of meeting held January 13 and 14, 1994, National Institutes of Health, Bethesda, MD. Pediatrics 93:814–819.
248. Wolff L, Parkinson J, White PD (1930) Bundle-branch block with short P-R interval in healthy young people prone to paroxysmal tachycardia. Am Heart J 5:685–704.
249. Woolley PV (1945) Mechanical suffocation during infancy. J Pediatr 26:572–575.
250. Yeats WB (1889) The Ballad of Moll Magee. In: The wanderings of Oisin and other poems, 1st edn. Kegan Paul & Co, London.

Techniques and Criteria in Anatomic and Forensic Pathology of Sudden Infant and Perinatal Unexplained Death

2

SIDS and sudden unexplained perinatal death are tragic events, still representing the most common form of death within the first year of life despite the progress in the field of maternal and infant health care [5, 36]. These deaths remain unexplained after the usual gross and microscopic examination, and are referable to similar underlying cardiac and neurophysiological mechanisms, as frequent alterations of the autonomic nervous system, both central and peripheral, have been reported [33, 34, 44, 50, 54, 77]. Malignant arrhythmias are known to be a substrate of unexpected infant and perinatal death, especially following accessory atrio-ventricular pathways [40, 73, 84–88]. Therefore, an accurate examination of the cardiac conduction system, again under the control of the nervous system, is also mandatory. These structural alterations are mainly of a congenital nature and therefore represent a common morphological substrate in both perinatal and infant sudden death. In view of the *post mortem* pathological findings [29–34, 38–54, 67–77], the need to perform an in-depth study of the cardiac conduction and autonomic nervous systems, following the guidelines reported below, is self-evident. Because this examination is not routinely performed, detailed indications are given in this protocol of the sampling, processing, cutting and staining procedures.

Each case of suspected SIDS or unexplained perinatal death should be referred to a pathologist or medical examiner who performs an extensive clinical and pathological investigation, including a detailed review of the clinical history and death scene, followed by a detailed postmortem examination, carried out according to the herein described protocol.

This diagnostic protocol includes an anatomo-pathologic examination of all the organs, including the thymus. In particular, in fetuses, the adnexa – placenta, umbilical cord and membranes – must be examined according to the usual procedure.

The need to submit the young victims to necropsy procedures is unanimously recognized and the chance of preventing SIDS and perinatal unexpected death relies

G. Ottaviani, *Crib Death - Sudden Infant Death Syndrome (SIDS): Sudden Infant and Perinatal Unexplained Death: The Pathologist's Viewpoint*,
DOI 10.1007/978-3-319-08347-6_2

mainly on a better knowledge of the underlying alterations of organs and etiopathogenetic mechanisms. Similarly, for diagnostic and epidemiological purposes, an accurate and careful examination of the circumstantial, environmental and familial situation where the death occurred is mandatory.

2.1 Clinical and Pathological Information

The procedure for the accurate anatomo-clinical study of each case of infant and perinatal unexplained death includes a review of the clinical history and of the death scene, as well as the anatomo-pathological examination. Thus, the guidelines for investigation include:

- A review of the clinical history;
- A detailed description of the death scene and circumstances, such as position of the baby in the crib, characteristics and consistency of the mattress, presence of pillow, etc.
- The anatomo-pathological protocol, to include the gross and histological description of the organs and of the developmental data, and particularly an exhaustive study of the autonomic nervous system, the cardio-respiratory system, the upper digestive pathways, the lungs, and the cardiac conduction system.

For each case of suspected SIDS and unexplained perinatal death as much clinical information as possible is collected. The review of clinical and epidemiological data, as well as a complete necropsy study, are performed according to the protocol devised by the University of Milan, Italy [53, 58, 60, 63].

In 1996, the bill "*Post mortem* regulation on the Sudden Infant Death Syndrome (SIDS) victims" was presented to the Italian House of Representatives. Since 2000, the former Institute of Pathology, University of Milan, has been the coordinating center for a project approved by the Lombardy Region which has the aim of "reduction of the risk of sudden infant death and unexpected fetal death". In 2002, a Lombardy Region Decree (DGR n° 11693 of 06-20-2002) required all regional hospitals to perform an autopsy on SIDS infants according to a specific protocol and to refer all the organs to the former Institute of Pathology, now the "Lino Rossi" Research Center for the study and prevention of unexpected perinatal death and SIDS, University of Milan, Italy [4, 58].

The form used to record the clinical and pathological information in each case is shown in Fig. 2.1.

Recently, the Centers for Disease Control and Prevention (CDC) [6], in response to numerous requests, has published the reporting form for the investigation of Sudden Unexplained Infant Death (SUID) which can be completed electronically, available for personal computer download and is modifiable based upon different jurisdictional needs.

CLINICO-PATHOLOGICAL QUESTIONNAIRE FOR THE EVALUATION OF THE RISK FACTORS OF SIDS AND UNEXPECTED PERINATAL DEATH

The present form, in double copy, is integral part of the hospital chart and with it should be completed by the Hospital personnel and must be submitted along with the case to be analyzed.

1. REGISTRY/INVESTIGATION DATA

Referred from (Hospital/Depart.)____________________
Referring physician____________________
Ref.# (Hospital Record/Autopsy Record)____________________
DATE (mm/dd/yyyy):____/____/____

LAST NAME:__________FIRST NAME__________MIDDLE NAME __________
DATE OF BIRTH (mm/dd/yyyy):____/____/____ AGE__________
PLACE OF BIRTH__________STATE__________COUNTRY__________
GENDER: ☐ M ☐ F____Gestational age__________
Postocnceptional age____(gestational age______+ postnatal age______)
Weeks of gestation __________
BIRTH WEIGHT (gms)__________ APGAR score:__________
DATE OF DEATH (mm/dd/yyyy):____/____/____ TIME__________
INFANT'S PRIMARY RESIDENCE:
Street____________________Zip code__________
City__________Province/State__________Country__________
INCIDENT'S ADDRESS
Street____________________Zip code__________
City__________Province/State__________Country__________
RACE/ETHNICITY:
☐ Caucasian/white non-hispanic ☐ White Hispanic/Latino ☐ Black/African American
☐ East Asian ☐ South Asian ☐ American Indian ☐ Alaskan Native ☐ Other, specify________
SOCIAL SECURITY#____________________

2. INFANT MEDICAL HISTORY

Born as ☐ Singleton ☐ Twin ☐ Triplet ☐ Quadruplet ☐ Other, specify__________
COMPLICATIONS PRIOR TO BIRTH, specify____________________
COMPLICATIONS AT BIRTH, specify____________________
COMPLICATIONS AFTER BIRTH, specify____________________

LENGTH at birth__________cms
WEIGHT at birth__________gms
FEEDING ☐ breast ☐ formula ☐ mixed
When did the formula feeding start?____________________
DID THE BABY USE THE PACIFIER? ☐ No ☐ Yes____________________
Date of last PEDIATRIC VISIT (mm/dd/yyyy):____/____/____
DATE OF THE LAST VACCINATION (mm/dd/yyyy):____/____/____
TYPE OF THE LAST VACCINATION ____________________

ANTENATAL DISEASES____________________

Fig. 2.1 Clinical and pathological information for cases of suspected SIDS or sudden perinatal unexplained death. Fill in the form and submit it along with the case to be analyzed

DISEASES AT BIRTH____
POSTNATAL DISEASES____

____

SIGNS AND SYMPTOMS prior to death:

☐ Abnormal growth ☐ Allergies ☐ Apnea ☐ Birth defects ☐ Cardiac abnormalities
☐ Choking ☐ Cold ☐ Cough ☐ Cyanosis ☐ Diarrhea ☐ Difficult feeding ☐ Eczema
☐ Exanthema ☐ Excessive sweating ☐ Fever ☐ Fussiness or excessive crying
☐ Gastroesophageal reflux ☐ Lethargy ☐ Stool changes ☐ Vomiting ☐ Weight gain
☐ Weight loss ☐ Other, specify____

THERAPIES____

ELECTROCARDIOGRAMS (ECG) performed on________________at______________________
*Attach to this form ECG and copy of the hospital chart including information on the resuscitative maneuvers.

3. FAMILY HISTORY

MOTHER
LAST NAME____________________FIRST NAME_________________MIDDLE NAME_________
DATE OF BIRTH (mm/dd/yyyy):______/_____/________ AGE____________
PLACE OF BIRTH_________________________STATE________________COUNTRY_________
RACE/ETHNICITY:
☐ Caucasian/white non-hispanic ☐ White Hispanic/Latino ☐ Black/African American
☐ East Asian ☐ South Asian ☐ American Indian ☐ Alaskan Native ☐ Other, specify

____

MARITAL STATUS: ☐ Single ☐ Married ☐ Long term Relationship ☐ Divorced ☐ Widowed
ADDRESS: ☐ same as above
Street____Zip code________________
City___________________________Province/State________________Country_______________
Preferred phone number:____
Email address:________________________@____
WORK/OCCUPATION____
PREGNANCY/BIRTH HISTORY
Was this child adopted? ☐ No ☐ Yes
If Yes, describe____
Was this child conceived through a medically assisted procedure? ☐ No ☐ Yes
If Yes, describe____
Where was prenatal care received?

____

____

LABOR/DELIVERY ☐ Vaginal delivery ☐ Inducted ☐ Cesarean delivery
describe:____
PREGNANCY COURSE____
First prenatal check-up (gestational week)____

Fig. 2.1 (continued)

Number of check-ups during pregnancy________________________________
Ultrasound ☐ normal ☐ abnormal, specify________________________________
Weight gain________________________________
Nutrition________________________________
Exercise________________________________
PARITY________________________________
PREVIOUS DELIVERIES________________________________
N° living births__________ N° stillborn__________ N° spontaneous abortion__________
N° voluntary abortions________________Dates________________
Date of the last previous delivery (mm/dd/yyyy):_____/____/________________
BIRTH CONTROL, specify________________
____

CIGARETTE SMOKING before pregnancy: ☐ No ☐ Yes
passive smoke exposure at home/work ☐ No ☐ Yes
describe:________________________________
Cigarettes smoked/day: ☐ 1-5 ☐ 6-10 ☐ 11-20 ☐ > 20
At what age did you start to smoke?________________________________

CIGARETTE SMOKING during pregnancy: ☐ No ☐ Yes
At what gestational week did you stop smoking?________________________________
passive smoke exposure at home/work ☐ No ☐ Yes
describe:________________________________
Cigarettes smoked/day: ☐ 1-5 ☐ 6-10 ☐ 11-20 ☐ > 20

CIGARETTE SMOKING after pregnancy: ☐ No ☐ Yes
passive smoke exposure at home/work ☐ No ☐ Yes
describe:________________________________
Cigarettes smoked/day: ☐ 1-5 ☐ 6-10 ☐ 11-20 ☐ > 20
Where do you smoke? ☐ indoor ☐ outdoor: ☐ balcony________________________________
ALCOHOL ☐ No ☐ Yes, specify________________________________
ILLICIT DRUGS ☐ No ☐ Yes, specify________________________________
COFFEE (n° cups/day)________________________________
MEDICATIONS ☐ No ☐ Yes, specify________________________________

MOTHER'S DISEASES________________________________
Infections
☐ HIV ☐ HBV ☐ HCV ☐ Syphilis ☐ CMV ☐ Rubella ☐ Herpes
☐ Pelvic inflammatory disease ☐ Endometriosis ☐ Chlamydia ☐ Gonorrhea
☐ Vaginal infections ☐ Other, specify________________________________
Hypertension ☐ No ☐ Yes ▫ gestational ▫ pre-gestational
Diabetes ☐ No ☐ Yes ▫ gestational ▫ pre-gestational
Hemoglobin alterations ☐ No ☐ Yes, specify ________________________________
Autoimmune diseases ☐ No ☐ Yes, specify________________________________
Other, specify________________________________

SCREENING TESTS FOR CHROMOSOMAL ABNORMALITIES
____

Fig. 2.1 (continued)

PRENATAL INVASIVE TESTS
Chorionic villus sampling (CVS): ☐ normal ☐ abnormal, specify_______________
Amniocentesis: ☐ normal ☐ abnormal, specify_______________
Funicolocentesis: ☐ normal ☐ abnormal, specify_______________
Fetoscopy: ☐ normal ☐ abnormal, specify_______________

FETAL ABNORMALITIES
☐ heart ☐ CNS ☐ abdominal wall ☐ gastrointestinal tract
☐ single umbilical artery ☐ muscle/bones ☐ Other, specify_______________

PLACENTA ABNORMALITIES:
☐ premature detachment ☐ previa ☐ vasa previa ☐ infarction
☐ accreta-percreta ☐ Other, specify_______________

UTERUS ABNORMALITIES:

PAST MEDICAL HISTORY_______________
☐ Arthritis ☐ Asthma ☐ Blood Transfusions ☐ Bronchitis ☐ Diabetes ☐ Eating Disorder
☐ Emphysema ☐ Epilepsy ☐ Gallstones ☐ Heart disease ☐ HIV+ ☐ Hypertension
☐ Kidney Disease ☐ Liver Disease ☐ Thyroid disease ☐ Other, specify

FAMILY HISTORY_______________

Other cases of sudden death in the family, specify_______________

FATHER
LAST NAME__________FIRST NAME__________MIDDLE NAME__________
DATE OF BIRTH (mm/dd/yyyy):____/____/______ AGE__________
PLACE OF BIRTH__________STATE__________COUNTRY__________
RACE/ETHNICITY:
☐ Caucasian/white non-hispanic ☐ White Hispanic/Latino ☐ Black/African American
☐ East Asian ☐ South Asian ☐ American Indian ☐ Alaskan Native ☐ Other, specify

MARITAL STATUS:
☐ Single ☐ Married ☐ Long term Relationship ☐ Divorced ☐ Widower
ADDRESS: ☐ same as above
Street__________Zip code__________
City__________Province/State__________Country__________
Preferred phone number:__________
Email address:__________@__________
WORK/OCCUPATION__________
CIGARETTE SMOKING (before, during and after pregnancy) ☐ No ☐ Yes
from__________to__________
Cigarettes smoked/day: ☐ 1-5 ☐ 6-10 ☐ 11-20 ☐ > 20

Fig. 2.1 (continued)

At what age did you start to smoke?______________________________

ALCOHOL ☐ No ☐ Yes

describe:______________________________

ILLICIT DRUGS ☐ No ☐ Yes

describe:______________________________

COFFEE (n° cups/day)______________________________

MEDICATIONS ☐ No ☐ Yes

describe:______________________________

CURRENT DISEASES______________________________

PAST MEDICAL HISTORY______________________________

☐ Arthritis ☐ Asthma ☐ Blood Transfusions ☐ Bronchitis ☐ Diabetes ☐ Eating Disorder

☐ Emphysema ☐ Epilepsy ☐ Gallstones ☐ Heart disease ☐ HIV+ ☐ Hypertension

☐ Kidney Disease ☐ Liver Disease ☐ Thyroid disease ☐ Other, specify

____

FAMILY HISTORY______________________________

____

Other cases of sudden death in the family, specify ______________________________

SIBLINGS

N° ______ GENDER______________________________

AGE______________________________

HEALTH STATUS______________________________

4. DEATH SCENE

DATE OF DEATH (mm/dd/yyyy):_____/_______/______________

TIME OF DEATH/WHEN THE BABY WAS FOUND DEAD______________________________

When was the last time the baby was seen alive? ______________________________

WHO DID FIND THE BABY DEAD?______________________________

Was anyone sleeping with the infant? ______________________________

When was the last MEAL administered?______________________________

RECOVERY/DEATH PLACE: ☐ HOSPITAL

☐ HOME: ☐ crib/pram ☐ parents' bed ☐ stroller, seat, car seat ☐ in parents' arms

POSITION:

In which position was the infant FOUND? ☐ prone ☐ supine ☐ on the side

In which position was the infant last PLACED? ☐ prone ☐ supine ☐ on the side

What was the infant USUAL position? ☐ prone ☐ supine ☐ on the side

What was the infant wearing?

Which of the following ITEMS were within the infant's reach?

☐ Blankets ☐ Toys ☐ Pillows ☐ Pacifier ☐ Stuffed animals ☐ Positional supports

☐ Other, specify ______________________________

What was the room TEMPERATURE? ______________________________

WITNESS INTERVIEW:

Are you the usual infant's caregiver? ☐ No ☐ Yes______________________________

Relationship to the deceased:

Fig. 2.1 (continued)

☐ Birth Mother ☐ Birth Father ☐ Grandmother ☐ Grandfather ☐ Adoptive or foster parent ☐ Physician
☐ Other, specify ____________

LAST NAME:____________FIRST NAME____________MIDDLE NAME ____________
DATE OF BIRTH (mm/dd/yyyy):______/______/______ AGE____________
PLACE OF BIRTH____________STATE____________COUNTRY____________
GENDER: ☐ M ☐ F___
ADDRESS: ☐ same as above
Street____________Zip code____________
City____________State/Province____________Country____________
SOCIAL SECURITY#____________
Preferred phone number:____________
Email address:____________@____________
WORK/OCCUPATION____________

5. AUTOPSY GROSS EXAMINATION
WEIGHT (gms)____________ CROWN-RUMP LENGTH (cm)____________
CROWN-HEEL LENGTH (cm)____________ HEADCIRCUMFERENCE (cm)____________
CHEST CIRCUMFERENCE (cm)____________ABDOMINAL CIRCUMFERENCE (cm)____________
FEET LENGTH (cm) ____________

WEIGHT OF THE ORGANS (gms): **REMARKS**
PLACENTA ____________
HEART ____________
BRAIN ____________
LIVER ____________
SPLEEN ____________
RIGHT LUNG ____________
LEFT LUNG____________
RIGHT KIDNEY____________
LEFT KIDNEY____________
RIGHT ADRENAL GLAND ____________
LEFT ADRENAL GLAND____________
THYMUS____________
**Attach copy of autopsy report.
Name of the attending pathologist who performed the autopsy and contact information
____
____
____
Form completed by: printed name ____________signature ____________
____
Preferred phone number:____________
Email address:____________@____________
Date:____________

Fig. 2.1 (continued)

2.2 *Post Mortem* Regulation on SIDS and Sudden Perinatal Unexplained Death

The honorable Dr. R. Calderoli, presented to the House of Representatives the bill n° 396 of July 5, 2001 "*Post mortem* regulation on SIDS and unexpected fetal death victims", later approved by the Senate of the Italian Republic [4, 48].

The problem of SIDS and unexplained fetal death after the 25th week of gestation (unexplained stillbirth) is of great scientific complexity, and the need is therefore clear for anatomo-pathological research performed at institutes and departments of pathology, designated as regional referral centers, according to a specific predefined protocol. In every region, the institutes and departments of pathology that are to be referral centers will be designated by special decree. These centers will examine the material and enhance research activity related to this issue. Furthermore, courses should be made available to physicians working in institutes and departments of pathology. Such courses are aimed at ensuring the uniformity and reproducibility of autopsy techniques and the associated research. Official campaigns to raise public awareness of the SIDS issue have been conducted involving the dissemination of appropriate material and the use of the mass media.

The Lombardy Region was the first Italian region to approve the "Project for the reduction of the risk of sudden infant death and of fetal unexpected death" (Deliberation of the Regional Government n° 11693 of 06-20-2002). My research group proposed a remedy for this difficult situation by providing an internationally innovative text in four simple articles at no additional cost to the tax payer. The Italian national Law n° 31 of 02-02-06 "*Disciplina del riscontro diagnostic sulle vittime della syndrome della morte improvvisa del lattante (SIDS) e di morte inaspettata del feto*"/"Regulations for diagnostic *post mortem* investigation in victims of sudden infant death syndrome (SIDS) and of unexpected fetal death" [7] designates the former Institute of Pathology of the University of Milan as the national referral center for all cases of suspected SIDS and unexplained perinatal death (Figs. 2.2 and 2.3). This law has represented a revolutionary innovation and milestone in health politics providing measures information and awareness campaigns, training programs, promotion of research-clinical anatomical, genetic and epidemiological projects and psychological support to the families of victims, in order to significantly reduce the loss of human lives. According to this Law n° 31, all Italian Regions should identify local reference centers for diagnostic examination of infants who died suddenly within one year of life and of unexplained fetal death after the 25th week of gestation, according to the diagnostic guidelines devised by the Institute of Pathology of the University of Milan [50, 53, 58, 60].

Following the deactivation of the Institute of Pathology of the University of Milan (quoted in the arts. 1 and 3 of the Law) in 2008, the Italian Ministry of Health has designated the "Lino Rossi" Research Center of the University of Milan as the new national reference Center for the application of the above mentioned national law.

In 2008, then US Senator Barack Obama introduced the Preventing Stillbirth and Sudden Unexpected Infant Death Act, which will enhance public health activities related to understanding and preventing stillbirth and sudden unexpected infant deaths [80].

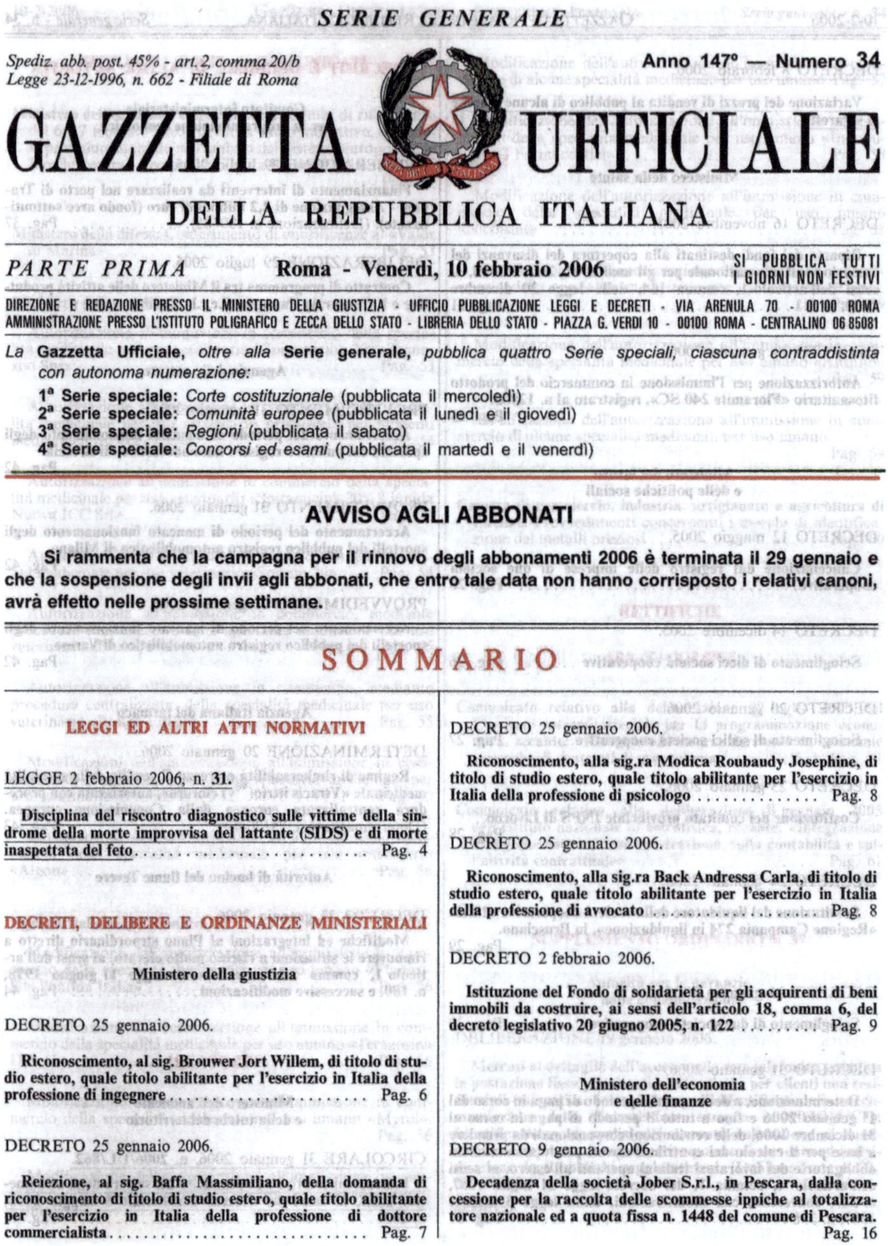

SERIE GENERALE

Spediz. abb. post. 45% - art. 2, comma 20/b
Legge 23-12-1996, n. 662 - Filiale di Roma

Anno 147° — Numero 34

GAZZETTA UFFICIALE

DELLA REPUBBLICA ITALIANA

PARTE PRIMA **Roma - Venerdì, 10 febbraio 2006** SI PUBBLICA TUTTI I GIORNI NON FESTIVI

DIREZIONE E REDAZIONE PRESSO IL MINISTERO DELLA GIUSTIZIA - UFFICIO PUBBLICAZIONE LEGGI E DECRETI - VIA ARENULA 70 - 00100 ROMA
AMMINISTRAZIONE PRESSO L'ISTITUTO POLIGRAFICO E ZECCA DELLO STATO - LIBRERIA DELLO STATO - PIAZZA G. VERDI 10 - 00100 ROMA - CENTRALINO 06 85081

La **Gazzetta Ufficiale,** *oltre alla* **Serie generale,** *pubblica quattro Serie speciali, ciascuna contraddistinta con autonoma numerazione:*

1ª **Serie speciale:** *Corte costituzionale* (pubblicata il mercoledì)
2ª **Serie speciale:** *Comunità europee* (pubblicata il lunedì e il giovedì)
3ª **Serie speciale:** *Regioni* (pubblicata il sabato)
4ª **Serie speciale:** *Concorsi ed esami* (pubblicata il martedì e il venerdì)

AVVISO AGLI ABBONATI

Si rammenta che la campagna per il rinnovo degli abbonamenti 2006 è terminata il 29 gennaio e che la sospensione degli invii agli abbonati, che entro tale data non hanno corrisposto i relativi canoni, avrà effetto nelle prossime settimane.

SOMMARIO

LEGGI ED ALTRI ATTI NORMATIVI

DECRETI, DELIBERE E ORDINANZE MINISTERIALI

Ministero della giustizia

Ministero dell'economia e delle finanze

Fig. 2.2 Gazzetta Ufficiale of February 10, 2006. In the Table of Contents there is Italian law n°. 31 of 02-02-2006 [7] (Courtesy of the Istituto Poligrafico e Zecca dello Stato, Rome)

LAW N. 31 of 2-02-2006

Regulations for Diagnostic *Post Mortem* Investigation in Victims of the Sudden Infant Death Syndrome (SIDS) and of Unexpected Fetal Death

Art. 1.

1. Infants that die suddenly within one year of life without any apparent cause, and fetuses that die after the twenty-fifth week of gestation without any apparent cause, must be rapidly submitted, with the consent of both parents, to diagnostic *post mortem* investigation to be performed in authorized centers, according to the criteria specified in article 2, to which their organs must be sent. Information about the pregnancy, fetal development and delivery and, in the case of sudden infant death syndrome (SIDS), about the environmental and familial situation where the death occurred, must be collected during family interviews, accurately recorded and, to complete the *post mortem* investigation and for scientific research purposes, assessed by the obstetrician-gynecologist, the neonatologist, the pediatrician involved in the case and the pathologist, in accordance with the international protocols.

2. The *post mortem* investigation to be set up as in comma 1 are performed according to the diagnostic protocol drawn up by the Institute of Pathological Anatomy, First Chair, University of Milan. To be applicable, the above protocol must be approved by the Ministry of Health.

Art. 2.

Within one hundred eighty days of adoption of the decree as in comma 1, the regions are called upon to individuate in their relative territory, the scientific centers, of University or Hospital appurtenance, that will take on the function of reference centers for the *post mortem* investigation of infants that die suddenly without any apparent cause within one year of life and of fetuses that die after the twenty-fifth week of gestation, without any apparent cause.

Art. 3.

The results of the *post mortem* investigation performed as in article 1 will be communicated by the authorized centers to the of the Institute of Pathological Anatomy, First Chair, University of Milan, that will, while fully respecting the norms for the treatment of personal data, set up a national data bank and send the collected data to the competent region, to the general practitioner and pediatricians, and to the relatives of the victim.

Art. 4.

1. The national and regional Health Authorities will be responsible, within the context of the ordinary budget allocation, for:

a) promoting campaigns to ensure awareness and prevention, promulgating correct information about the problems associated with SIDS and unexpected fetal death without any apparent cause;

b) setting up appropriate multidisciplinary research programs carrying out studies of cases from the anamnestic, clinical, laboratory, anatomo-pathological, histological standpoints.

Fig. 2.3 Text of Italian law n° 31 of 02-02-2006 "Regulations for diagnostic *post mortem* investigation in victims of sudden infant death syndrome (SIDS) and of unexpected fetal death" [7]

Art. 5.

1. To the charges inherent to the present law, equal to 67.000 Euros annually, starting in the year 2006, it is provided by correspondent reduction of the enrolled appropriation, for of the triennial budget 2005–2007, within the anticipatory base of current "special fund" of the Office of the economy and the finances for the 2006, to the purpose partially using the related Ministry budget.

2. The Ministry of the economy and finances is authorized to bring, with own decrees, the required variations of budget.

Fig. 2.3 (continued)

2.3 Necropsy Procedure

Infants and fetuses after the 25th week of gestation dying suddenly and unexpectedly are submitted to a complete necropsy examination starting 24 h after death has occurred, as required by the Italian law. The pathologist, before starting the autopsy, should check the validity of the autopsy consent, signed by both parents at the coroner's office.

Multiple samples from all organs are fixed in 10% phosphate-buffered formalin, processed and embedded in paraffin, and 5-μm sections are stained with Hematoxylin-Eosin (H&E). The brain, after fixation, is sectioned in the coronal plane. Multiple samples of the various lobes are fixed and processed, and 5-μm sections are stained with H&E. For the common myocardium, 5-μm sections are stained with H&E and trichromic Heidenhain (Azan) stains.

In fetuses after the 25th week of gestation considered in our study, the autopsy examination includes a systemic gross and microscopic evaluation of the body, the placental disk, the umbilical cord and membranes. Signs of hypoxic suffering are evaluated using specific criteria based on the presence of subpleural hemorrhagic petechiae, second-degree depletion of the thymus, marked hepatic erythropoiesis and stress-response pseudofollicular changes of the adrenal gland [10, 44, 96].

In addition to the routine autopsy procedure, this autopsy protocol includes in particular the collection and study of the following structures:

- Cardiac conduction system [40, 68, 73];
- Central, peripheral and autonomic nervous systems
  - Brainstem
    - Medulla oblongata
    - Pons
    - Midbrain [27, 43, 60];
  - Spinal cord
    - Cervicothoracic tract [53];
  - Cerebellum [31, 32];
  - Sympathetic ganglia
    - Stellate ganglion
    - Superior cervical ganglion;

- Carotid bifurcation
  Carotid glomus
  Carotid sinus [85];
- Ganglionic and paraganglionic mediastinal plexuses situated in the fibroadipose tissue between the ascending aorta/aortic arch and the bifurcation of the pulmonary artery [81, 85].

2.4 Cardiac Sampling and Study of the Conduction System

2.4.1 Cardiac Sampling

At the general autopsy, before analysis of the heart's conduction system, any extracardiac cause of death should be ruled out. At autopsy, the heart is removed in the usual way, but taking the utmost care to sever the great vessels very close to the pericardial reflections. In particular, the superior vena cava should be cut about two cm above the pericardial sac to ensure the ability to examine a possibly "high" sinoatrial node (SAN) and of many ganglia of the SAN nerve plexus which extend to the caval funnel adventitia [82–84] (Fig. 2.4).

Determination of the size and weight of the heart should not be omitted, and the values should be compared with normal values for infants of the same age and weight [15, 94, 97]. Pericardial and fat tissues should be dissected and removed. After the presence of gross cardiac malformations has been excluded, the origin of the coronary arteries should be carefully inspected. The heart is systematically examined for pathological changes in the atria, septa, ventricles, pericardium, endocardium and coronary arteries. Samples of the myocardium are stained with H&E and trichromic Heidenhain (Azan) stains.

Considering that the pre-atherosclerotic reversible lesions have been reported to start in fetal age [45, 47, 49], histological examination of the coronary arteries should be carried out according to the following procedure. The major epicardial coronary arteries and branches (left main, anterior descending, left circumflex, right main, posterior descending, right marginal) are excised transversely to their longitudinal axis in segments of approximately 3–4 mm. Each segment is labeled sequentially from either its aortic ostium or its origin from the left main coronary artery. The segments are dehydrated, embedded in paraffin, and sections are stained with H&E and Azan for histological examination, alcian blue at pH 0.5 and 2.5 for analysis of acid mucopolysaccharides, and Weigert's resorcin-fuchsin stain for identification of elastic fibers. In selected cases, the cells of the walls of the coronary arteries and of the cardiac conduction arteries are immunophenotyped using the immunoperoxidase technique with the following primary antibodies (Dako reagents): anti-α-smooth muscle actin to identify smooth muscle cells (SMCs), anti-CD68 to identify monocytes, anti-CD20 and anti-UCHL-1 to identify B- and T-lymphocytes, respectively [45, 47, 49, 55, 61].

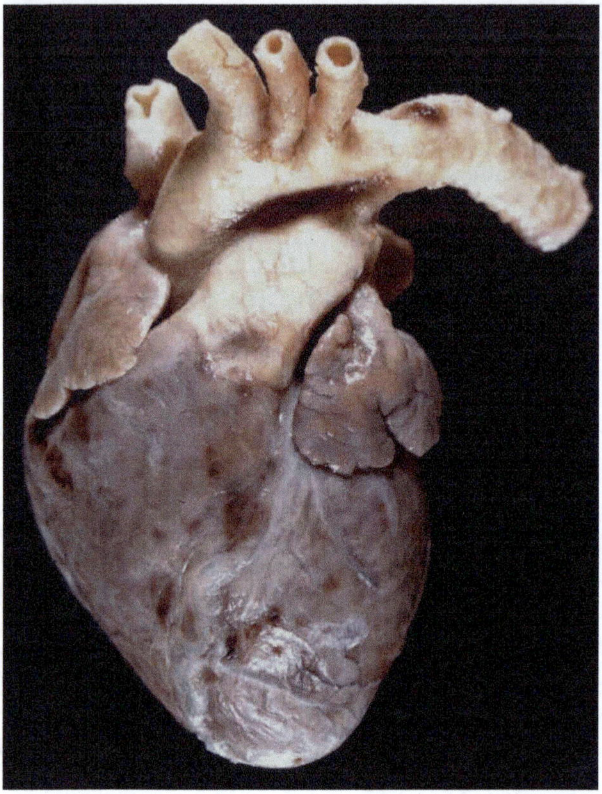

Fig. 2.4 At autopsy, the heart should be removed together with a significant length of the great vessels. Determination of the size and weight of the heart should not be omitted, and the values should be compared with normal values for infants of the same age and weight. After the presence of gross cardiac malformations have been excluded, the origin of the coronary arteries should be carefully inspected

2.4.2 Removal of the Cardiac Conduction System Blocks

Histological observations are focused on the cardiac conduction system, which, though fairly constant in layout and structure, shows noteworthy individual variations [37, 85]. Therefore, histological examination of serial sections would be expected to provide the necessary information concerning both topography and pathology of the specialized tissue [53]. The cardiac conduction system is removed in two blocks for paraffin embedding. It is important, in order to "save the pacemaker", to avoid the customary incision to open the right atrium heart margin cutting directly the intercaval bridge between the superior and inferior venae cavae. Instead, the incision should be driven laterally towards the superior vena cava, dividing lengthwise the intercaval bridge. Indeed, using the customary incision, the SAN may be slashed diagonally, together with the *crista terminalis*. The aorta should always be opened by cutting the mitral aortic valve [83]. Another heart dissection procedure that should be avoided is to perform a single longitudinal cut to exposes all the heart chambers of both sides of the heart, like a "sandwich".

According to the sampling technique devised by Rossi [82–90], two blocks of heart tissue should be removed for paraffin embedding.

Block 1 contains the SAN, its atrial approaches and the *crista terminalis*, and the SAN ganglionar plexus. The main visual reference for removal is centered upon the *sulcus–crista terminalis*. The incisions to be made are the following:

- The first incision is made longitudinally, parallel to the *sulcus-crista terminalis*, through the atrial wall, from the inferior vena cava along the AV margin. This incision is extended to the right auricula in the midline.
- The second incision is also made longitudinally, parallel to the *sulcus-crista terminalis*, through the atrial wall, this time from the AV margin to the superior vena cava.
- These two longitudinal incisions are made parallel to the *sulcus-crista terminalis* line through the atrial wall, with medial extension on the right side to encompass the anterior aspect of the inlet of the superior vena cava. On the left side, one has to section very medially the cava–cava bridge and extend the incision to the superior vena cava wall. Of the two transverse incisions, the superior one is oriented to remove as much as possible of the cava funnel.
- The third incision is carried out at the level of the inferior portion of the right atrium and removes, more or less distally according to the atrial volume, the fan of the pectinate muscles that radiate from the *crista terminalis*.
  The procedure for the excision of block 1 is illustrated in Fig. 2.5.

Block 2 contains the atrioventricular (AV) system – atrioventricular node, bundle of His, bifurcation of bundle of His, bundle branches, Purkinje cells – with its atrial approaches. The reference points for the excision are, on the right side, the outlet of the coronary sinus and the *pars membranacea septi*. Holding the already opened heart so as to expose the interventricular septum against a fairly intense light source, one can clearly see the transparent area of the *pars membranacea*, which can then be grasped between thumb and index finger. One then proceeds to excise the interventricular septum together with the central fibrous body, the lowermost part of the atrial septum and the adjacent segments of the AV fibrous annuli. The incisions to be made are as follows:

- A longitudinal incision (a) through the posterior part of the septum, across the AV fibrous annulus and up to the superior margin of the coronary sinus ostium.
- A longitudinal incision (b) a through the superior part of the septum extending to the aortic valvular ring.
- Two incisions perpendicular to (a) and (b) to take away the tissue block, with its upper (atrial-aortic) margin about 1.5 cm above the AV ring and its lower (ventricular apex) margin encompassing the base of the medial tricuspid papillary muscle and possibly the moderator band.

The procedure for the excision of block 2 is illustrated in Fig. 2.6. After removal, block 2 can be trimmed to regularize its shape by removing the valvular leaflets with the chordae, and the useless tracts of aortic wall and pulmonary conus muscle, well above the *pars membranacea*.

Some investigators [92, 93] have adopted a technique very similar to the one described above for the excision of tissue block 2, but involving further subdivision of the block into a number of minor fragments which are mounted and sectioned separately. The only advantage of this method is that smaller blocks are presented

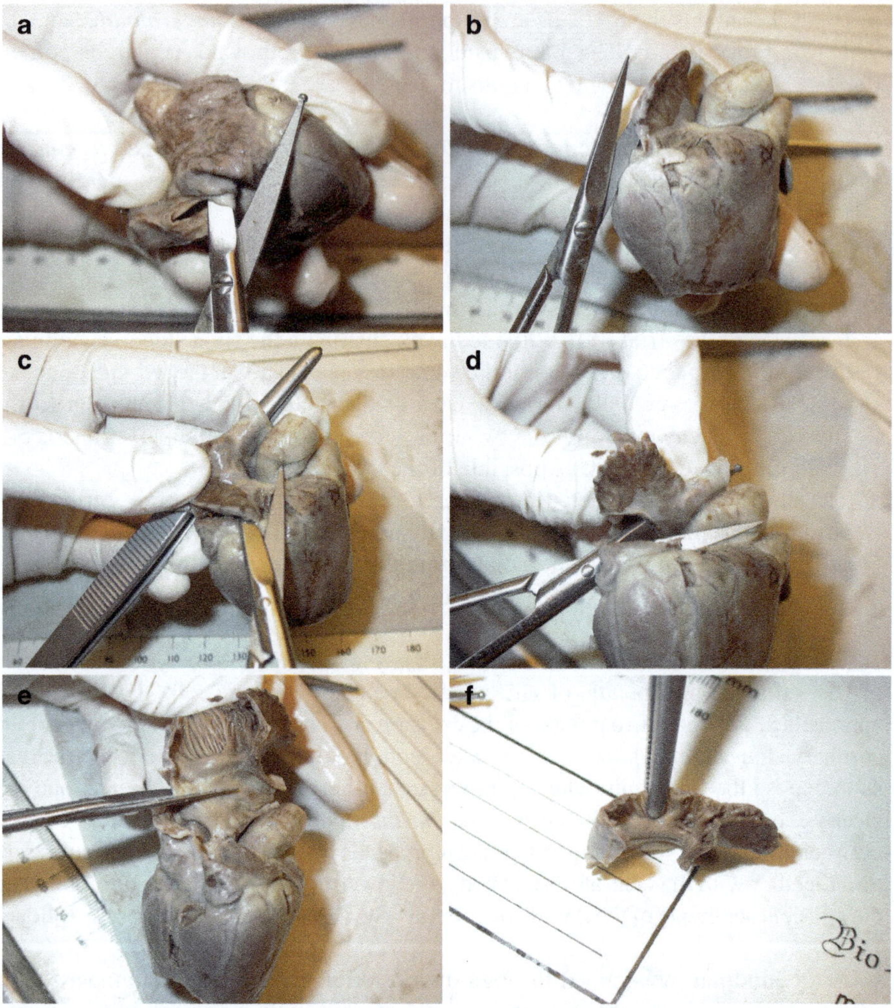

Fig. 2.5 Excision of block 1 for the study of the cardiac conduction system. (**a**) The first incision is made from the inferior vena cava along the AV margin. (**b**) This first excision is extended to the right auricular in the midline. (**c**) A second incision is made from the AV line to the superior vena cava. (**d**) An incision parallel to the *crista terminalis* is then made. (**e**) A cut parallel to the *crista terminalis* is then made. (**f**) The block obtained contains the SAN, its atrial approaches, the *crista terminalis*, and the SAN ganglionar plexus. The main visual reference for the removal is centered upon the *sulcus–crista terminalis*

to special microtomy more suitable for serial sectioning; however, this instrumental advantage is obtained at the cost of occasionally interfering with the fundamental histopathological understanding of the exact extension and layout of damage along the spatially reconstructed AV system and of interfering with the search for mediate accessory AV pathways. It is indeed extremely difficult, if not impossible, to make sections from different fragments coincide with one another in three dimensions, which, in turn, is one of the prerequisites for understanding the arrhythmological pathology of the conduction system.

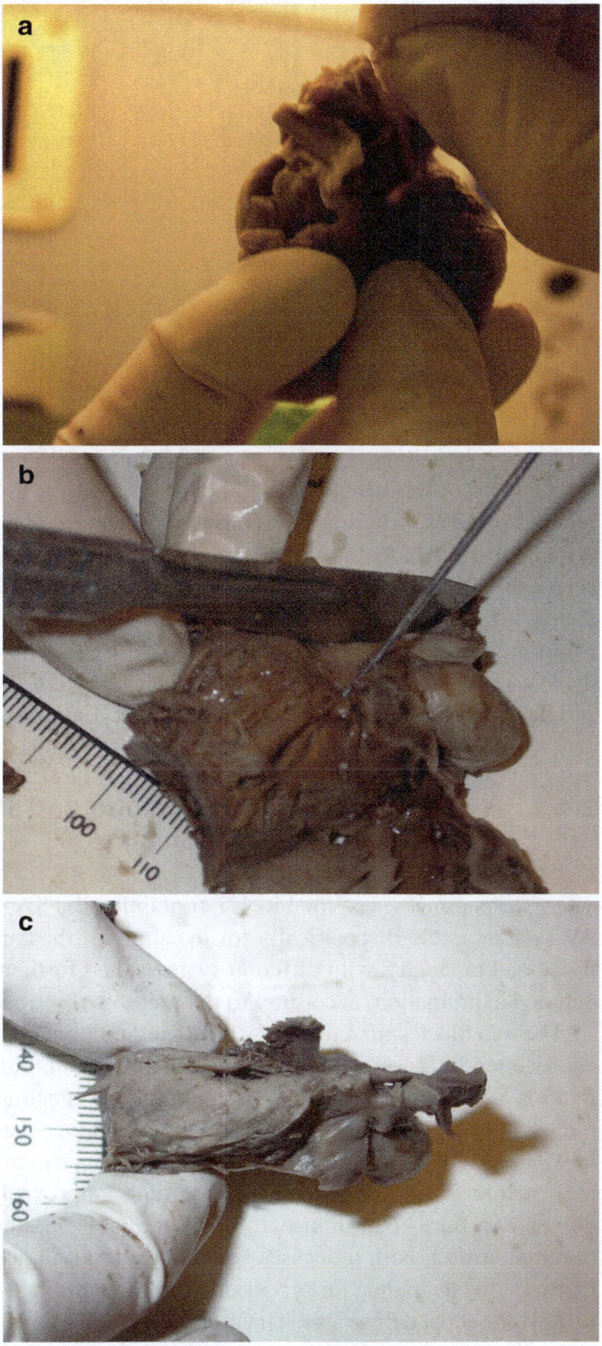

Fig. 2.6 (**a**–**c**) Excision of block 2 for the study of the cardiac conduction system. (**a**) Holding the already opened heart so as to expose the interventricular septum against a fairly intense light source, the transparent area of the *pars membranacea* can be clearly identified. (**b**) The interventricular septum is then excised together with the central fibrous body, the lowermost part of the atrial septum and the adjacent segments of the AV fibrous annuli. A longitudinal incision through the posterior part of the septum, across the AV fibrous annulus and up to the superior margin of the coronary sinus ostium is made. (**c**) Block 2 contains the AV system with its atrial approaches. The reference points of the excision are, on the right side, the outlet of the coronary sinus and the *pars membranacea septi*

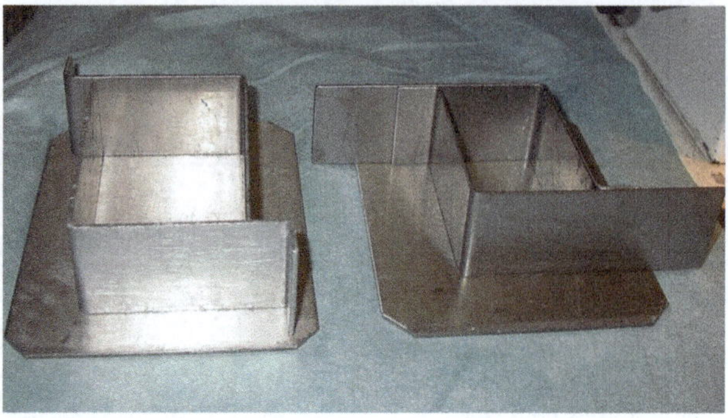

Fig. 2.7 The two tissue blocks for the study of the cardiac conduction system after dehydration are embedded in paraffin using metallic molds for oversized specimens

Accessory pathways of James and Mahaim type, together with any medial/septoseptal direct Kent bundles, are included in block 2. Other direct AV accessory bundles of Kent, bridging the AV rings elsewhere, require the examination of both AV annuli in their entirety, with the adjacent muscle, as follows: radial incisions, perpendicular to the plane of the AV ostia, will subdivide the fibrous ring into fragments 1.5–2 cm thick, together with the muscle attached to the ring on both sides; trimming away the free valvular leaflets is suggested. This technique for studying the AV junctional tissue and its atrial approaches in the triangle of Koch involves serial sectioning in a plane parallel, i.e. tangential, to the endocardial surface.

2.4.3 Fixation, Processing, Sectioning, and Staining of the Cardiac Conduction Blocks

The two specimens, i.e., the block 1 containing the SAN and block 2 containing the AV system, excised specifically for the study of the cardiac conduction system are processed manually, with different systems, and further sectioned in series to allow detailed examination, according to the method described by Rossi [83–90].

The two blocks are reduced by removing redundant tissue (papillary muscles and chordae tendinae, etc.) and fixed in 10% phosphate-buffered formalin [1, 9]. Once fixation is complete (3–20 days depending on specimen volume), the formalin is removed under running tap water for about 20 min. The material is then dehydrated in 95% ethanol for 24 h followed by four passages in pure dioxan (diethylene dioxide) each for 12 h. The tissue is then partially impregnated in a mixture of one-third dioxan/two-thirds paraffin (melting point 56–58 °C) and, finally, total impregnated in pure paraffin, both processes being carried out in an oven. Dioxan is the crucial factor in this technique for processing the conduction system since it is both a paraffin solvent and a dehydrator. The more commonly used ethylic dehydration tends to cause the material to become too hard so it breaks upon microtome sectioning [3]. After dehydration, paraffin embedding is carried out using metallic molds for oversized specimens (Fig. 2.7).

The two blocks must be precisely orientated. For the SAN block, the reference points are the pectinati muscles, that should stand upwards. For the AVN block the aortic semilunar valves should be placed opposite the cut surface. The blocks should be stored in a freezer. The surface paraffin is first removed from each block, and a scalpel is used to mold all around the block to facilitate sectioning in the microtome and to allow better distension in warm water. The paraffin blocks are better if they are made fairly tall so that they can be caught high in the microtome vice, avoiding the wood or plastic base that tends to become loose.

Serial sectioning is an essential part of the investigation of the conduction system, since it allows a further three-dimensional reconstruction of the examined conducting tissue [53, 88, 91]. Depending on the specimen's size, sectioning should be carried out at intervals every 20–40 μm for SAN blocks and every 40–60 μm for AVN blocks, collecting three 8-μm sections at each level [40, 53, 63].

Microscopic evaluation of the slides will enable one to decide whether or not the investigation can be considered ended, in which case the remaining paraffin block can be stored for possible further investigation. The serial sectioning itself can be carried out using a normal manual sledge microtome adapted for tall specimens. The sections obtained can be expanded in warm water at 40–50 °C in twin baths, one containing Sta-On tissue section adhesive (Surgipath) for histochemistry, the other without for immunohistochemistry. The sections for immunohistochemistry are collected onto slides pretreated with 3-aminopropyl triethoxysilane (silanized). The slides are previously countersigned and labeled with the number of the case, the paraffin block and the sequence level, and whether silanized or not, and then put in an oven at 37 °C overnight. The slides destined for further staining for apoptosis are replaced in the oven at 60 °C for 4 h to enhance the adherence of the section to the glass slide.

For prescreening, it is not necessary to stain specimens from all the levels (70–100 levels for the SAN, 100–130 for the AVN); it may be enough to stain selected specimens from five or six levels alternately with H&E and Azan (azocarmine aniline blue stain of Heidenhain).

To obtain good results, before applying the aniline blue, myofibril conducting muscle should be overstained in Azan, developed slowly and blocked with acetic acid, followed finally by the application of phosphotungstic acid as mordant. These Azan solutions are also prepared in the laboratory. Unstained slides are archived for eventual follow-up of the investigations. Various so-called "secondary" stainings are also utilized according to the abnormalities demonstrated.

The histochemical alcian-blue stain, pH 2.5, and periodic acid-Schiff (PAS) stain for acid polysaccharides are used to stain the cartilaginous hypermetaplasia of the heart's central fibrous body from SIDS victims. Alcian blue is also used to stain for circulating and tissue mast cells [1, 3, 35]. Mallory's phosphotungstic acid hematoxylin (PTAH) stain, that we apply with the Armed Forces Institute of Pathology (AFIP) [35] modification with satisfactory results, is similar to Azan and is particularly indicated for morphometric studies and/or for the central nervous system since it stains muscle, elastic fibers, neuroglia, erythrocytes, fibrin and cartilage deep blue, myelin light blue, and cytoplasm, collagen, elastic and reticular fibers, basal membranes and osteoid tissue orange or light-brown. Weigert's method is used specifically for elastic fibers as it stains black or deep brown over a yellow-red background due to Van Gieson's stain for gross connective and muscle tissue. We usually avoid contrast staining with Van Gieson's stain since it fades and disappears in a matter of ten years, preferring the resorcin-fuchsin method that is known to give quite favorable results. The "slow eosin" method using very dilute eosin (a couple of drops in a beaker of water) gives good results as a differential stain for leukocytes in "critical" preparations, for example in eosinophilic myocarditis. The silanized blank sections can be processed for immunohistochemistry, for example the detection of apoptosis by the TUNEL method for staining fragmented DNA and by PCNA staining, and DAKO S-100 and GFAP for staining neurofibrils [41].

For each heart, the average number of histological sections stained and examined is about 200. The cardiac conduction system can be reconstructed in three dimensions from the series of two-dimensional slides. The same procedure is applicable to study the cardiac conduction system in adults [62, 67, 69, 85].

2.5 Brainstem Sampling

There is a continuity between SIDS and unexplained perinatal loss as common developmental abnormalities, mainly hypoplasia and neuronal immaturity, have been detected in the brainstem nuclei of regulation of the vital functions. Therefore, the histopathological evaluation of the brainstem focuses on the arcuate nucleus, the hypoglossus nucleus, vagal dorsal motor nucleus, nucleus of the solitary tract, ambiguus nucleus, reticular ventrolateral formation, the pre-Bötzinger nucleus, the inferior olivary nucleus in the medulla oblongata; the locus coeruleus, and the parabrachial Kölliker-Fuse complex, and the parafacial nucleus in the pons and midbrain [13, 21, 22, 24–26, 42–44].

The aim of the histopathological investigation of the human brainstem is to provide basic information on the cardiocirculatory and respiratory central neuronal circuits in order to provide an increasing understanding of the inherent histopathological parameters in SIDS/SNUD/SIUD cases.

The brainstem sampling techniques described here, complete and simplified, could allow the pathologist to cope using a systematic approach with the central neuropathology of SIDS and unexpected perinatal death or to preserve suitable material for further investigation by specialists, which is much needed to help to provide a better understanding of SIDS and sudden unexpected perinatal death.

The examination of the brainstem in SIDS, sudden unexpected perinatal deaths and controls has underlined a remarkable variability, particularly of the arcuate nucleus (ARCn), in both size and neuronal density [26, 42]. Therefore, the complete evaluation of the brainstem and its possible abnormalities requires its examination on serial sections or, in the simplified procedure, the individualization of defined and constant section levels, identifiable through anatomic reference points [46, 53, 60].

In all cases it is important to avoid removing the leptomeninges by tearing, in order to avoid a discontinuity of the ventral medullary surface. The time required for fixation of the brainstem in 10% phosphate-buffered formalin varies from 3–4 days to several days, based on the number of gestational weeks or age of the fetus or infant.

2.5.1 Complete Examination of the Brainstem

In the procedure for complete examination, the brainstem is entirely processed and serially sectioned throughout its entire length. This includes cranially the lower third of the midbrain and caudally the medulla oblongata sectioned some millimeters distally from the lower pole of the inferior olivary nucleus.

In the stillborn and in the newborn the brainstem specimen is processed in its entirety, while in infants, because of its greater size, the brainstem is divided into two parts:

1. The first specimen comprises the medulla oblongata. The upper incision is made some millimeters proximal to the border between the medulla oblongata and the pons; the lower incision is made some millimeters below the lower pole of the olivary body.
2. The second specimen comprises the pons and the lower third portion of the midbrain.

The brainstem specimen or specimens after fixation is/are dehydrated in ethanol at increasing concentrations and embedded in paraffin with a melting point of 56–58 °C. These passages in ethanol and then in paraffin, to optimize the results, are done manually, varying the times according to the specimen size. The number of serial sections through the entire brainstem varies in relation to the age of the victim. In the fetus, from the 25th week of gestation, the average number of sections is 360, while in the fetus at term and/or in the newborn it is 600. In SIDS victims of 3–4 months and over 6 months of age it is 900 and 1,400, respectively. This procedure allows a detailed evaluation of all the other brainstem nuclei, apart from the ARCn.

In order to apply the appropriate histological staining (H&E, Klüver-Barrera, or trichromic Heidenhain stains) and to perform further histochemical investigations (i.e. Glees-Marsland silver stain for neurons and neurofibrils, Bielschowsky's silver stain for axons and dendrites, Mallory's PTAH stain for glia) and immunohistochemical tests (to study apoptosis, various neuroreceptor structures, the expression of specific genes, etc.), groups of 12 sections are prepared, three of which are used for the histological methods and the other nine saved and stained as deemed necessary for further investigations. Therefore, the number of groups of 12 serial sections varies from 30 in the fetus at the 25th week of gestation (corresponding to 360 sections) to 120 in SIDS victims over 6 months of age (corresponding to 1,400 sections). Therefore, for each case analyzed, and according to the age of the subject, between 90 and 360 sections are stained with H&E, Klüver-Barrera and trichromic Heidenhain stains, and between 270 and 1,080 unstained sections are kept and stained as necessary.

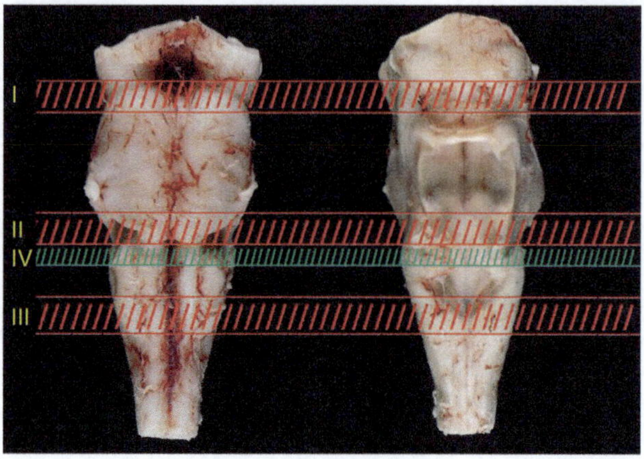

Fig. 2.8 Ventral (*left*) and dorsal (*right*) surfaces of the brainstem showing the location of the sample blocks I–IV

This process represents four weeks of work by a histotechnician. Although having the merits of completeness and accuracy, it is not routinely applicable in all histopathological laboratories, for the obvious reason that it requires additional technical personnel [46].

2.5.2 Simplified Examination of the Brainstem

The simplified procedure for the examination of the brainstem of an infant or of the term fetus or newborn requires a much lower number of sections. The cranial, intermediate and caudal portions of the nuclei can be examined, and the technique is applicable in every laboratory. However, this method requires careful and precise sampling.

The brainstem is divided into the following three blocks, as shown in Fig. 2.8:

Block I The cranial block, includes the pontomesencephalic junction;

Block II The intermediate block, includes the pontobulbar junction;

Block III The caudal block, includes the medulla oblongata corresponding to the submedian area of the inferior olivary eminence; has the obex as a reference point and extends 2–3 mm above and below the obex.

A fourth block (block IV), just below block II, can be excised and submitted for genetic analysis [58].

2.5.3 Fixation, Processing, Sectioning, and Staining of the Brainstem Blocks

The brainstem specimens, after fixation, are dehydrated in ethanol at increasing concentrations and embedded in paraffin with a melting point of 56–58 °C. These passages in ethanol and then in paraffin, to optimize the results, are done manually, varying the times according to the specimen size.

Each block is sectioned transversely at intervals of 30 μm (levels). For each level, twelve 5-μm sections are obtained, three of which are routinely stained for histological examination alternately with H&E, Bielschowsky's and Klüver-Barrera stains, and the other nine are saved and stained as deemed necessary for further investigations. The number of levels and consequently of serial sections through the entire brainstem varies in relation to the age of the victim. In fetuses, from the 30th week of gestation, the average number of sections is 360 (corresponding to 30 groups of 12 serial sections), while in term fetuses and newborns, 600 sections may be obtained (30 groups). From infants of 3–4 months and over 6 months of age an average of 900 and 1,400 sections are obtained from 75 and 120 levels, respectively. The important nuclei are demonstrated, namely the ARCn, the hypoglossal nucleus, the dorsal motor vagal nucleus, the solitary tract nucleus, the ambiguous nucleus and the trigeminal tract nucleus, and the ventrolateral reticular formation in the medulla oblongata, together with the locus coeruleus and the parabrachial/Kölliker-Fuse complex in the pons [53, 60].

Two expanding baths are advised, one with Sta-On adhesive and the other without, both at 40–45 °C. Each level requires 12 sections, i.e., one for H&E staining, one for Klüver-Barrera staining, six unstained, and four on silanized slides. All are accurately countersigned and put in an oven 37 °C overnight. In the morning the H&E stained sections are screened in order to decide upon further processing. For morphometry, Klüver-Barrera staining is needed, whereas for apoptosis a prior 4-h incubation in an oven at 60 °C is needed.

H&E staining is advised in all cases. Another method advised is the silver impregnation method of Bielschowsky for axons, dendrites, and nerve cells which are stained black–violet, and in which the "photographic" reduction is obtained by formol, with a final fixing with sodium thiosulfate that renders the silver impregnation permanent. Another method we employ, particularly for the brainstem, is the silver impregnation method of Glees and Marsland for neuronal bodies and neurofibers which are stained black or brown on a bronze-brown lighter background. Mostly in the brainstem the Klüver-Barrera stain is employed for myelin and neurons. It utilizes Luxol fast blue which is derived from tetrabenzotetrazo-porphyrin. The Luxol stain binds with phospholipidic myelin components such as lecithin and sphingomyelin. The Luxol is chromatically contrasted with cresyl violet, which makes it possible to obtain evidence also of cytoplasmic Nissl substance. Mallory's PTAH is also a satisfactory stain for glia, and Azan can be used to show glomic neuroreceptors [1, 3, 35].

2.5.4 Morphometric Analysis

Morphometric analysis is performed with an image analyzer (Image-Pro Plus, Media Cybernetics, Silver Spring, Maryland, USA). For each brainstem nucleus, in particular, the ARCn and the parabrachial/Kölliker-Fuse complex, the neuronal cell body areas, neuronal density, transverse section areas and volume are evaluated, using serial sections stained with Klüver-Barrera stain. Only those neurons with an obvious nucleus and nucleolus are included in the measurements. The profile area of the neuronal bodies is expressed in microns squared, and the transverse sectional area, after delineation of the outer boundaries, in millimeters squared. The neuronal density is evaluated in transverse sections as the number of neurons per millimeter squared. For two-dimensional reconstruction, a computer program developed by Voxblast (Vaytek, Fairfield, Iowa, USA) is used to digitize and align the anatomic boundary tracings in the serial sections [25, 42].

2.6 Cerebellum Sampling

It is essential to perform an accurate examination of the cerebellum, in view of its role in controlling the respiratory muscles and of the observation of developmental anomalies of the cerebellum cortex and cerebellar deep nuclei in cases of perinatal and infant unexpected death [32–34, 60]. In order to examine both the cerebellar cortex and the four deep cerebellar nuclei, i.e., the dentate, emboliform, globose, and fastigii nuclei, samples of hemisphere extending all along the major diameter should be obtained. The cerebellum is excised from the brainstem by cutting through the cerebellar peduncles before proceeding to the horizontal sections. The cerebellar hemispheres are cut in the sagittal plane in serial parallel sections at 0.5 cm intervals, beginning at the vermis and then proceeding to the right and left of the midline [31].

2.7 Study of the Carotid Bifurcation, Ganglia and Paraganglia

2.7.1 Carotid Bifurcation

The carotid bifurcation – right and left – is located at the level of the superior edge of the thyroid cartilage (C4) and is flattened into a Y shape (Fig. 1.7). Two receptors at the carotid bifurcation provide feedback to the vasomotor and respiratory centers of the brain: the carotid body and the carotid sinus.

The carotid body or glomus is a highly vascular area located between the two bifurcation carotid branches. It is found in the carotid bifurcation area, on the internal carotid artery side, close to the "swelling" of the carotid sinus (Fig. 1.7). The carotid body is a differentiated chemoreceptor paraganglion, formed principally by cells of neuronal origin whose cytoplasm is rich in argyrophilic granules of catecholamine neurotransmitter. These cellular elements, gathered in glomeruli ("zellballen") are surrounded by sustentacular cells of schwannian type. The organelle is in strict connection with the adventitia of arterioles of carotid derivation and with mixed glossopharyngeal nervous plexuses which are vagal and less frequently sympathetic. The carotid body functions as a chemoreceptor sensitive to blood oxygen concentration (pO2) and, to lesser extent, blood pH and the partial pressure of carbon dioxide (pCO2).

The carotid sinus is located a little above the bifurcation, just at the root of the internal carotid artery. The carotid sinus delineates an anatomic area inside the arterial media (outer layer), wherein many nerve endings (also Krause's club-like) lie. However, even in this area (well outside the carotid body) some small glomera can be recognized microscopically. For this reason it is better not to draw too clear-cut topographic boundaries between chemoreceptors (paraganglia) and baro- or mechanoreceptors (intercarotid nerve endings). The carotid sinus is a fusiform dilatation that functions as a baroreceptor to monitor blood pressure [85, 88, 90].

The carotid bifurcations are separately embedded in paraffin and serially sectioned.

2.7.2 Mediastinal Ganglionic and Paraganglionated Plexuses

The soft adipose fibrous (fascial) tissue between the aortic and pulmonary trunk (intertruncal plexuses), and between the aortic arch and the pulmonary hili, is removed. Sectioning the fragments in series reveals the cardiac plexus ganglia and paraganglia. The left coronary artery neuroglomic plexus should be sought at the root of the artery; sometimes the tiny intertruncal artery can be glimpsed. The plexuses are embedded well, compressing the fatty tissue on the cutting surface. The structures to be examined are invisible to the naked eye, so the maximal surface needs to be examined in each section [53, 56, 81].

2.7.3 Cervical Sympathetic Ganglia

In term fetuses and in infants, while taking out an "generous" intercarotid block of tissue, the superior cervical ganglion can be found; the middle cervical ganglion is inconstant, while the stellate ganglion (inferior cervical often fused with the first thoracic) can be found close to the branching of the subclavian and vertebral arteries. The ganglia can be embedded complete, or can be divided longitudinally.

The carotid bifurcation, mediastinal and aorticopulmonary ganglia and paraganglia, adequately labeled, are fixed in buffered formalin. In infants, we recommend that the excision of these structures be carried out on already fixed material. The material should be washed in tap water immediately after fixation. The dehydration of these tissues is different from that used for the conduction system study [1]. The ablated fragments have a soft consistency and it is better to use a dehydration that will harden up the specimens. Ethylic alcohol is used at increasing concentrations (70%, 95% in two changes, 100% in two changes) and then xylol in two changes, which is followed by embedding in two changes of pure paraffin at a melting point of 56–58 °C in the oven. The changes are best carried out manually because of the different times required depending on the specimen dimensions. The embedded material is serially sectioned [58].

2.8 Lung Evaluation of the Stage of Development

In each case of infant and perinatal unexpected death the stage of pulmonary development is evaluated on the basis of the autopsy macroscopic criterion of the ratio between lung weight and body weight (LW/BW), and according to the microscopic criterion of the radial alveolar count (RAC). Determination of the RAC involves examining at least ten fields for each case with a 40× lens, in order to estimate the number of alveoli transected by a perpendicular line drawn from the center of the most peripheral bronchiole – recognized by being incompletely covered by epithelium – to the pleura or the nearest interlobular septum. For this examination, samples of the lungs sectioned parallel to the frontal plane and passing through the hilus are obtained.

According to the macroscopic criterion, the normal reference values for the lLW/BW ratio are >0.012 for LW/BW. According to the microscopic criterion, the normal range values for RAC vary at different ages [2, 11, 12, 44, 75].

2.9 Immunohistochemistry and Other Techniques

In selected cases, immunohistochemistry studies are performed on sections of the cardiac conduction system, brainstem, and coronary arteries.

2.9.1 Apoptosis

The sections are deparaffinized and incubated with 20 μg/ml proteinase K (Sigma, St. Louis, MO, USA). After blocking the endogenous peroxidase with 3% H2O2, deoxynucleotidyl transferase (TdT 0.3 U/ml) is used to add digoxigenin-conjugated deoxyuridine (dUTP 0.01 mM/ml) to the ends of DNA fragments. The signal of TdT-mediated dUTP nick end labeling (TUNEL) is then detected by an anti-digoxigenin antibody conjugated with peroxidase (ApopTag peroxidase in situ apoptosis detection kit; Oncor, Gaithersburg, MD, USA). Apoptotic nuclei are identified by the presence of dark-brown staining. Counterstaining is performed by immersing the slides in methyl green for 10 min. The apoptotic index (AI) is defined as the number of apoptotic cells divided by the total number of cells counted, expressed as a percentage [41, 65].

2.9.2 Proliferating Cell Nuclear Antigen (PCNA)

Paraffin sections are cut and mounted on glass slides and air-dried at room temperature overnight. Sections are deparaffinized and immersed in Tris-HCl buffered saline solution (TBS, pH 7.6). After blocking the endogenous peroxidase with 3% H2O2, the sections are immunostained with the monoclonal PC10 antibody (dilution 1:200) using the avidin biotin (ABC) complex method with overnight incubation.

Diaminobenzidine is used as a chromogen, and a light hematoxylin counterstain is used. Biotinylated rabbit anti-mouse IgM is used as a secondary antibody (Vectastain ABC kit; Vector Laboratories, Burlingame, CA, USA). All incubations are carried out in a humidified chamber at room temperature, and, after each incubation, the slides are extensively washed with three changes of TBS. Inflamed palatine tonsils are used as positive controls for PCNA. The PCNA labeling index (PCNA-LI) is defined as the number of cells with strong unequivocal nuclear staining, divided by the total number of cells counted, expressed as a percentage [23, 64].

2.9.3 c-Fos

Sections are deparaffinized in xylene and rehydrated. Endogenous peroxidase is blocked by incubation with 3% hydrogen peroxide for 5 min. After washing in phosphate-buffered saline (PBS), the sections are incubated with 10% normal goat serum and then with 1:100 diluted polyclonal anti-c-fos antibody (SC-52P, Santa Cruz Biotechnology, CA, USA) at room temperature for 1 h. After washing in PBS for 5 min, the sections are incubated with biotinylated goat anti-rabbit IgG antibody supplied in the kit for 30 min, incubated with streptavidin-peroxidase for 30 min, stained with 3,3′-diaminobenzidine tetrahydrochloride (DAB, Sigma) solution (30 mg DAB and 0.5 ml 0.3% hydrogen peroxide in 100 ml 0.05 M Tris-HCl, pH 7.6) and counterstained with cresyl violet. In order to confirm the specificity of c-fos immunostaining, sections from every case are also treated with a blocking peptide (final concentration 10 μg/ml, SC-52P; Santa Cruz Biotechnology), coincubated with the anti-c-fos antibody and then treated in the same way.

In selected cases, the nuclei of the medulla oblongata (in particular the hypoglossal, dorsal motor vagal, solitary tract, ambiguous, arcuate and inferior olivary nuclei) are examined for c-fos immunoreactivity. Neurons are defined as positive when a clear brown staining is present, which is stronger than in the surrounding interstitium. To evaluate the distribution of c-fos immunostaining in the nuclei of the medulla oblongata, a qualitative rating system is used at each level examined (rostral, intermediate and caudal, respectively), ranging from – to +++. Briefly, the scoring system for each brainstem nucleus is: –, no c-fos-positive cells; +, a few dark c-fos-positive cells (<10%); ++, a moderate number of c-fos-positive cells ranging from 10 to 50%; and +++, a high number of c-fos-positive cells (>50%) [24].

2.9.4 Glial Fibrillar Acidic Protein (GFAP)

To reveal the reactive astrocytes, the sections were stained by the indirect immunoperoxidase method with antibody to the GFAP (bovine GFAP, Novocastra, Newcastle, Tyne, UK). The GFAP dilution was 1:200; the time of incubation 1 h. Sections were then counterstained with Mayer's hematoxylin. Astrocytes were counted if they displayed a GFAP-positive cytoplasm and counterstained nucleus. For all the immunohistochemical methods, negative controls are prepared by replacing the respective primary antibodies with PBS in the incubation. As regards to gliosis, the density and the ratio of reactive astrocytes in braistem and cerebellum sections are evaluated. A case is considered as positive when a percentage higher than 25% of immunopositive cells is detected.

2.9.5 Engrailed-2 (*En-2*)

En-2 gene expression is detected by means of the monoclonal antibody Mab 4D9 that specifically recognizes engrailed En-2 proteins. Four- μm tissue sections are washed in 0.01 M PBS at pH 7.4 for 5 min and then rinsed in 3% hydrogen peroxide in PBS for 15 min in order to inactivate endogenous peroxidase. After peroxide treatment, tissue sections are washed three times for 5 min each in PBS and then incubated in 10% normal rabbit serum in PBS for 1 h followed by overnight incubation at 4°C with the monoclonal primary antibody 4D9 directed against the En-2 protein, diluted 1:75 in PBS. Following incubation with the primary antibody, the sections are washed three times in PBS. For visualization of the En-2 protein, the sections are incubated for 1 h in biotinylated goat anti-rabbit immunoglobulin G diluted 1:400 in PBS. After another three rinses for 5 min each in PBS, the site of the antigen–antibody reaction was revealed with anti-mouse immunoglobulin followed by peroxidase–antiperoxidase complex. The unlabeled antiserum was placed on the sections for 2 h, diluted 1:200 at room temperature. The sections were then exposed to the peroxidase–antiperoxidase complex for 2 h at 1:200 dilution. The sites of peroxidase activity are visualized with 0.3% hydrogen peroxide in buffer containing 0.04% diaminobenzidine tetrahydrochloride and 0.5 g nickel ammonium sulfate. Slides are rinsed, dehydrated, mounted and examined by light microscopy [27, 29].

2.9.6 Tyrosine Hydroxylase (TH)

For TH immunostaining, the sections are rinsed three times in 0.1 M Trizma buffered saline (TBS) followed by a 48-h incubation at 4 °C with a 1/500 dilution of primary rabbit antiserum to TH (Novocastra Laboratories, Newcastle, UK). The dilutions are prepared with a solution of 1% normal goat serum (NGS) and 0.25% Triton X-100 in 0.1 M Tris–saline. This was followed by a 2.5-h incubation with biotinylated goat anti-rabbit immunoglobulin G (IgG) (Vector Laboratories, Burlingame, CA, USA) diluted 1/200 with 1% NGS in Tris–saline. The tissue is then incubated for 2 h with the avidin–biotin complex diluted 1/100 with 1% NGS in Tris–saline (Vector). Between each incubation, the sections are rinsed three times with 1% NGS in Tris-saline. The sections are then treated for 6 min with a 0.05% solution of 3,3′diamino–benzidine and 0.01% hydrogen peroxide, rinsed in phosphate buffer, mounted on gel-coated slides, cleared in xylene and coverslipped with Depex mounting medium. To evaluate the immunoreactivity for TH protein the

following rating system based on the examination of all the immunostained sections along the caudorostral extension of the brainstems is adopted. Only neurons with intense brown staining are considered to be positive. The scoring for each brainstem nucleus follows:
– No positive neuron, or presence of weakly immunostained neurons;
+ A number of positive neurons ≤30% (moderate positivity);
++ A number of positive neurons >30% (strong positivity) [27].

2.9.7 Somatostatin (SS)

To neutralize endogenous peroxidase, sections are pretreated with a solution of 0.3% hydrogenase peroxide for 20 min. After rinsing in buffer, sections are exposed for 48 h to the specific primary antiserum (Novocastra Laboratories, Newcastle, UK) diluted 1:150 at 25 °C. After 10 min in buffer, the site of antigen–antibody reaction is revealed with anti-rabbit immunoglobulin followed by peroxidase–anti-peroxidase complex. The unlabeled antiserum was placed on the sections for 2 h, diluted 1:200 at room temperature. The sections are then exposed to peroxidase–antiperoxidase complex for 2 h at a dilution of 1:200 [27].

2.9.8 α-Actin

In coronary arteries, to identify neointimal cells as smooth muscle cells (SMCs), additional immunohistochemical staining with the avidin-biotin method is performed with a monoclonal antibody against α-actin (Renner, Dannstadt, Germany) [47, 51, 61].

2.9.9 Fluorescence In Situ Hybridization (FISH)

In selected cases, coronary and carotid arteries are studied using FISH.

An α-satellite DNA probe is used, specific for the centromeric region of chromosome 7, labeled with biotin (Oncor). The centromeric probe is prepared by mixing 1.5 µl of the probe with 30 µl of Hybrisol VI (Oncor). The probe is applied to the prepared air-dried slides (15 µl) and coverslipped. Both probes and target DNAs are denatured by placing the slides on a hot-plate at 67 ± 2 °C for 5 min followed by incubation overnight in a prewarmed humidified chamber at 37 °C. The hybridized signals are detected using a commercial kit (FITC avidin detection kit, Oncor). An antifade solution containing propidium iodide 2.5 µg/ml is used for counterstaining. A Leitz Orthoplan with a Ploemopak incident-light fluorescence microscope, equipped with ultraviolet excitation filter sets, is used for scoring. Only interphase cell nuclei with intact morphology are scored. The number of hybridization spots in each cell is determined [28].

2.10 Cases Analyzed

From 1987 to 2008, at the Institute of Pathology and the "Lino Rossi" Research Center, University of Milan, many cases of sudden infant and fetal death have been analyzed, as the Reference Center for the Lombardy Region for SIDS and late unexplained fetal death (DGR n° 11693 of 06-20-2002). Furthermore, the Institute of Pathology/"Lino Rossi" Research Center has been the National Referral Center for the Study of Sudden Unexpected and Unexplained Infant and Perinatal Death, according to Italian law n° 31 of 02-02-2006 "Regulations for diagnostic *post mortem* investigation in victims of sudden infant death syndrome (SIDS) and unexpected fetal death" [7].

From an even larger number of cases, a total of 120 SIDS victims, 37 infant controls, 63 unexplained stillbirths, 16 unexplained neonatal death victims, and 19 perinatal controls were analyzed, based on the completeness of clinical and postmortem finding data availability, and after exclusion of violent causes of death.

2.10.1 SIDS Cases

The cases are classified as SIDS victims when the death of an infant under one year of age was sudden and remained unexplained after a thorough case investigation, including performance of a complete autopsy, examination of the death scene, and review of the clinical history [98]. SIDS victims eligible for this study were those who died suddenly and unexpectedly and whose autopsy findings did not have any other explanation than SIDS [95]. The SIDS group considered in this study comprised 81 males (67.5%) and 39 females (32.5%) (Fig. 2.9), ranging in age from 3 to 416 days (mean ± SEM 91.90 ± 9.55 days).

For the study of the cardiac conduction system, since SIDS occurs most commonly between two and four months of age [16, 17, 57] and postnatal morphogenesis of the cardiac conduction system is age-related [18–20], the SIDS infants were divided into three subgroups: (1) from 3 to 60 days, (2) from 61 to 120 days, and (3) from 121 to 365 days.

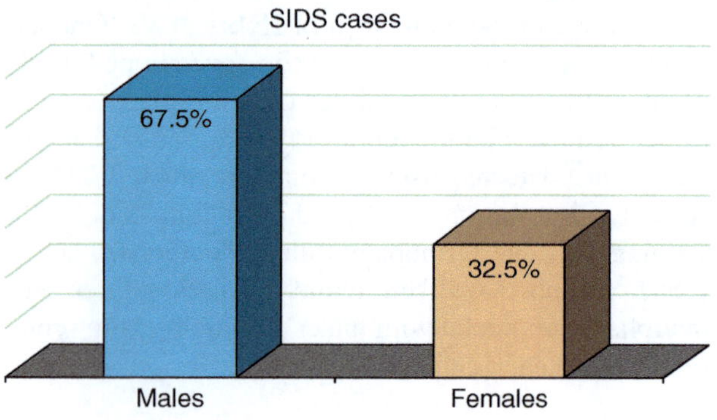

Fig. 2.9 The SIDS cases were 81 males (67.5%) and 39 females (32.5%)

For each case of suspected SIDS analyzed, the purposes were to verify the diagnosis of SIDS, whether there were any common pathological findings among the SIDS victims, and to suggest areas for further research.

2.10.2 SIUD Cases

A case is classified as sudden intrauterine unexplained death (SIUD) when the feutus dies before complete expulsion or removal of the fetus from the mother ≥22 weeks of gestation or ≥500 gm body mass which is unexpected by history and is unexplained after a thorough pathological exam of the fetus and the fetal adnexa [8, 14, 73].

In the analyzed unexplained stillborn fetuses, the brainstem and the cardiac conduction system were investigated in serial sections. The coronary arteries were also studied.

2.10.3 SNUD Cases

A case is classified as Sudden Neonatal Unexplained Death (SNUD) when the newborn dies suddenly with no explained cause, from birth to the end of the first postnatal month of life [75, 78, 79].

2.10.4 "Grey Zone"/Borderline Cases

A case is classified as SIDS/SNUD/SIUD "grey zone" or borderline when the infant/newborn/fetus dies suddenly and unexpectedly following a concomitant pathological event, itself not deadly – such as a mild leptomeningitis, a bronchus pneumonic infection or a chorionamnionitis – that acts as a triggering phenomenon in particularly vulnerable individuals, i.e., suffering from undetected preexisting nervous autonomic or cardiac conduction alterations [38, 39, 59, 72, 74].

2.10.5 Explained Death Cases

The control group was represented by term fetuses, newborns and infants who had died of various documented causes, including in particular, accidental cranial trauma, generalized sepsis, necrotizing enterocolitis, hypertrophic cardiomyopathies, etc.

In some cases submitted to the Institute of Pathology of the University of Milan with a clinical and sometimes even *post mortem* diagnosis of SIDS, the study of the cardiac conduction system and brainstem on serial sections had instead disclosed a precise cause of death [66]. For the study of the cardiac conduction system, the control infants, in a similar manner to the SIDS victims, were divided into three subgroups, according to age: (1) from 3 to 60 days, (2) from 61 to 120 days, and (3) from 121 to 365 days.

2.11 Statistical Analysis

Quantitative data were expressed as means ± SEM. The significance of differences between group parameters was evaluated by Student-t test, chi-square test or Fisher's test. In case of skewed distribution, a nonparametric Whitney rank sum test was used. One-way ANOVA was used for quantifying and partitioning variance between groups. Statistics were compiled using SigmaStat and plotted using Sigma Plot (SPSS Inc, Chicago, IL). The selected level of significance was $p < 0.05$, two-tailed.

2.12 Review Questions

This test, composed of 10 multiple-choice questions, is designed to measure knowledge about the contents of this chapter on Techniques and Criteria in Anatomic and Forensic Pathology of Sudden Infant and Perinatal Death. Questions have only one correct answer and cover the major content areas of this chapter. Check the correct responses and score your test using the answer keys on pages 92–93.

11. How is the heart dissected for the study of the cardiac conduction system?
    - □ A. Open the right atrium cutting directly the intercaval bridge between the superior and inferior venae cavae.
    - □ B. Perform a single longitudinal cut to exposes all the heart chambers of both sides of the heart, like a "sandwich".
    - □ C. Two blocks of heart tissue should be removed for paraffin embedding: one containing the sinoa-trial node and one containing the atrio-ventricular node, His bundle, His bifurcation and bundle branches.
    - □ D. Two blocks of heart tissue should be removed fresh, not for paraffin embedding: one containing the sinoa-trial node and one containing the atrio-ventricular node, His bundle, His bifurcation and bundle branches.
    - □ E. Three blocks of heart tissue should be removed for paraffin embedding: one containing the sinoa-trial node, one containing the atrio-ventricular node and His bundle, and one containing the His bifurcation and bundle branches.
12. Where is the ambiguus nucleus located?
    - □ A. in the medulla oblongata
    - □ B. in the cerebellum
    - □ C. in the pons only
    - □ D. in the midbrain only
    - □ E. in both pons and midbrain
13. Where is the Kölliker Fuse nucleus located?
    - □ A. in the medulla oblongata
    - □ B. in the cerebellum
    - □ C. in the pons only
    - □ D. in the midbrain only
    - □ E. in both pons and midbrain

14. How is the brainstem dissected for the study of the nuclei regulating the cardio-respiratory and arousal regulatory functions?
    - □ A. Three samples of brainstem are removed, one at the level of the ponto-mesencephalic junction, one at the level of the pontobulbar junction, and medulla oblongata.
    - □ B. Two samples of brainstem are removed, one at the level of the ponto-mesencephalic junction and one at the level of the pontobulbar junction.
    - □ C. One sample of brainstem is removed, including the medulla oblongata.
    - □ D. Three samples of brainstem are removed, one at the level of the midbrain, one at the level of the pons, and one at the level of the medulla oblongata.
    - □ E. Two samples of brainstem are removed, one consists of pons and one consists of medulla oblongata.
15. In each case of perinatal and infant sudden unexpected death, how is the lung stage of development evaluated?
    - □ A. according to the macroscopic criterion of the ratio between the lung weight and the body length.
    - □ B. according to the macroscopic criterion of the ratio between the lung weight and the body weight.
    - □ C. according to the microscopic criterion of the radial alveolar count.
    - □ D. according to the microscopic criterion of the peripheral alveolar count.
    - □ E. according to the macroscopic criterion of the ratio between the lung weight and the body weight, and according to the microscopic criterion of the radial alveolar count.
16. The coronary arteries should be carefully inspected and sampled, as initial pre-atherosclerotic reversible lesions have been reported to start at what age?
    - □ A. in infancy.
    - □ B. in adult age.
    - □ C. in elderly.
    - □ D. in term fetuses.
    - □ E. in newborns.
17. The initial pre-atherosclerotic lesions detected in perinatal age should be analyzed *post mortem* in coronary and cardiac conduction system arteries cut:
    - □ A. on a single section.
    - □ B. on serial sections.
    - □ C. N/A as the initial atherosclerotic lesions have not been reported in perinatal age.
18. The guidelines for the study of the sudden unexplained infant and perinatal death include:
    - □ A. the study of the brainstem on serial sections throughout the one to three sampled blocks, depending on fetus/infant's age.
    - □ B. the study of the cardiac conduction system on serial sections throughout the two sampled blocks containing respectively the sino-atrial node (block 1) and the atrio-ventricular node, bundle of His, bifurcation of bundle of His, bundle branches, Purkinje cells (block 2).

□ C. the study of both the brainstem and of the cardiac conduction system on serial sections throughout the sampled blocks of tissue.
□ D. the study of the brainstem on a single section for each of the sampled tissue blocks.
□ E. the study of the cardiac conduction system on a single section for each of the two sampled blocks of tissue containing respectively the sino-atrial node (block 1) and the atrio-ventricular node, bundle of His, bifurcation of bundle of His, bundle branches, Purkinje cells (block 2).

19. When is a case classified as SIDS?
□ A. A case is classified as SIDS when the death of an infant under two years of age is sudden, and remains unexplained after a thorough case investigation, including a complete autopsy, examination of the death scene, and review of the clinical history.
□ B. A case is classified as SIDS when the death of an infant under one year of age is sudden, and remains unexplained after a thorough case investigation, including a complete autopsy, examination of the death scene, and review of the clinical history.
□ C. A case is classified as SIDS when the death of an infant under three years of age is sudden, and remains unexplained after a thorough case investigation, including a complete autopsy, examination of the death scene, and review of the clinical history.
□ D. A case is classified as SIDS when the death of an infant under one month of age is sudden, and remains unexplained after a thorough case investigation, including a complete autopsy, examination of the death scene, and review of the clinical history.

20. When is a SIDS case classified as grey zone or borderline?
□ A. when the infant's death is non-natural.
□ B. when the fetus or newborn dies suddenly and unexplainedly following a concomitant pathological event, itself not deadly that acts as a triggering phenomenon in particularly vulnerable individuals.
□ C. when the SIDS has not been submitted to in-depth investigations of the brainstem and cardiac conduction system.
□ D. when the SIDS occurs in a fetus or newborn.
□ E. when the infant dies suddenly and unexpectedly following a concomitant pathological event, itself not deadly that acts as a triggering phenomenon in particularly vulnerable individuals.

2.13 Answer Keys

Block 2 (Questions 11–20)

11. C
12. A
13. E

14. A
15. E
16. D
17. B
18. C
19. B
20. E

References

1. Alfonsi G, Crippa M (1994) Tecniche istologiche e immunoistochimiche di seriatura e colorazione del sistema di conduzione e nervoso cardiaco. Pathologica 86:444–449.
2. Askenazi SS, Perlman M (1979) Pulmonary hypoplasia: lung weight and radial alveolar count as criteria of diagnosis. Arch Dis Child 54:614–618.
3. Bancroft J, Stevens A (1982) Theory and practice of histological techniques, 2nd edn. Churchill Livingstone, New York.
4. Calderoli R, Martini F, Galli S, Matturri L (2002) Post mortem discipline on the sudden infant death syndrome (SIDS) and of unexpected late fetal stillbirth victims. In: Proceedings of the 7th SIDS International Conference, Florence, p 135.
5. Centers for Disease Control and Prevention (CDC) (2014) Linked birth/infant death records, 2007–2009 Results. http://wonder.cdc.gov/lbd-current.html. Accessed July 26, 2014.
6. Centers for Disease Control and Prevention (2014) Sudden unexplained infant death investigation reporting form. http://www.cdc.gov/sids/suidrf.htm. Accessed July 26, 2014.
7. Constitution of the Italian Republic, February 2, 2006, Law n° 31. Regulations for diagnostic post mortem investigation in victims of sudden infant death syndrome and unexpected fetal death. Official Gazette of the Italian Republic General Series 2006;34:4. http://users.unimi.it/giuliaottaviani/pdf/legge.pdf. Accessed July 26, 2014.
8. Cotzias CS, Paterson-Brown S, Fisk NM (1999) Prospective risk of unexplained stillbirth in singleton pregnancies at term: population based analysis. BMJ 319:287–288.
9. Crippa M, Alfonsi G (1991) Tecniche di studio del sistema di conduzione cardiaco. BIO-Informazioni, BIO-OPTICA, Milan, pp 55–58.
10. de Sa DJ (1978) Stress response and its relationship to cystic (pseudofollicular) change in the definitive cortex of the adrenal gland in stillborn infants. Arch Dis Child 53:769–776.
11. Emery JL, Mithal A (1960) The number of alveoli in the terminal respiratory unit of man during late intrauterine life and childhood. Arch Dis Child 35:544–547.
12. Emery JL, Mithal A (1969) The weight of the lungs. In: Emery J (ed) The anatomy of the developing lung. Heinemann Medical, London, pp 203–205.
13. Filiano JJ, Kinney HC (1992) Arcuate nucleus hypoplasia in the sudden infant death syndrome. J Neuropathol Exp Neurol 51:394–403.
14. Frøen JF, Arnestad M, Vege A, Irgens LM, Rognum TO, Saugstad OD, Stray-Pedersen B (2002) Comparative epidemiology of sudden infant death syndrome and sudden intrauterine unexplained death. Arch Dis Child Fetal Neonatal Ed 87:F118–F121.
15. Gilbert-Barness E, Kapur RP, Oligny LL, Siebert JR (2007) Potter's pathology of the fetus and infant, 2nd edn. Mosby, Philadelphia.
16. Haas JE, Taylor JA, Bergman AB, Van Belle G, Felgenhauer JL, Siebert JR, Benjamin DR (1993) Relationship between epidemiologic risk factors and clinicopathologic findings in the sudden infant death syndrome. Pediatrics 91:106–112.
17. Hoffman HJ, Damus K, Hillman L, Kangrad E (1988) Risk factors for SIDS. Results of the National Institute of Child Health and Human Development SIDS cooperation epidemiological study. Ann N Y Acad Sci 533:13–30.

18. James TN (1968) Sudden death in babies: new observation in the heart. Am J Cardiol 22:479–506.
19. James TN (1970) Cardiac conduction system: fetal and postnatal development. Am J Cardiol 25:213–226.
20. James TN (1983) The Mikamo lecture. Structure and function of AV junction. Jpn Circ J 47:1–47.
21. Kinney HC, Filiano JJ, Harper RM (1992) The neuropathology of the sudden infant death syndrome. A review. J Neuropathol Exp Neurol 51:115–126.
22. Kinney HC, Filiano JJ, Panigraphy A, Rava LA, White WF (1995) Anatomic and neurochemical studies of the ventral medulla oblongata in early life. Observation relevant to the sudden infant death syndrome. In: Trouth CO, Millis RH, Kiwull-Schone H, Schlafke ME (eds) Ventral brainstem mechanisms and control respiration and blood pressure. Dekker, New York, pp 589–609.
23. Lavezzi AM, Ottaviani G, De Ruberto F, Fichera G, Matturri L (2002) Prognostic significance of different biomarkers (DNA content, PCNA, karyotype) in colorectal adenomas. Anticancer Res 22:2077–2082.
24. Lavezzi AM, Ottaviani G, Matturri L (2003) Identification of neurons responding to hypoxia in sudden infant death syndrome (SIDS). Pathol Int 53:769–774.
25. Lavezzi AM, Ottaviani G, Ballabio G, Rossi L, Matturri L (2004) Preliminary study on the cytoarchitecture of the human parabrachial/Kölliker-Fuse complex, with reference to sudden infant death syndrome and sudden intrauterine unexplained death. Pediatr Dev Pathol 7:171–179.
26. Lavezzi AM, Ottaviani G, Mauri M, Matturri L (2004) Hypoplasia of the arcuate nucleus and maternal smoking during pregnancy, in perinatal and infant sudden unexpected death. Neuropathology 24:284–289.
27. Lavezzi AM, Ottaviani G, Matturri L (2005) Adverse effects of prenatal tobacco smoke exposure on biological parameters of the developing brainstem. Neurobiol Dis 20:601–607.
28. Lavezzi AM, Ottaviani G, Matturri L (2005) Biology of the smooth muscle cells in human atherosclerosis. APMIS 113:112–121.
29. Lavezzi AM, Ottaviani G, Mauri M, Terni L, Matturri L (2005) Involvement of the EN-2 gene in normal and abnormal development of the human arcuate nucleus. Int J Exp Pathol 86:25–31.
30. Lavezzi AM, Ottaviani G, Mingrone R, Matturri L (2005) Analysis of the human locus coeruleus in perinatal and infant sudden unexplained deaths. Possible role of the cigarette smoking in the development of this nucleus. Brain Res Dev Brain Res 154:71–80.
31. Lavezzi AM, Ottaviani G, Mauri M, Matturri L (2006) Alterations of biological features of the cerebellum in sudden perinatal and infant death. Curr Mol Med 6:429–435.
32. Lavezzi AM, Ottaviani G, Terni L, Matturri L (2006) Histological and biological developmental characterization of the human cerebellar cortex. Int J Dev Neurosci 24:365–371.
33. Lavezzi AM, Ottaviani G, Mauri M, Matturri L (2007) Biopathology of the dentate-olivary complex in sudden unexplained perinatal death and sudden infant death syndrome related to maternal cigarette smoking. Neurol Res 19:525–532.
34. Lavezzi AM, Ottaviani G, Matturri L (2007) Ontogenesis of human cerebellar cortex and biopathological characterization in sudden unexplained fetal and infant death. Virchows Arch 450:31–40.
35. Luna LG (1973) Manual of histologic staining methods of the Armed Force Institute of Pathology, 3rd edn. McGraw-Hill, New York.
36. MacDorman MF, Kirmeyer SE, Wilson EC (2012) Fetal and perinatal mortality, United States, 2006. Natl Vital Stat Rep 60:1–23. www.cdc.gov/nchs/data/nvsr/nvsr60/nvsr60_08.pdf. Accessed July 26, 2014.
37. Massing GK, James TN (1976) Anatomical configuration of the His bundle and bundle branches in the human heart. Circulation 53:609–621.
38. Matturri L, Ottaviani G, Biondo B, Ramos SG, Rossi L (1998) Discrete T-lymphocytic leptomeningitis of the ventral medullary surface in a case of sudden unexpected infant death. Adv Clin Path 2:313–316.

39. Matturri L, Ottaviani G, Rossi L (1999) Sudden and unexpected infant death due to an hemangioendothelioma located in the medulla oblongata. Adv Clin Path 3:29–33.
40. Matturri L, Ottaviani G, Ramos SG, Rossi L (2000) Sudden infant death syndrome (SIDS). A study of cardiac conduction system. Cardiovasc Pathol 9:137–145.
41. Matturri L, Ottaviani G, Lavezzi AM, Turconi P, Cazzullo A, Rossi L (2001) Expression of apoptosis and proliferating cell nuclear antigen (PCNA) in the cardiac conduction system of crib death (SIDS). Adv Clin Path 5:79–86.
42. Matturri L, Biondo B, Suàrez-Mier MP, Rossi L (2002) Brain stem lesions in the sudden infant death syndrome: variability in the hypoplasia of the arcuate nucleus. Acta Neuropathol (Berl) 194:12–20.
43. Matturri L, Minoli I, Lavezzi AM, Cappellini A, Ramos S, Rossi L (2002) Hypoplasia of medullary arcuate nucleus in unexpected late fetal death (stillborn infants): a pathological study. Pediatrics 109:E43.
44. Matturri L, Lavezzi AM, Minoli I, Ottaviani G, Cappellini A, Rubino B, Rossi L (2003) Association between pulmonary hypoplasia and hypoplasia of arcuate nucleus in stillbirth. J Perinatol 23:328–332.
45. Matturri L, Lavezzi AM, Ottaviani G, Rossi L (2003) Intimal preatherosclerotic thickening of the coronary arteries in human fetuses of smoker mothers. J Thromb Haemost 1:2234–2238.
46. Matturri L, Ottaviani G, Alfonsi G, Crippa M, Rossi L, Lavezzi AM (2004) Study of the brainstem, particularly the arcuate nucleus, in sudden infant death syndrome (SIDS) and sudden intrauterine unexplained death (SIUD). Am J Forensic Med Pathol 25:44–48.
47. Matturri L, Ottaviani G, Corti G, Lavezzi AM (2004) Pathogenesis of early atherosclerotic lesions in infants. Pathol Res Pract 200:403–410.
48. Matturri L, Ottaviani G, Lavezzi AM (2004) Autoptic examination in sudden infant death syndrome and sudden intrauterine unexpected death: proposal of a national law. J Matern Fetal Neonatal Med 16(Suppl 2):43–45.
49. Matturri L, Ottaviani G, Lavezzi AM, Rossi L (2004) Early atherosclerotic lesions of the cardiac conduction system arteries in infants. Cardiovasc Pathol 13:276–281.
50. Matturri L, Ottaviani G, Benedetti G, Agosta E, Lavezzi AM (2005) Unexpected perinatal death and sudden infant death syndrome (SIDS): anatomopathologic and legal aspects. Am J Forensic Med Pathol 26:155–160.
51. Matturri L, Ottaviani G, Lavezzi AM (2005) Natural history of perinatal coronary atherosclerosis. In: Proceedings of the "6th International Congress on Coronary Artery Disease: from Prevention to Intervention". Monduzzi Editore, MEDIMOND Srl publishing company, Bologna, pp 67–70.
52. Matturri L, Ottaviani G, Lavezzi AM (2005) Sudden infant death triggered by dive reflex. J Clin Pathol 58:77–80.
53. Matturri L, Ottaviani G, Lavezzi AM (2005) Techniques and criteria in pathologic and forensic-medical diagnostics in sudden unexpected infant and perinatal death. Am J Clin Pathol 124:259–268.
54. Matturri L, Ottaviani G, Lavezzi AM (2005) Unexpected sudden death related to medullary brain lesions. Acta Neuropathol (Berl) 109:554–555.
55. Matturri L, Ottaviani G, Lavezzi AM, Grana D, Milei J (2005) Madres fumadoras y aterosclerosis prenatal. Rev Argent Cardiol 73:366–369.
56. Matturri L, Ottaviani G, Lavezzi AM, Ramos SG (2005) Peripheral chemoreceptors and sudden infant death syndrome: a wide open problem. Curr Cardiol Rev 1:65–70.
57. Matturri L, Ottaviani G, Lavezzi AM (2006) Maternal smoking and sudden infant death syndrome: epidemiological study related to pathology. Virchows Arch 449:697–706.
58. Matturri L, Giuliani P, Lavezzi AM, Ottaviani G, Minoli I, Colombi R, Nespoli L, Agosti M, Bulgheroni C, Cannatelli G, Farneti A, Lodi F, Cappellini A, Cattoretti G, Vergani P, Tagliabue P, Mosca F, Boffi R, Malaguti E, Merlino L, Lucchina C (2007) Protocollo diagnostico. Indagine anatomo-patologica e medico legale sulle vittime della sindrome della morte improvvisa del lattante (SIDS) e della morte inaspettata del feto. Regione Lombardia Sanità, Milan.

59. Matturri L, Ottaviani G, Mingrone R, Lavezzi AM, Fulcheri E (2007) Sudden Intrauterine Unexplained Death (SIUD) «Gray Zone» or borderline. 8th World Congress of Perinatal Medicine. Florence, Italy. J Perinat Med 35(Suppl):210.
60. Matturri L, Ottaviani G, Lavezzi AM (2008) Guidelines for neuropathologic diagnostics of perinatal unexpected loss and sudden infant death syndrome (SIDS) – a technical protocol. Virchows Arch 452:19–25.
61. Milei J, Ottaviani G, Lavezzi AM, Grana DR, Stella I, Matturri L (2008) Perinatal and infant early atherosclerotic coronary lesions. Can J Cardiol 24:137–141.
62. Ottaviani G (2006) Histopathological study of the cardiac conduction system in systemic lupus erythematosus. J Postgrad Med 52:10.
63. Ottaviani G (2006) How to sample the cardiac conduction system. "SIDS e ALTE Aggiornamento 2005. Primo Corso Teorico Pratico di Anatomia-Patologica in casi di Sospetta SIDS e di morte inaspettata fetale", Parma, Italy. Acta Biomed Ateneo Parmense 77:50.
64. Ottaviani G, Lavezzi AM, De Ruberto F, Fichera G, Matturri L (1999) The prognostic value of cell proliferation in colorectal adenomas assessed with tritiated thymidine and anti-proliferating cell nuclear antigen (PCNA). Cancer Detect Prev 23:57–63.
65. Ottaviani G, Lavezzi AM, Rossi L, Matturri L (1999) Proliferating cell nuclear antigen (PCNA) and apoptosis in hyperacute and acute myocardial infarction. Eur J Histochem 43:7–14.
66. Ottaviani G, Rossi L, Ramos SG, Matturri L (1999) Pathology of the heart and conduction system in a case of sudden death due to a cardiac fibroma in a 6-month-old child. Cardiovasc Pathol 8:109–112.
67. Ottaviani G, Rossi L, Matturri L (2002) Histopathology of the cardiac conduction system in a case of metastatic pancreatic ductal adenocarcinoma. Anticancer Res 22:3029–3032.
68. Ottaviani G, Matturri L, Rossi L, James TN (2003) Crib death: further support for the concept of fatal cardiac electrical instability as the final common pathway. Int J Cardiol 92:17–26.
69. Ottaviani G, Matturri L, Rossi L, Jones D (2003) Sudden death due to lymphomatous infiltration of the cardiac conduction system. Cardiovasc Pathol 12:77–81.
70. Ottaviani G, Lavezzi AM, Rossi L, Matturri L (2004) Sudden unexpected death of a term fetus in a anticardiolipin positive mother. Am J Perinatol 21:31–35.
71. Ottaviani G, Matturri L, Rossi L, Lavezzi AM, James TN (2004) Multifocal cardiac Purkinje cell tumor in infancy. Europace 6:138–141.
72. Ottaviani G, Matturri L, Bruni B, Lavezzi AM (2005) Sudden infant death syndrome "gray zone" disclosed only by a study of the brain stem on serial sections. J Perinat Med 33:165–169.
73. Ottaviani G, Matturri L (2008) Histopathology of the cardiac conduction system in sudden intrauterine unexplained death. Cardiovasc Pathol 17:146–155.
74. Ottaviani G (2008) Sudden Intrauterine Unexplained Death (SIUD) «gray zone» or borderline. Neurosci Imaging 2:127–133.
75. Ottaviani G, Mingrone R, Lavezzi AM, Matturri L (2009) Infant and perinatal pulmonary hypoplasia frequently associated with brainstem hypodevelopment. Virchows Arch 454:451–456.
76. Ottaviani G (2009) The role of post-mortem investigations in determining the cause of sudden unexpected death in infancy. Arch Dis Child 94:170–171.
77. Ottaviani G (2011) Sudden infant and perinatal unexplained death: are we moving forward yet? Cardiovasc Pathol 10:302–306.
78. Ottaviani G (2011) Sudden unexplained neonatal deaths. Arch Dis Child Fetal Neonatal Ed. http://fn.bmj.com/content/96/6/F440/reply. Accessed July 26, 2014.
79. Ottaviani G (2011) Sudden deaths in term infants within 24 hours of birth. Pediatrics. http://pediatrics.aappublications.org/content/127/4/e869/reply. Accessed July 26, 2014.
80. Preventing Stillbirth and SUID. Act of 2008, Bill introduced in the Senate of the United States, June 17, 2008 by Mr. Reid (for Mr. Obama). S3142 IS. 110th Congress, 2nd Session, S. 3142. http://www.thomas.gov/cgi-bin/query/z?c110:S.3142. Accessed July 26, 2014.

81. Ramos SG, Matturri L, Biondo B, Ottaviani G, Rossi L (1998) Hyperplasia of the aorticopulmonary paraganglia: a new insight into the pathogenesis of sudden infant death syndrome? Cardiologia 43:953–958.
82. Rossi L (1969) Histopathologic features of cardiac arrhythmias. Casa Editrice Ambrosiana, Milan.
83. Rossi L (1978) "Salvage the pacemaker" at autopsy. Am Heart J 95:540–541.
84. Rossi L (1983) The pathologic basis of cardiac arrhythmias. Cardiol Clin 1:13–17.
85. Rossi L, Matturri L (1990) Clinicopathological approach to cardiac arrhythmias. A color atlas. Centro Scientifico Torinese, Turin.
86. Rossi L, Matturri L (1991) Anatomohistological features of sudden infant death. New Trends Arrhyt 6:135–142.
87. Rossi L, Matturri L (1995) Anatomo-histological features of the heart's conduction system and innervation in SIDS. In: Rognum TO (ed) Sudden infant death syndrome: new trends in the nineties. Scandinavian University Press, Oslo, pp 207–212.
88. Rossi L, Matturri L (1995) Cardiac conduction and nervous system in health disease and sudden death: an anatomoclinical overview. Osp Maggiore 89:239–257.
89. Rossi L, Thiene G (1983) Arrhythmologic pathology of sudden cardiac death. Casa Editrice Ambrosiana, Milan.
90. Rossi L, Matturri L, Lotto A (1988) Cardiac conduction blocks and pacemaking. An anatomoclinical color atlas. Clas International, Brescia.
91. Rossi L, Pozzato R, Matturri L (1991) L'anatomia patologica della morte cardiaca oggi. Riv Ital Med Leg 13:93–110.
92. Suàrez-Mier MP, Aguilera B (1998) Histopathology of the conduction system in sudden infant death. Forensic Sci Int 93:143–154.
93. Suàrez-Mier MP, Gamallo C (1998) Atrioventricular node fetal dispersion and His fragmentation of the cardiac conduction system in sudden cardiac death. J Am Coll Cardiol 32:1885–1890.
94. Valdés-Dapena M, Huff D (1983) Perinatal autopsy manual. Armed Forces Institute of Pathology, Washington, DC.
95. Valdès-Dapena M, McFreeley PA, Hoffman HJ, Damus KH, Franciosi RR, Allison DJ, Jones M, Hunter JC (1993) Histopathology atlas for the sudden infant death syndrome. Armed Forces Institute of Pathology, Washington, DC.
96. Van Baarlen J, Schuurman HJ, Huber J (1988) Acute thymus involution in infancy and childhood: a reliable marker for duration of acute illness. Hum Pathol 19:1155–1160.
97. Weller U, Jorch G (1993) Current percentile curves for body weight, body length and head circumference of newborn infants after the 25th week of pregnancy. Monatsschr Kinderheilkd 141:665–669.
98. Willinger M, James LS, Catz C (1991) Defining the sudden infant death syndrome (SIDS): deliberations of an expert panel convened by the National Institute of Child Health Development. Pediatr Pathol 11:677–684

Pathological and Related Epidemiological Findings in Sudden Infant and Perinatal Unexplained Death

3

3.1 Epidemiological Results

The risk factors investigated for SIDS and sudden perinatal unexplained death (SPUD) whenever applicable were:

- Infant factors: gender, age, prematurity, low birth weight, family association with SIDS, season, sleep prone position (Table 1.1);
- Maternal factors: cigarette smoking, drugs, alcohol, age, marital status, socio-economic status (Table 1.1).

3.1.1 Age Distribution

The age distribution of the SIDS infants is shown in Fig. 3.1. In particular, 21% of deaths occurred in the 2nd month of life, 22% in the 3rd month, 13% in the 4th month, and 10% in the 5th month.

Regarding the SPUD victims, based on the age of the analyzed cases, it could be established that a higher frequency of SNUD occurs in the two first days of postnatal life, with a peak at the first day; SIUD is more frequent in the last weeks of gestation, i.e., 37th–41st gws.

3.1.2 Gender Distribution

The SIDS group consisted of 67.5% males and 32.5% females, ranging in age from 3 to 416 days (mean ± SEM 91.90 ± 9.55 days). The remarkable prevalence of the male gender is self evident (Fig. 2.9).

G. Ottaviani, *Crib Death - Sudden Infant Death Syndrome (SIDS): Sudden Infant and Perinatal Unexplained Death: The Pathologist's Viewpoint*,
DOI 10.1007/978-3-319-08347-6_3

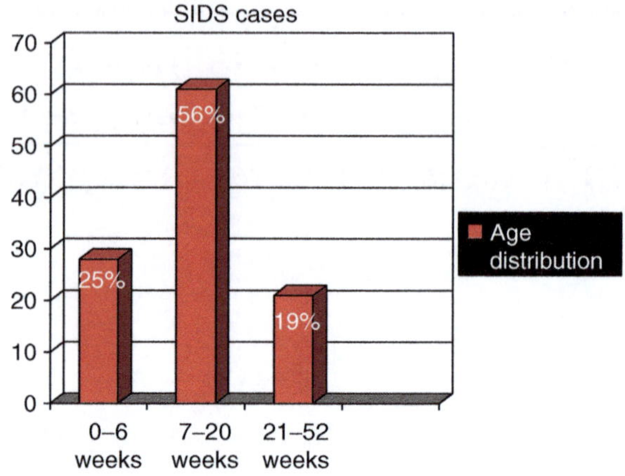

Fig. 3.1 Age distribution of SIDS victims

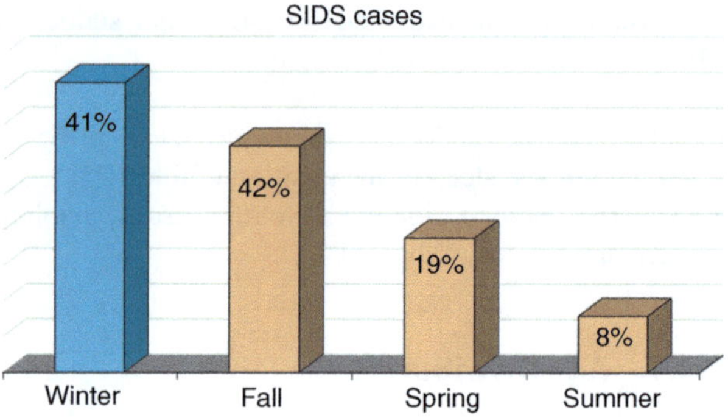

Fig. 3.2 SIDS occurred more frequently in winter and fall

3.1.3 Season of Death

SIDS occurred more frequently in winter, as shown in Fig. 3.2. The distribution of SIDS according to the month was: 16% in January, 10% in February, 8% in March, 4% in April, 12% in May, 5% in June, 5% in July, 1% in August, 4% in September, 9% in October, 12% in November, and 14% in December. The highest peak of SIDS incidence was in January and the lowest in August.

3.1.4 Time of Death

Most of the SIDS infants died between 10.00 p.m. and 8.00 a.m. (62%); 47% died between 8.00 a.m. and 2.00 p.m., 7% between 2.00 p.m. and 6.00 p.m., and 9% between 6.00 p.m. and 10.00 p.m.

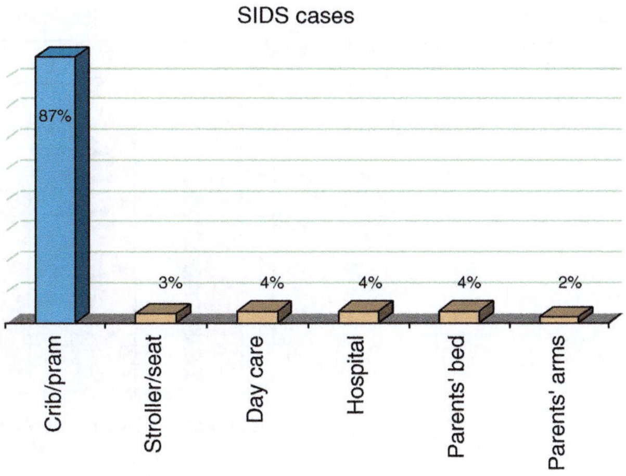

Fig. 3.3 SIDS distribution according to the place of death

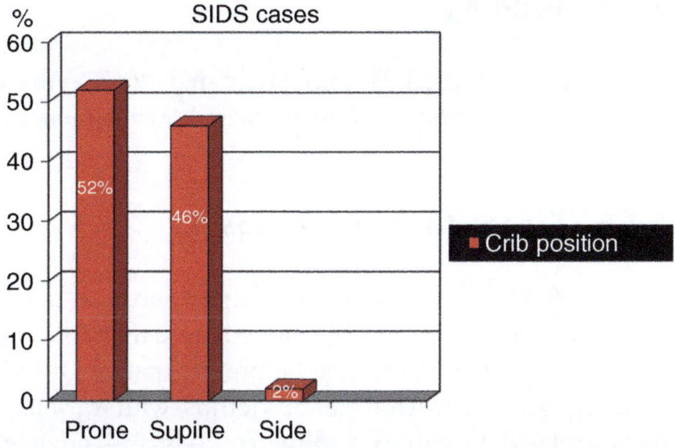

Fig. 3.4 SIDS distribution according to position in the crib

3.1.5 Death Scene: Place of Death

Most of the SIDS infants were found dead in the crib or pram (87%); 3% were in a stroller, seat or car seat, 4% at day care, 4% in hospital, 4% in the parents' bed, and 2% in the parents' arms. The places of death were not mutually exclusive, and infants found dead in the crib or pram were at kindergarten (4 %) (Fig. 3.3).

3.1.6 Death Scene: Position in the Crib

Most of the SIDS infants died in a prone position (52%); 46% were in a supine position and 2% were lying on their side (Fig. 3.4).

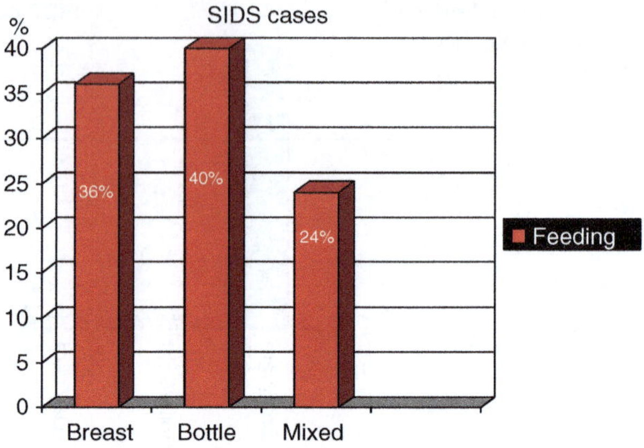

Fig. 3.5 Feeding: 36% of SIDS infants were breast-fed, 40% were formula-fed, and in 24% feeding was mixed (about 50% formula and 50% human milk)

3.1.7 Feeding

Of the SIDS infants, 36% were breast-fed, 40% were formula-fed, and in 24% feeding was mixed (about 50% formula and 50% human milk) (Fig. 3.5).

3.1.8 Cigarette Smoke Exposure

In about 55% of SIDS and unexplained perinatal death victims, at least one parent was a smoker and, generally, smoked more than five cigarettes a day. In the mothers, the smoking habit had started before pregnancy [14, 47]. In 94% of SIDS and 85% of unexplained perinatal death victims with various anomalies of the brainstem nuclei related to cardio-respiratory control – arcuate nucleus hypodevelopment, somatostatin positivity of the hypoglossus nucleus, tyrosine hydroxylase negativity in the locus coeruleus, strong brainstem diffuse gliosis, hypoglossus nucleus hypoplasia – at least one parent was a smoker [19, 47]. The arcuate nucleus hypodevelopment included bilateral hypoplasia, monolateral hypoplasia, partial hypoplasia, delayed neuronal maturation, decreased neuronal density [14, 47]. In about two-third of SIDS cases, breast feeding was combined with cigarette smoking by one or both parents [38, 41]. Maternal smoking during pregnancy resulted to be the most important preventable risk factor for SIDS, related to morphological and/or functional alterations of brainstem centers [47].

3.2 Cardiac Conduction Findings

Victims of sudden unexpected infant and perinatal death do not show any abnormality of the ordinary myocardium, while the cardiac conduction system, where the cardiac rhythm arises and spreads, shows some abnormalities [31, 54].

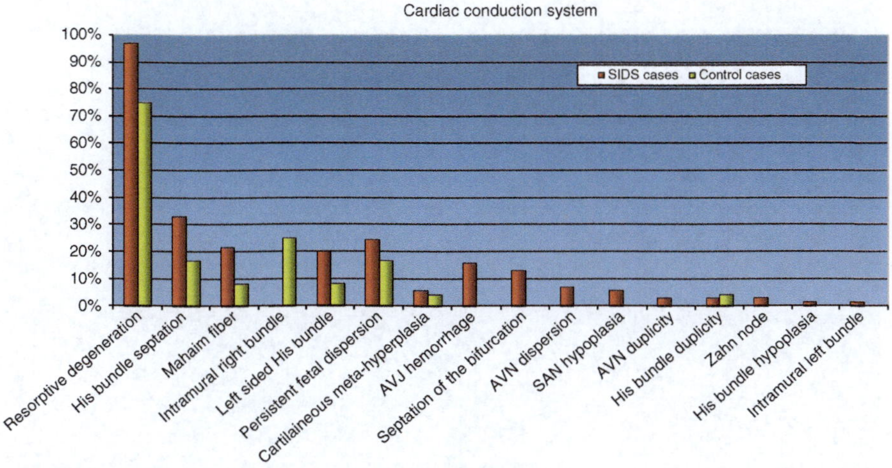

Fig. 3.6 Cardiac conduction system findings in SIDS infants and controls

No significant differences were found between SIDS/unexplained perinatal death victims and the control explained death groups and subgroups with regard to the mean ages (Student's *t* test), nor were there significant differences between sexes ($\chi 2$ test).

The demographic data of the infants and cardiac conduction histological findings for the two groups are presented in Fig. 3.6.

More than one cardiac conduction change was present in the same infant or term fetus, but no unusual combined cardiac anomalies [3] were observed.

3.2.1 Resorptive Degeneration

Areas of abnormal resorptive degeneration were observed in 97% of the SIDS infants and in 75% of the age-matched controls (Fig. 3.6). Statistical analysis showed a significant difference between the two groups ($p < 0.05$). In the resorptive degeneration areas clusters of young fibroblasts depositing collagen caught in the central fibrous body were observed, sometimes isolated from the overdeveloped specialized structures, and sometimes adjacent to them [5, 49]. In these areas there were no associated inflammation nor any massive necrosis or hemorrhage. Macrophages were sometimes present adjacent to the small foci of degeneration, acting eventually as scavenger cells [7, 31, 54] (Fig. 3.7).

In the SPUD victims, areas of resorptive degeneration were observed in 55% of cases and in 47% of the perinatal death controls, without statistically significant differences [59, 60].

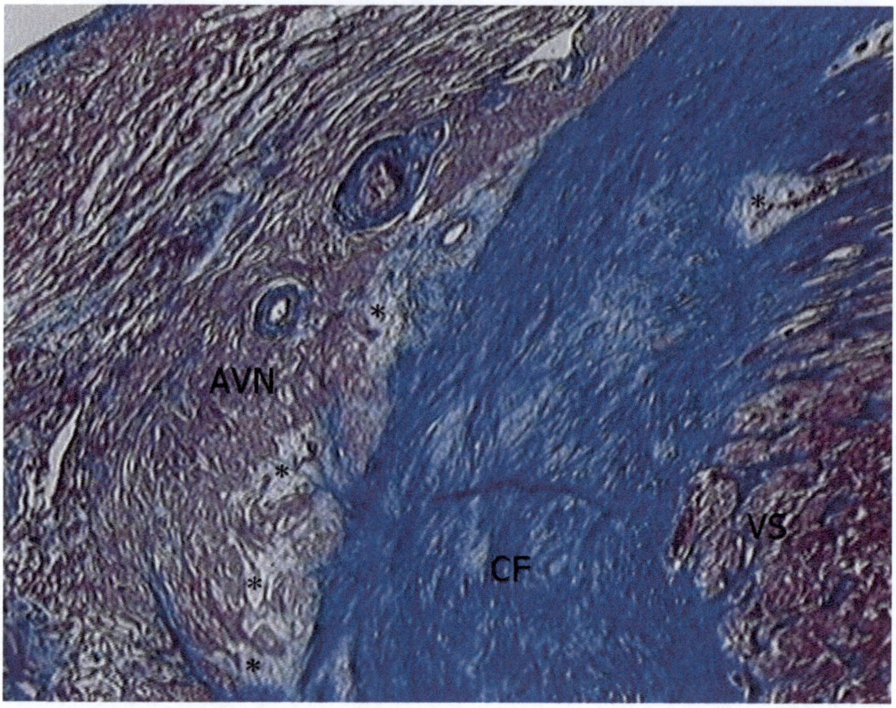

Fig. 3.7 Cardiac conduction system. Areas of resorptive degeneration (*asterisks*), located at the periphery of the atrioventricular node (*AVN*) and embedded in the central fibrous body (*CF*) (*VS* interventricular septum; trichromic Heidenhain, ×25)

3.2.2 Atrioventricular Node and Bundle of His Dispersion/Septation

Dispersion or septation of the bundle of His [70, 71], characterized by fragmentation of the main bundle within the central fibrous body [31, 54, 75], was observed in 33% of SIDS infants and in 17% of the controls, without a statistically significant difference ($p > 0.05$) (Fig. 3.6).

Atrioventricular node (AVN) dispersion or septation [31, 50, 54] was present in 7% of SIDS infants, while it was not detected in the controls.

Dispersion or septation of the AV junction was observed in 64.5% of SPUD victims and in 53% of the control cases, with no statistically significant difference [59, 60].

3.2.3 Persistent Fetal Dispersion

Islands of conduction tissue in the central fibrous body, designated as persistent fetal dispersion [9, 75], were found in 25% of SIDS infants and in 17% of infant controls, and in 80% of SIUD versus 73% of inherent controls, without statistically

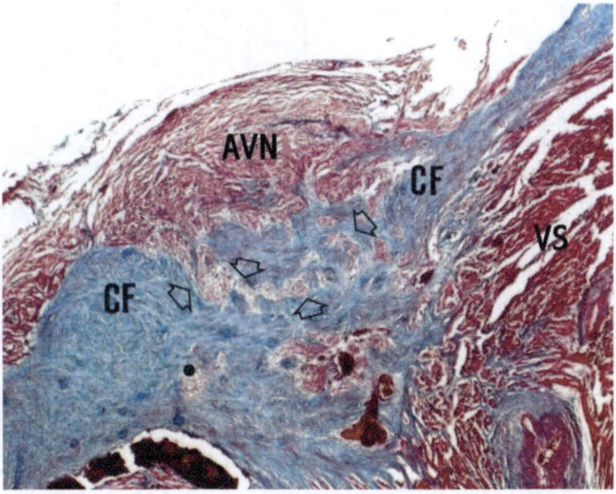

Fig. 3.8 SIDS case. Persistent fetal dispersion. *Arrows* point to islands of junctional tissue separated from the atrioventricular node (*AVN*), dispersed in the central fibrous body (*CF*), some of which are undergoing resorptive degeneration (•) (*VS* interventricular septum; trichromic Heidenhain, ×25)

significant differences (p>0.05). In such cases we observed islands of conduction tissue separated from the AVN and bundle of His, dispersed in the central fibrous body, resembling the normal fetal pattern [6, 9, 54] (p>0.05) (Fig. 3.8).

3.2.4 Accessory Pathways

Mahaim fibers, specialized connections between the AV junction and the upper ventricular septum [26, 69–71], were detected in 23% of SIDS infants and in 8% of controls, without statistically significant difference (p>0.05) (Figs. 3.6 and 3.9). In the SIUD group, Mahaim fibers were detected in 20% of cases while were absent in the age-matched control cases [60].

James fibers, defined as atriohissian accessory pathways connecting the right atrium directly with the bundle of His [4, 8], were also observed in 4% of SIDS infants, but were not detected in sudden unexplained perinatal death victims nor in age-matched controls [59, 60].

Kent fibers, defined as direct accessory pathways outside the AV junction [10], are the morphological substrate for the Wolff-Parkinson-White (WPW) syndrome [73, 74, 77, 78]. They were detected in 2% of SIDS infants, but were not detected in sudden unexplained perinatal death victims nor in age-matched controls [59, 60].

3.2.5 Cartilaginous Meta/Hyperplasia

Cartilaginous meta/hyperplasia of the central fibrous body [54, 70] was present in 6% of SIDS infants and in 4% of infant controls, in 20% of SPUD victims versus 18% of age-matched controls, without statistically significant differences (p>0.05) [60] (Figs. 3.6 and 3.10).

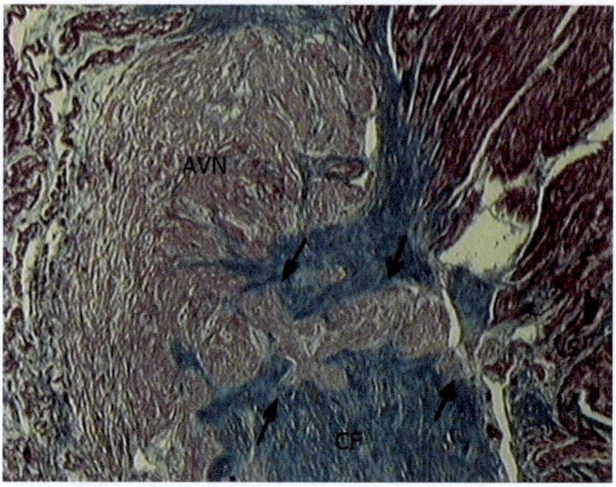

Fig. 3.9 Nodoventricular accessory Mahaim fibers (*arrows*) likely residual from defective resorptive degeneration, bridging the atrioventricular node (*AVN*) and the ventricular septum (*VS*) through the central fibrous body (*CF*) (Trichromic Heidenhain, ×25)

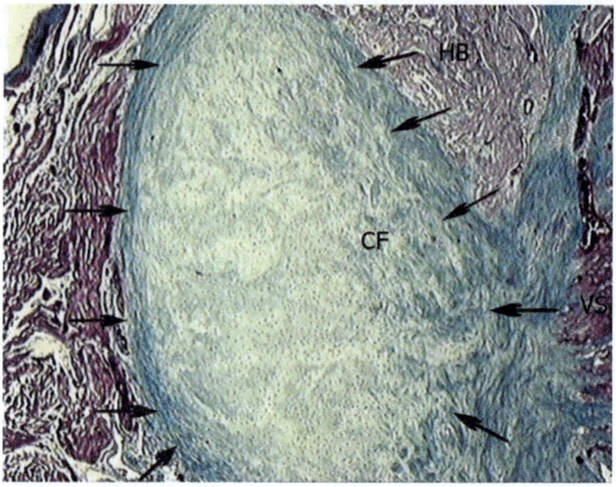

Fig. 3.10 Cartilaginous hypermetaplasia (*CM*) within the central fibrous body (*CF*, *arrows*) (*HB* bundle of His, *VS* interventricular septum; trichromic Heidenhain, ×25)

3.2.6 Hemorrhage of the Cardiac Conduction System

Hemorrhage of the AV junction characterized by red blood cells seen in the intercellular spaces [68] was present in 16% of SIDS infants, in 7% of SPUD victims and in 9% of the age-matched controls. In some cases the red cells were widely dispersed over an area of the conducting tissue, and in other cases discrete clumps of red cells were present enclosing several common as well as specialized myocardial fibers [54, 59, 60].

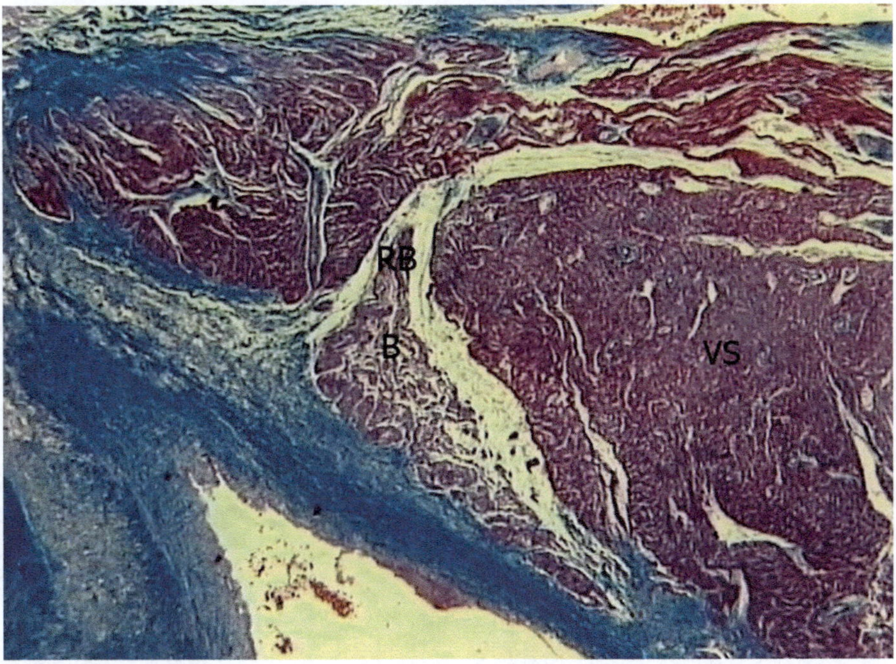

Fig. 3.11 Left sided bifurcation (*B*) and intramural right bundle branch (*RB*) (*VS* interventricular septum; trichromic Heidenhain, ×25)

3.2.7 Intramural Right Bundle Branch

An intramural right bundle branch [31] was present, respectively, in 20% of SIDS and in 25% of the control infants, in 6.5% of SPUD victims and in 5% of the age-matched controls. There were no statistically significant differences between the SIDS-SPUD and the inherent control groups ($p > 0.05$) [31, 59]. In SIDS infants dying from 3 to 60 days, an intramural right bundle was more frequent than in those dying from 61 to 120 days ($p = 0.01$) [31] (Figs. 3.6 and 3.11).

3.2.8 Left-Sided Bundle of His

A left-sided bundle of His [1, 27] was present in 20% of SIDS infants and in 8% of infants with explainable death, without statistically significant difference between the two infant groups ($p > 0.05$) [31]. In the SPUD victims, a left-sided bundle of His/His bifurcation was detected in 7% of cases and in none of the age-matched controls [60]. In 2% of SIDS cases, the bundle of His was left-sided and intramural (Figs. 3.6 and 3.12).

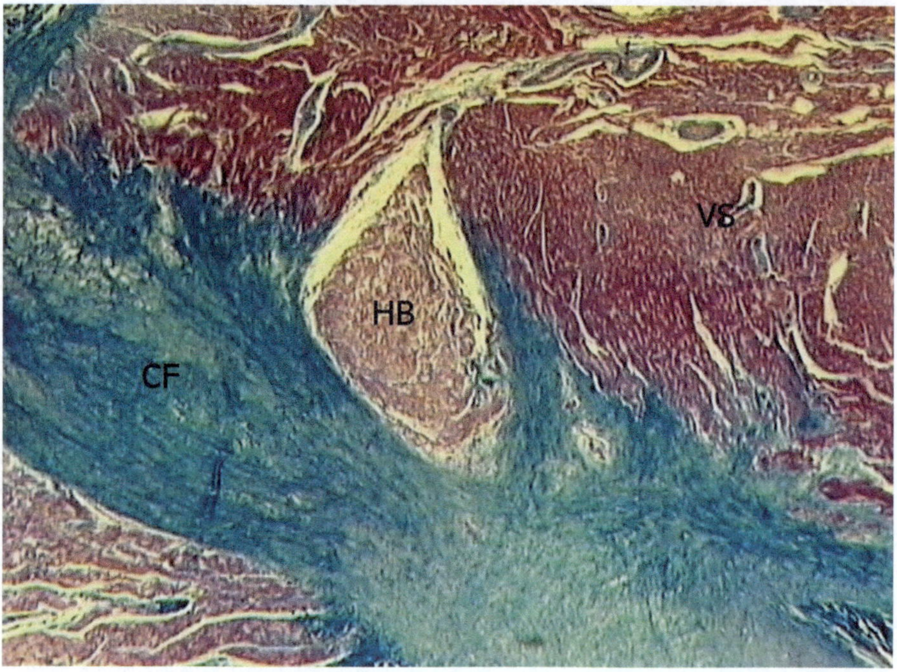

Fig. 3.12 Intramural left-sided bundle of His (*HB*) penetrating the interventricular septum (*VS*) (*CF* central fibrous body; trichromic Heidenhain, ×25)

3.2.9 Intramural Left Bundle Branch

Intramural left bundle [67] was observed in 2% of SIDS infants, and in none of the controls nor of the perinatal cases (Fig. 3.6).

3.2.10 Septation of the Bifurcation

Septation of the bifurcation, known also as anomalous bifurcation [31, 70], characterized by interposition of fibrous tissue of the central fibrous body, was detected in 13% of SIDS infants, and in none of the perinatal cases nor controls (Fig. 3.13).

3.2.11 Hypoplasia of the Cardiac Conduction System

Hypoplasia of the sinoatrial node (SAN) [1, 70] was present in 6% of SIDS infants (Fig. 3.6), in 3% of SPUD victims, while was absent in control fetuses and infants.

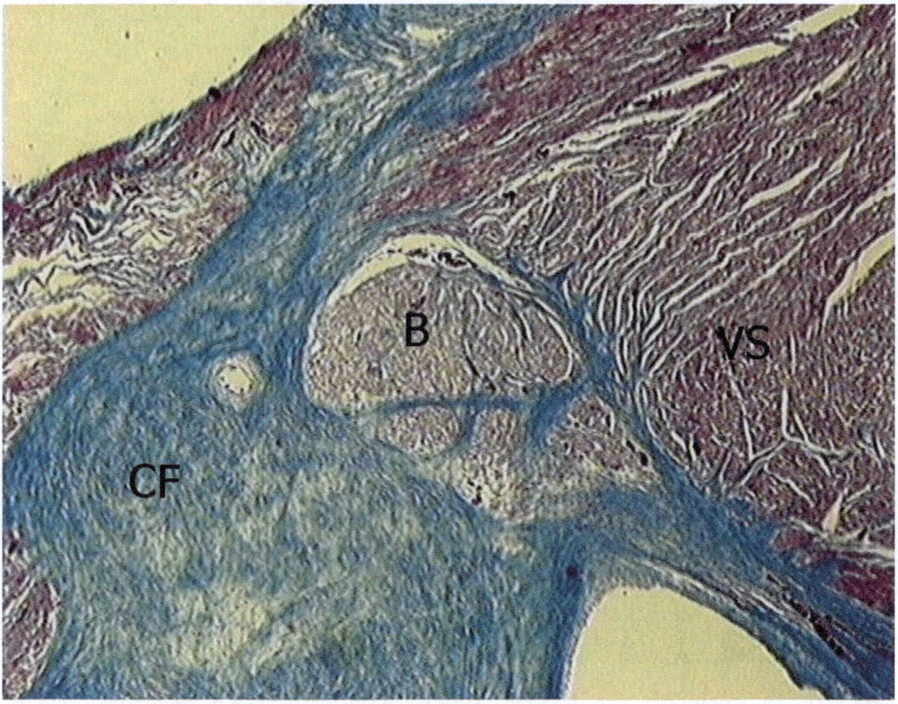

Fig. 3.13 Anomalous bifurcation (*B*) characterized by interposition of fibrous tissue of the central fibrous body (*CF*) (*VS* interventricular septum; trichromic Heidenhain, ×25)

Hypoplasia of the bundle of His was present in 5% of SIDS infants and in none of the controls (Fig. 3.6).

Hypoplasia of the central fibrous body [59, 60] was detected in 7% of the SPUD victims while it was absent in age-matched controls.

3.2.12 Atrioventricular Node/Bundle of His Dualism

A dualism/duplicity of the AVN or spli AVN was present in 3% of SIDS infants (Fig. 3.14), all in the SIDS subgroup who died between 3 and 120 days of life (Fig. 3.14) and in none of those with explainable death [31] (Fig. 3.6). A dualism of the AVN was also detected in 3% of SPUD victims and in non of the age-matched controls [59].

Dualism of the bundle of His or split bundle of His was present in 3% of SIDS infants and in 4% of the controls [31] (Fig. 3.6).

In these cases the AVN and/or the bundle of His appeared stratified into two portions by the interposition of a fibrous diaphragm [31, 51, 54] (Fig. 3.14).

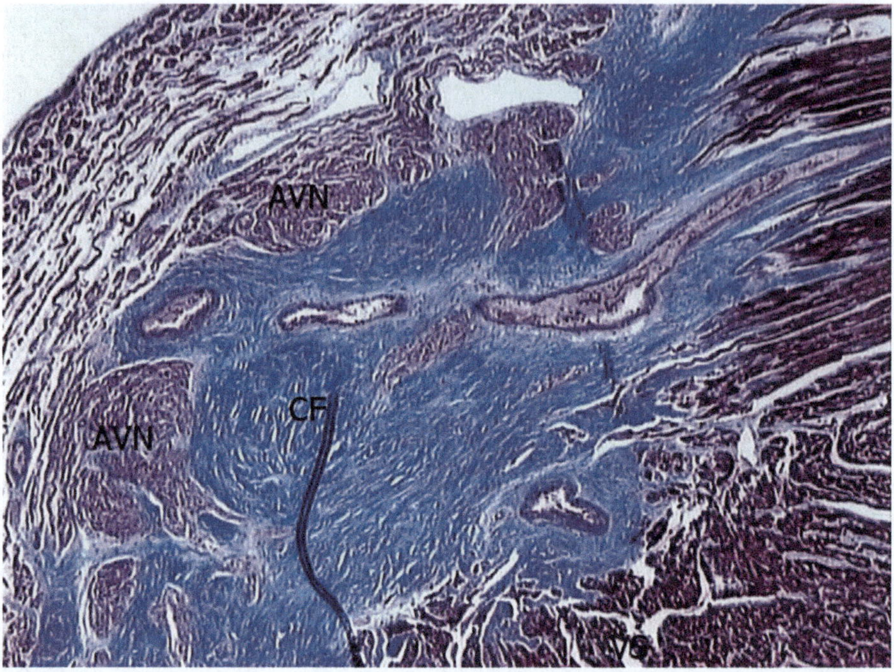

Fig. 3.14 The atrioventricular node (*AVN*) is subdivided into two portions by interposition of fibrous tissue of the central fibrous body (*CF*) (*VS* interventricular septum; trichromic Heidenhain, ×25)

3.2.13 Zahn Node

A Zahn node, also known as a coronary sinus node [28, 66, 76, 79], was present in 3% of the SIDS infants (Fig. 3.6), but in none of the perinatal unexplained death nor in control cases. The Zahn node was located close to the major axis of the AVN, and was identified as a formation composed of myocytes of small size and lengthened or stellate in shape arranged with a muscular network, morphologically definable as a small AVN. A typical feature of a Zahn node is a posterosuperior prolongation with a pseudohissian fascicle.

3.2.14 Fibromuscular Hyperplasia of the Conduction System Arteries

In 21% of SIDS and in 13% of SPUD victims a thickening of the SAN and/or AVN artery was observed. This thickening consisted of fibromuscolar hyperplasia of the cardiac conduction system arteries attributable to an initial preatherosclerotic process [42, 54].

The more diffuse initial preatherosclerotic lesions were seen in formula-fed babies with smoker parents. These lesions were marked by significant fragmentation of the elastic fiber system and deposits of amorphous material, mainly lipids, even in the innermost portion of the media [41, 42] (Fig. 3.15).

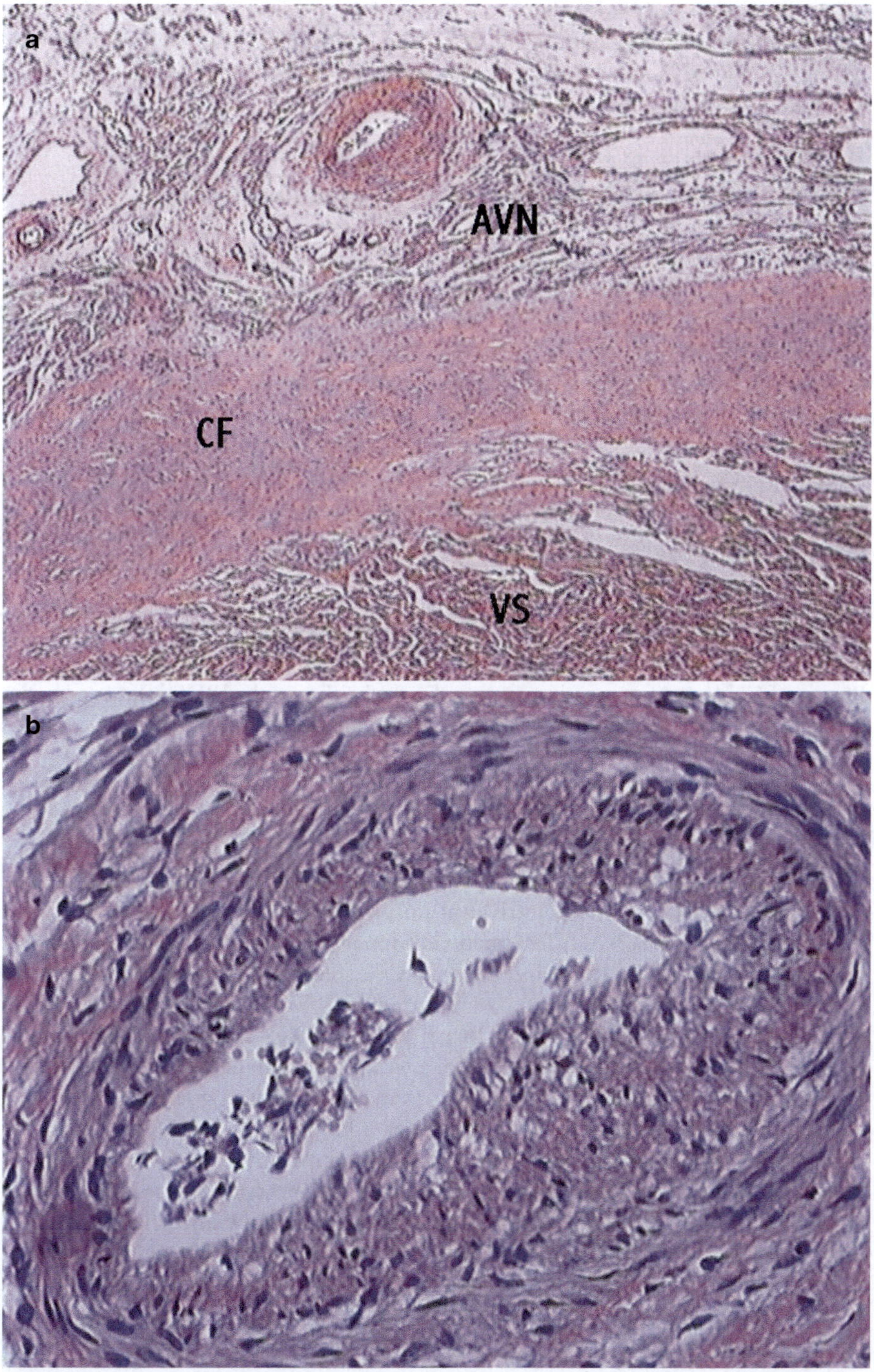

Fig. 3.15 (**a**, **b**) Myointimal thickness of the atrioventricular node artery in a 4-month-old child who died suddenly and unexpectedly. Note the increased amount of mucoid ground substance in the subendothelial connective tissue (*AVN* atrioventricular node, *CF* central fibrous body, *VS* interventricular septum; H&E, **a** ×25, **b** ×100)

A significant correlation between the initial preatherosclerotic lesions these lesions and parental cigarette smoking was found ($p<0.05$) [42]. The atherogenic effects of formula feeding were detectable after the 4th month of life, and worsened if the formula feeding was prolonged [41, 42].

3.2.15 Apoptosis Expression in the Conducting Tissue

The apoptotic indices (AI) in the cardiac conduction system of SIDS and SIUD cases and in age-matched controls showed no statistically significant differences ($p>0.05$; Student's *t* test), while in the resorptive degeneration areas the AI was found to be higher in the controls than in the SIDS infants ($p<0.05$; Student's *t* test), but not in SIUD cases. The SAN in both sudden death and control groups showed AI similar to those in the common myocardium. In almost all cases, TUNEL labeling was detected in the peripheral region of the AVN, close to the atrial myocardium (Fig. 3.16). The AI were higher in the AVN, the bundle of His, and in the initial tract of the bundle branches, than in the common myocardium ($p<0.05$; Student's *t* test) [32, 53, 60].

3.2.16 PCNA Expression in the Conducting Tissue

Positive PCNA immunoreactivity was not found either in the SIDS infants or in the controls, nor in the conducting system or the common myocardium.

3.2.17 ECG Findings

One or more ECG recordings were available in 15% of the SIDS infants. The ECGs recorded at the time of arrival at hospital when resuscitative efforts were attempted showed that five infants had ventricular fibrillation, and two had supraventricular tachycardia. In six infants the ECGs, recorded mostly soon after birth because of prematurity problems, were unremarkable; in two patients the ECGs showed the long QT syndrome [31]. In a 3-month-old boy dying of SIDS, who was submitted to external cardiac massage for a total of 90 min in two successive bouts, the heart resumed sporadic beating 16 h from the start of resuscitation attempts, aided by sporadic emergency maneuvers, for a few hours, with ECG findings of right branch block and downsloping of the ST segment, but no clear-cut sign of ischemia. The baby remained unconscious and was pronounced dead 26 h after hospitalization. At the *post mortem* examination, in the right sinoatrial area and in the uppermost ventricular septum there was a wide myofibrillary injury, similar to contraction band degeneration, typical of hyperacute infarction [39]. Another case of myocardial injury attributable to external cardiac massage in infants has been reported [57].

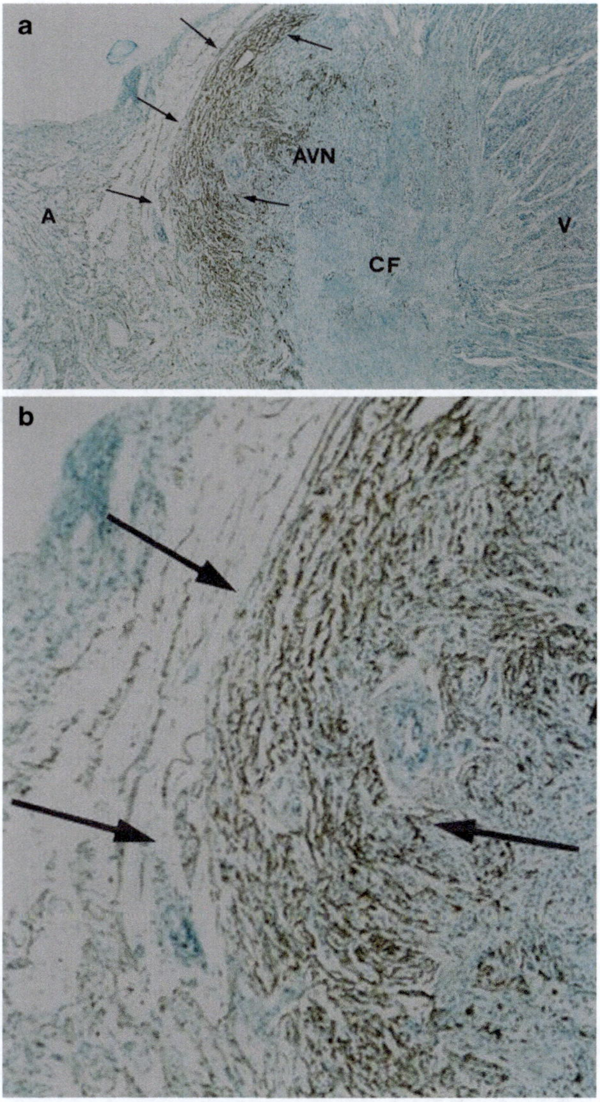

Fig. 3.16 (**a**, **b**) Apoptotic cells (*stained brown*, *arrows*) located at the periphery of the atrioventricular node (*AVN*) close to the atrial myocardium (*A*) (*VS* ventricular septum, *CF* central fibrous body; TUNEL, **a** ×20, **b** ×100)

3.2.18 Myocardial Damage attributable to Cardiac Massage

Compression of the heart between the spine and the sternum exerted during this emergency maneuver causes a direct vertical pressure perpendicular to both the atrial and ventricular septum, which badly stretches the AVN, the bundle of His, and the proximal bundle branches traveling therein [36, 39] (Fig. 3.17). The same concept applies to damage to the SAN region, which is located in the vulnerable

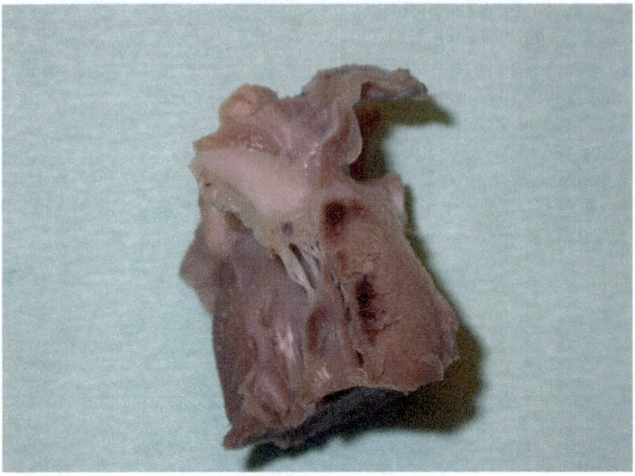

Fig. 3.17 During cardiac massage squeezing the heart between the spine and the sternum exerts a direct vertical pressure perpendicular to both the atrial and the ventricular septum. The interventricular septum (block 2 in the study of the cardiac conduction system) has brownish infarct-like areas attributable to excessive cardiac massage

anatomic junction between the superior vena cava and the thin right atrial wall, and which is associated with the risk of subsequent pacemaker impairment [68]. Such damage could be due to instant cardiac stretching, as well as to prolonged compressive resuscitative maneuvers. Thus, maneuvers involving external cardiac massage, if they are protracted beyond the time limits suggested by authoritative criteria [2], may be responsible for the findings of wide myofibrillary injury in the right sinoatrial area and in the uppermost ventricular septum. Such a lesion represents infarct-like damage, as in the patient described above and in many examples of myocardial biopsy [39, 57], following passive instrumental compression and overstretching of the cardiac muscle, that could interfere with the regional contractile activity (Fig. 3.18). While stressing that such a maneuver must obviously be carried out, we suggest that this should never be prolonged beyond a reasonable time according to the criteria suggested by Eisenberg and Mengert [2].

3.2.19 Coronary Artery Findings

3.2.19.1 Infants

Histological study of the coronary arteries of the SIDS victims showed a normal structure in 39% of cases. In 61% of SIDS infants there was thickening of varying severity in the artery walls. In 30.5% of cases the lesions were initial preatherosclerotic lesions, mostly located in the anterior descending branch of the left coronary artery, and in 30.5% of cases juvenile soft atherosclerotic plaques were observed in all the coronary branches, with narrowing of the lumen (Fig. 3.19).

A significant correlation was evident between preatherosclerotic lesions and both formula feeding and parental cigarette smoking ($p<0.05$). In infants in

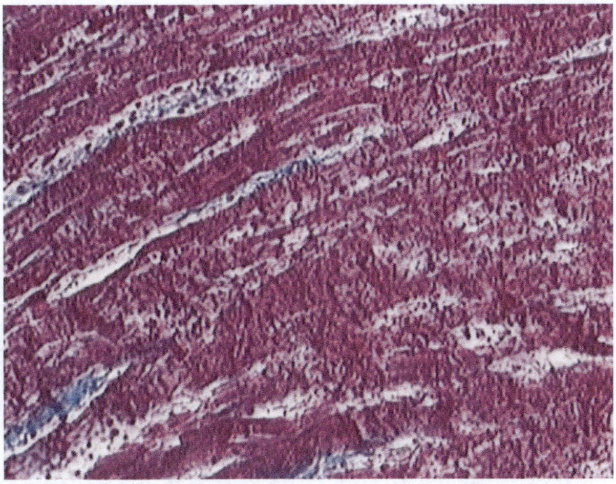

Fig. 3.18 Areas of contraction band necrosis in the ventricular septum indicating infarct-like damage (Trichromic Heidenhain, ×100)

whom the atherogenic factor was cigarette smoking, especially if the mother was a smoker, the lesions appeared early and were detectable in the first few months of life.

The histological picture varied according to the atherogenic factor. The preatherosclerotic lesions attributable only to the effects of cigarette smoke, observed in 62% of the breast-fed infants with at least one smoker parent, show an evident structural alteration of the tunica media, which appeared to be fragmented.

Marked cell proliferation was also present. The proliferating cells appeared to be arranged in columns with the axis perpendicular to the tunica itself. These elements appeared to infiltrate the intima together with acid mucopolysaccharide deposits, consisting of type A and C chondroitin sulfates and hyaluronic acid, probably synthesized by the smooth muscle cells (SMC) themselves. Low numbers of monocytes were present; B lymphocytes were generally absent.

While 8% of infants presented preatherosclerotic lesions despite having been breast-fed and having nonsmoker parents, soft plaques were not present [41].

3.2.19.2 Fetuses

No intimal proliferations were revealed by the histological examination of the coronary walls in 45% of fetuses deceased suddenly and unexpectedly, but in 55% all of whom died after 35 weeks of gestation, multifocal structural alterations of all the coronary arteries were detected, and these were more severe along the anterior descending branch of the left coronary artery. More specifically, in 32% of fetuses, foci of altered architecture of the media with thinning and fiber fragmentation were observed, even in fields far from the bifurcations.

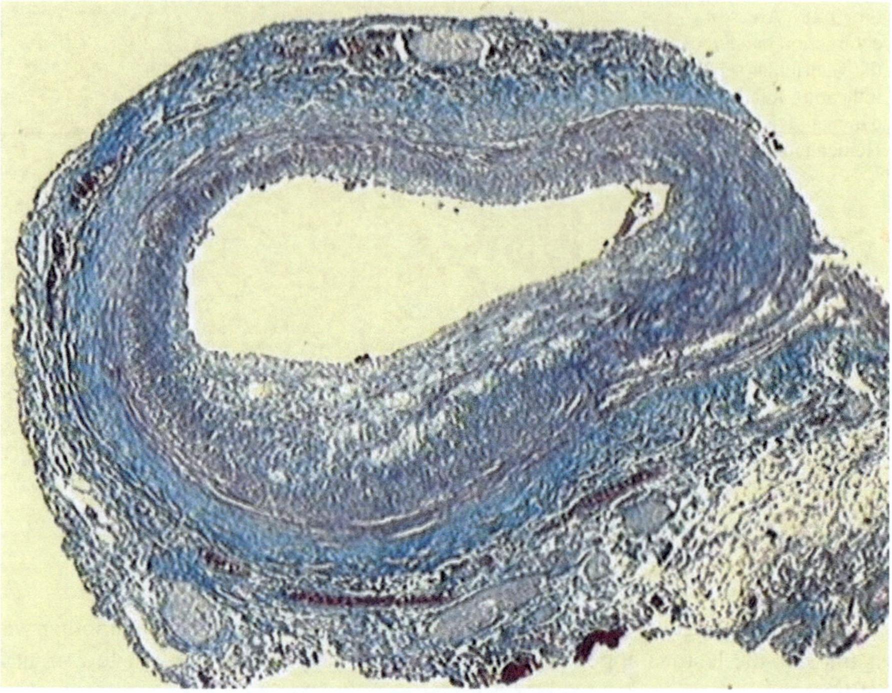

Fig. 3.19 Left main coronary artery of a 2-month-old SIDS victim with smoking parents. An early atherosclerotic lesion characterized by soft thickening with numerous foam cells is visible, narrowing the coronary lumen (Trichromic Heidenhain, ×25)

The SMCs showed loss of polarity, forming columns of myocytes located perpendicular to the axis of the media itself and infiltrating the subendothelial connective tissue. In 23% of fetuses, besides this intense reaction of the SMCs of the media, increased amounts of mucoid ground substance were observed in the subendothelial connective tissue, with formation of intimal preatherosclerotic lesions of proliferative aspect (Fig. 3.20). Such processes also seem to determine fragmentation and detachment of the internal elastic membrane. Sometimes SMCs appeared in the gaps of this lamina. The clinical data showed that the mothers of 83% of the fetuses with intimal thickenings were smokers before the start of their pregnancy.

In all the lesions, immunohistochemical study of the biological markers showed intense c-fos positivity of the SMCs, while PCNA-positive cells were not detected. The search for chromosome 7 alterations using the FISH technique gave negative results, showing only two normal hybridization spots per nucleus. Frequently, in these cases, apoptotic SMCs were present [20, 43].

A significant correlation ($p < 0.05$) was evident between the presence of intimal preatherosclerotic lesions, c-fos gene activation and maternal smoking. Indeed, in the 83% of the fetuses of smoker mothers, c-fos-positive preatherosclerotic lesions were present. Coronary wall alterations were seen in only 17% of fetuses of non-smoking mothers [38].

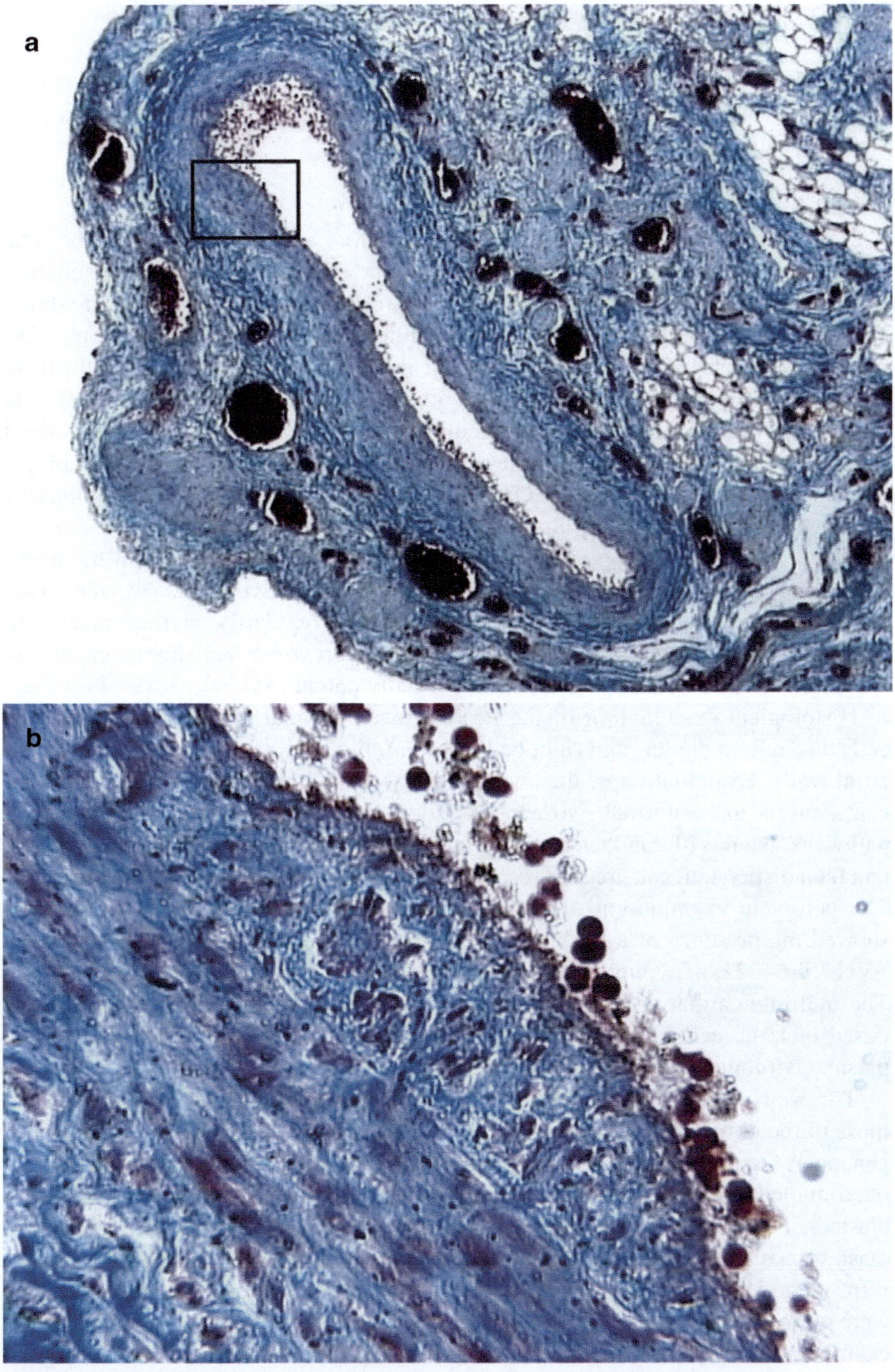

Fig. 3.20 (**a**, **b**) Left main coronary artery of a fetus of 37 weeks' gestation. The myointimal thickness shows increased amounts of mucoid ground substance in the subendothelial connective tissue (Trichromic Heidenhain, **a** ×40, **b** ×400)

3.2.20 "Grey Zone"/ Borderline Cases

A total of 7% of SIDS and 11% of SPUD victims were classified as "grey zone"/ borderline cases. Below, two examples of SIDS grey zone cases classified as such based on cardiac conduction findings are described.

3.2.20.1 Cardiac Purkinje Cell Tumor

A 2-month-old female infant with no known history of medical problems became unresponsive. The baby was taken to an emergency department where resuscitation was attempted without success until she was pronounced dead 20 min after admission. She was born at term, after an uncomplicated pregnancy. No previous ECG recordings were available. Little was known about her family history, since the baby was a gypsy, and her family moved to another country after her death, so that little clinical and family information was collected. Her death remained unexplained after a complete routine autopsy. The case was referred to the Institute of Pathology, University of Milan, for more specialized investigations, including study of the cardiac conduction system and brainstem in serial sections.

The heart weighed 46 g, and its dimensions were 4.5×5×3.8 cm in the transverse, longitudinal and anteroposterior directions, respectively. *Post mortem* gross cardiac examination revealed cardiomegaly with irregularity of the epicardium (Fig. 3.21). On dissection the myocardium was brownish and homogeneous in appearance. The coronary arteries were normally patent [55].

Histological examination of the heart showed nodular aggregates of Purkinje cells throughout the left and right endocardium, the interatrial septum and both the atrial walls. Examination of the conduction system showed the SAN and its adjacent ganglia to be normal. No abnormalities were detected along the internodal pathways. Islands of conduction tissue in the central fibrous body, known as persistent fetal dispersion, and areas of resorptive degeneration in the AVN were observed. The complete examination of the cardiac conduction system on serial sections showed the presence of a Purkinje cell tumor near the SAN, and another near the AVN (Fig. 3.22). The bundle of His and the bundle branches were unremarkable. The multiple cardiac lesions proved to be small myocardial tumor nodules composed of large cells, characterized by a pale, granular, slightly acidophilic cytoplasm. Cytological atypia was not observed.

The walls of the Purkinje cells varied in thickness and were more dense than those of the normal myocardial cells. In most groups the Purkinje cells were homogeneously distributed, but in some locations they were intermingled with a few other myocardial cells. There was no encasement or capsule about the Purkinje cell clusters. The Purkinje cells showed a moderate amount of strongly PAS- and PAS-diastase-positive granular material, typical of glycogen. Only occasional myofibrils were identified within these Purkinje cells. All of the uninvolved myocardial cells were normal in appearance. There was no evidence of myocarditis. The histological examination of the pericardium disclosed a fibrinous pericarditis. The histological examination of the brainstem revealed a mild bilateral hypoplasia of the ARCn. No other significant pathological changes were found.

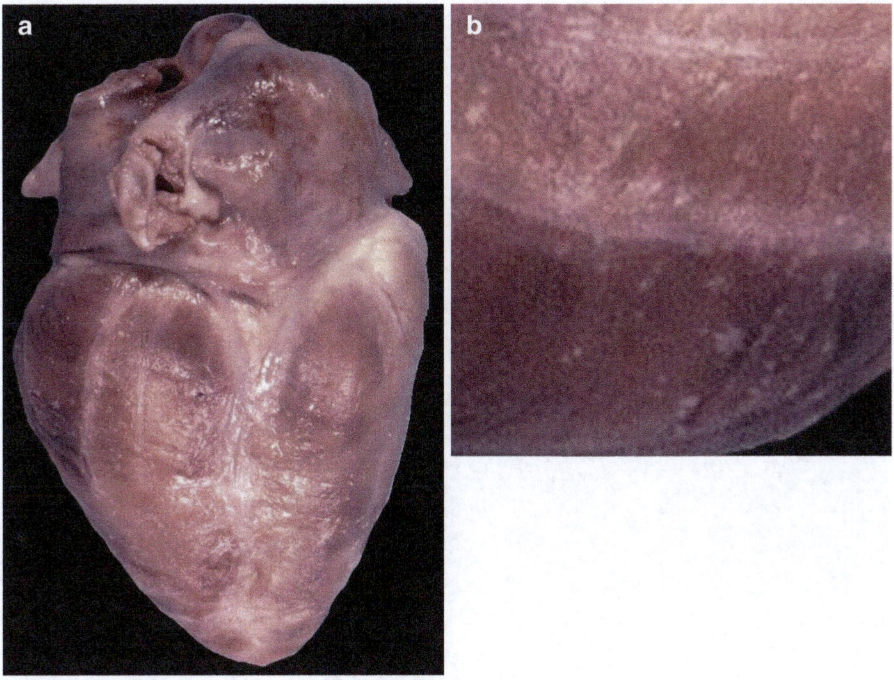

Fig. 3.21 (**a**, **b**) Cardiac Purkinje cell tumor. (**a**) Gross cardiac examination reveals generalized cardiac hypertrophy with irregularity of the epicardium. (**b**) Detail of the epicardium shows the gross aspect of fibrous pericarditis

The Purkinje cell tumor alone may or may not have accounted for the sudden death, but, in this vulnerable baby with hypoplastic ARCn, it could have played a triggering role in causing death in this baby. Therefore, this case was classified as SIDS grey zone or borderline [55, 56].

3.2.20.2 Myocardial Infarction and Mahaim Fibers

In a SIDS infant, an accessory Mahaim fiber was associated with acute myocardial infarction. The hypoxia was combined with severe tachycardia (240 beats/min) due to the accessory Mahaim fiber.

3.2.21 Non SIDS/Sudden Explained Death

3.2.21.1 Cardiac Fibroma

A 6-month-old white female with no known history of medical problems, died suddenly and unexpectedly. At autopsy there were no marks of violence. The lungs were congested and slightly edematous. The heart weighed 85 g (expected 31 g), and its dimensions were $6.5 \times 7 \times 4$ cm in the transverse, longitudinal and anteroposterior directions, respectively. *Post mortem* gross cardiac examination

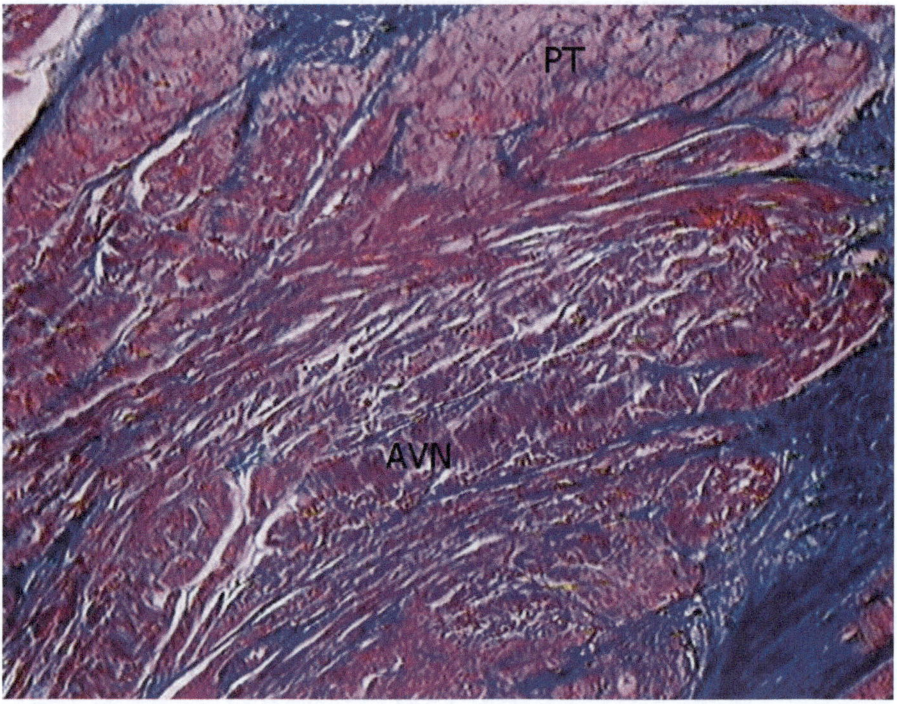

Fig. 3.22 Cardiac Purkinje cell tumor. Cluster of Purkinje cells tumor (*PT*) among normal myocytes, close to the atrioventricular node (*AVN*) (Trichromic Heidenhain, ×100)

revealed cardiomegaly with a localized bulge on the anterior left ventricular wall (Fig. 3.23a, b). Dissection of the heart showed a mass 4.5×4×3.5 cm in diameter which completely replaced the ventricular septum and encroached upon the left ventricular chamber, extending from the apex to the base of the heart. The left ventricular cavity, displaced posteriorly, was slit-like. The bulging interventricular septum compressed the infundibulum of the right ventricle. The mass encroached upon and distorted the mitral valve and the aortic outflow. The mass appeared as a single, circumscribed but nonencapsulated lesion; its cut surface was grayish-white, firm and solid and looked trabeculated (Fig. 3.23c).

Histological examination of the cardiac tumor showed a nonencapsulated proliferation of fibroblasts with regular nuclei and an abundant network of collagen and elastic fibers that dissociated and entrapped the myocytes. Van Gieson's stain confirmed the presence of collagen fibers which appeared red. These morphological features led to the diagnosis of primary cardiac fibroma [52]. Mitotic figures and cytological atypia were not observed. No foci of dystrophic calcification were present. The periphery of the tumor was more cellular and vascular, showing a sparse chronic inflammation basically comprising monocytes. The SAN, adjacent nerve plexuses and the internodal right atrial myocardium were free of alterations. Due to the gross thickening of the interventricular septum due to the tumor, the AVN and

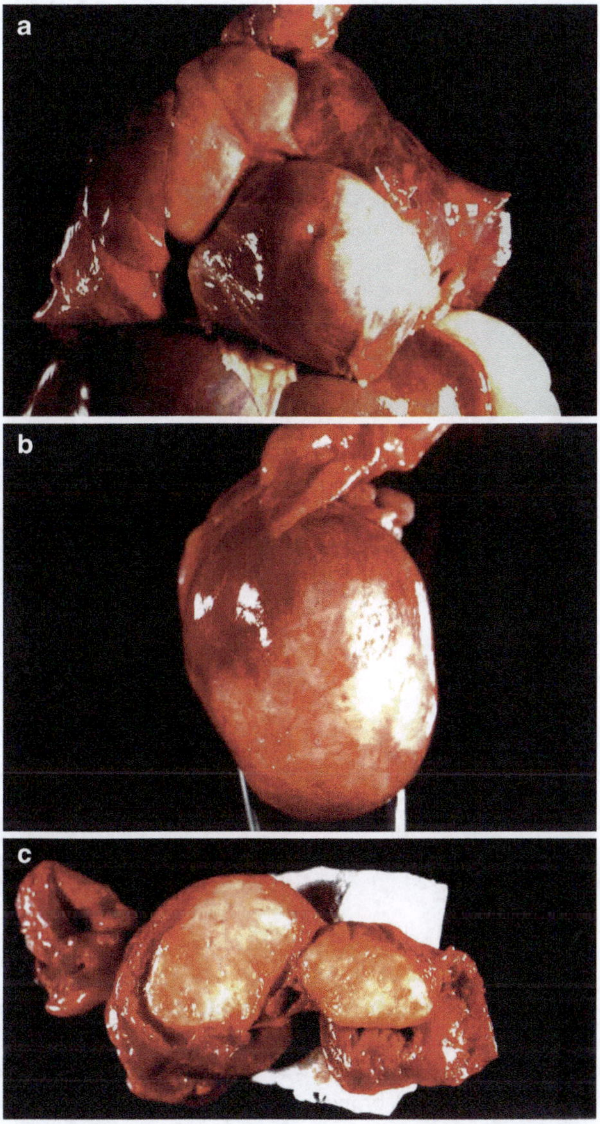

Fig. 3.23 (**a–c**) Explained sudden death caused by cardiac fibroma in a 6-month-old female baby. (**a**, **b**) Gross cardiac examination revealed cardiomegaly. (**c**) Dissection of the heart showed a mass 4.5×4×3.5 cm completely replacing the ventricular septum, extending from the apex to the base

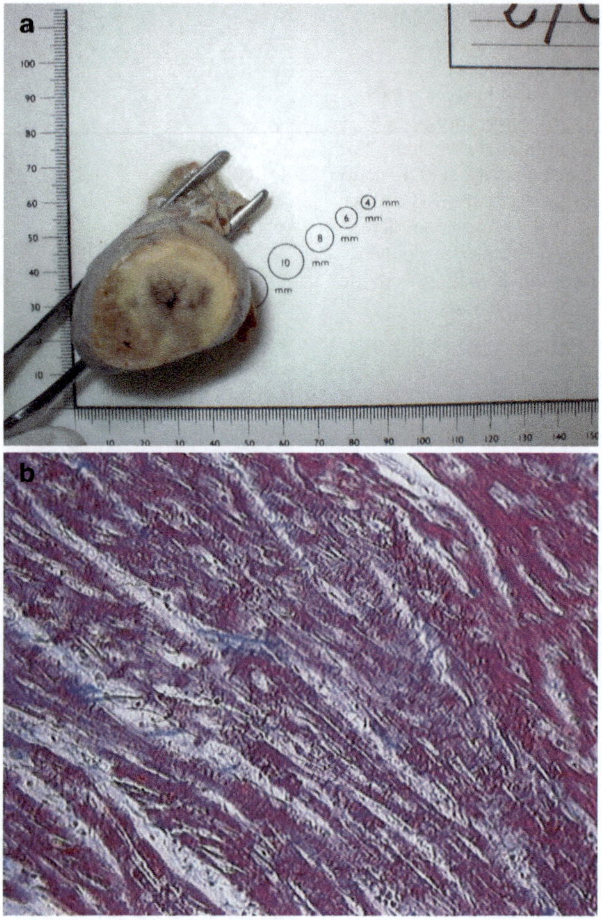

Fig. 3.24 (**a**, **b**) Explained sudden death in a 3-month-old boy. Massive left ventricular hypertrophy and dyschromic areas (**a**) in the ventricles and septum which was found (**b**) to be areas of contraction band degeneration (Trichromic Heidenhain, ×100)

its atrial approaches were overstretched horizontally, as well as the bundle of His which was localized on the right side of the pars membranacea septi. The bifurcation of the bundle of His was divaricated and located on the left side of the septal crest. Both bundle branches were found to be compressed. The tumor did not infiltrate the conduction system, which was severely crushed together at the tumor periphery. Sparse chronic inflammation was present at the junction of the tumor and in the common uninvolved myocardium.

3.2.21.2 Hypertrophic Cardiomyopathy

In several cases submitted to our institution with the clinical diagnosis of SIDS, a hypertrophic cardiomyopathy, complicated by ischemia or myocardial infarction, has been detected (Fig. 3.24). When a documented cause of death is documented, the case is classified as explained death.

3.3 Central and Autonomic Nervous System Findings

In victims of sudden unexplained infant or perinatal death, while the gross examination of the brain may not show any alterations, the histopathological study of the brainstem may show the following frequent congenital developmental anomalies: hypertrophic long dendritic spines, a marker of neuronal immaturity, hypoplasia and agenesis of the ARCn, of the reticular formation or of other brainstem nuclei [37, 45, 48, 58].

3.3.1 Hypoplasia and Agenesis of the Arcuate Nucleus

In SIDS victims, mono- or bilateral hypoplasia, or even agenesis, of the ARCn is particularly frequent. It was observed in 56% of SIDS cases, and was found to be bilateral diffuse in 26%, bilateral partial (two-thirds caudal) in 18%, and monolateral (right) in 12% of victims [14, 40] (Figs. 3.25 and 3.26).

ARCn hypoplasia has also been detected in 43% of unexplained perinatal deaths [14, 33, 37, 40].

Morphometric reconstruction allows the volume reduction and the neuronal depletion resulting from this abnormality to be quantified. In every brainstem analyzed, the cytoarchitectural and dimensional parameters of the ARCn were compared with those of the nearby olivary nucleus, since both these nuclei have the same embryological origin, arising from the basal lamina of the neuronal tube. The morphometric analysis was performed on serial sections with an image analyzer (Media Cybernetics, Silver Spring, MD, USA) evaluating the mean neuronal density (number of neurons per unit area, expressed as means ± SEM millimeters squared) and the mean section area of the neuronal cell bodies (expressed as means ± SEM microns squared). We further considered the shape of the cell body, nucleus and nucleolus [14, 33].

In control fetuses under the 25th week of gestation, the ARCn showed a high density of small undifferentiated neuroblasts, which were roundish and apolar with compact chromatin, a nucleolus not clearly identifiable, and scarce cytoplasm (mean cell density $246 \pm 14/\text{mm}^2$, mean cell body area 18 ± 26 μm^2). From the 28th to the 36th week of gestation, the neurons in the ARCn showed a polygonal aspect, and were bipolar with a big vesicular nucleus with loose chromatin (mean density $195 \pm 22/\text{mm}^2$, mean cell area 42 ± 18 μm^2). After birth, the neurons, often multipolar, were decreased in number (mean cell density $140 \pm 30/\text{mm}^2$). The nuclei were enriched with finely scattered chromatin and an evident nucleolus (mean cell body area 81 ± 8 μm^2). The same neuronal model of differentiation was found in the brainstem of SIDS victims with or without ARCn hypoplasia. In the 20% of SIDS victims with normal ARCn architecture an increase in neuronal density was observed (mean value $188 \pm 21/\text{mm}^2$), with smaller neurons (mean neuronal body area 28 ± 20 μm^2). Many of these were lengthened, with a flattened nucleus, compact chromatin, and a poorly evident nucleolus [34].

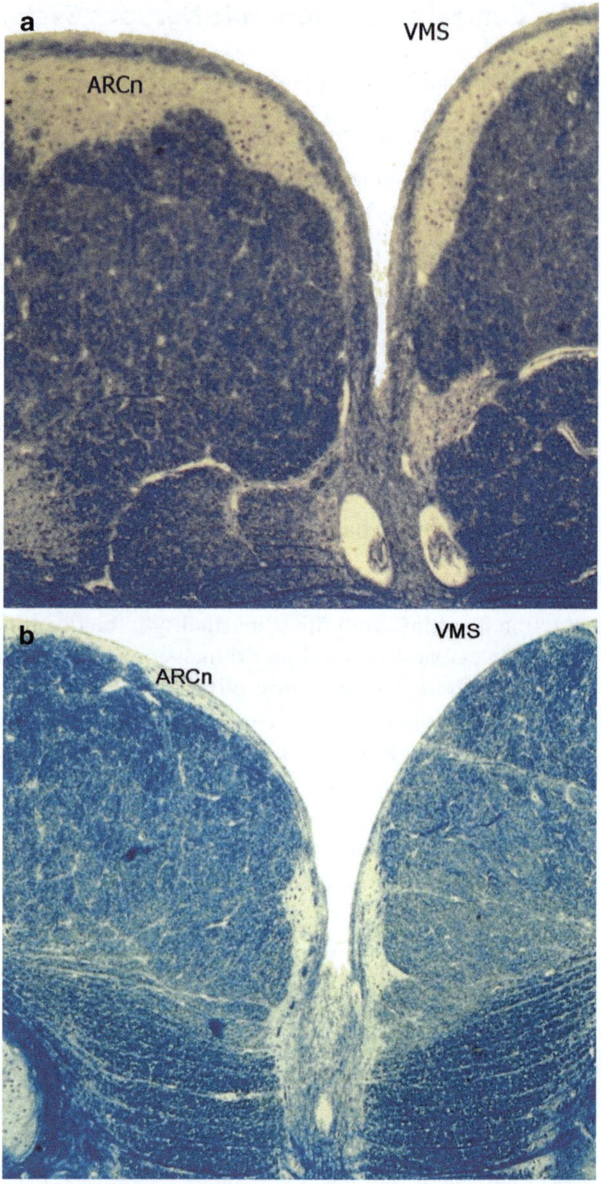

Fig. 3.25 (**a**, **b**) Sections of the brainstem showing the arcuate nucleus (*ARCn*) (**a**) in a 5-month-old infant as control and (**b**) in a 5-month-old SIDS victim with hypoplasia (*VMS* ventral medullary surface; Klüver-Barrera, ×25)

3.3.2 Combined Pulmonary and Arcuate Nucleus Hypoplasia

In 65% of unexplained stillbirths a bilateral pulmonary hypoplasia was observed, characterized by a decrease in volume and/or weight of the lungs, without lobulation anomalies, alteration of the indices of pulmonary development, with a LW/BW ratio below 0.022, a RAC index below 2.2 (Fig. 3.27) and the presence of

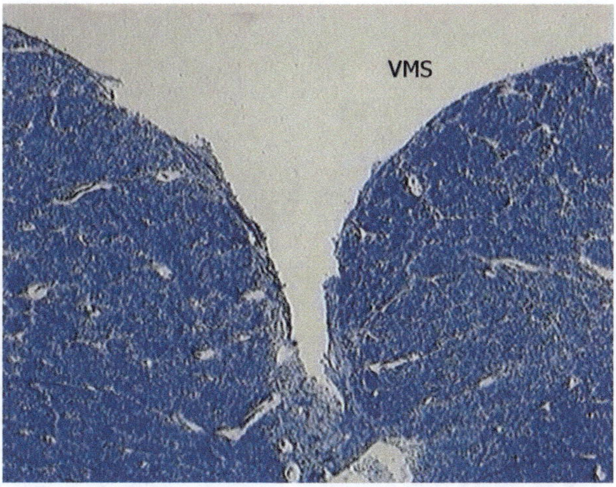

Fig. 3.26 Section of the brainstem showing agenesis of the arcuate nucleus in a SIDS victim, an infrequent finding (*VMS* ventral medullary surface; Klüver-Barrera, ×25)

cartilaginous bronchi up to the distal peripheral level. In 31% of cases, a microscopic examination of serial sections of the brainstem showed varying degrees of hypoplasia of the ARCn associated with the simultaneous presence of pulmonary hypoplasia. A significant correlation ($p<0.05$) between pulmonary hypoplasia and ARCn hypoplasia or agenesis was found [37].

The pulmonary hypoplasia was detected in 85% of SIDS cases and was significantly more frequent in the SIDS group compared to the sudden unexplained death group.

About 20% of cases presenting with both pulmonary hypoplasia and hypodeveloped brainstem nuclei had smoking parents [61].

3.3.3 Parabrachial/Kölliker-Fuse Complex Findings

The morphology of the parabrachial/Kölliker-Fuse (PB/KF) was homogeneous in all cases; therefore the precise structure of the three nuclei was described. The nucleus of the Kölliker-Fuse is made up of an area of clustered neurons (subnucleus compactus) and an adjacent area with dispersed neurons (subnucleus dissipatus) [11, 13].

3.3.3.1 Morphological Analysis of the Parabrachial/Kölliker-Fuse Complex

Comparative analysis of the serial histological sections obtained from the pons and mesencephalon of the SIUD and SIDS victims with those of the two control groups, made it possible to define the morphological features of the three principal nuclei of the human Parabracial/Kölliker-Fuse (PB/KF) complex: the lateral parabrachial nucleus (lPB), the medial parabrachial nucleus (mPB) and the KF nucleus. The PB/KF complex is located in the dorsolateral region of the rostral pons. Only the KF continues along the upper side in the caudal portion of the mesencephalon [13, 17].

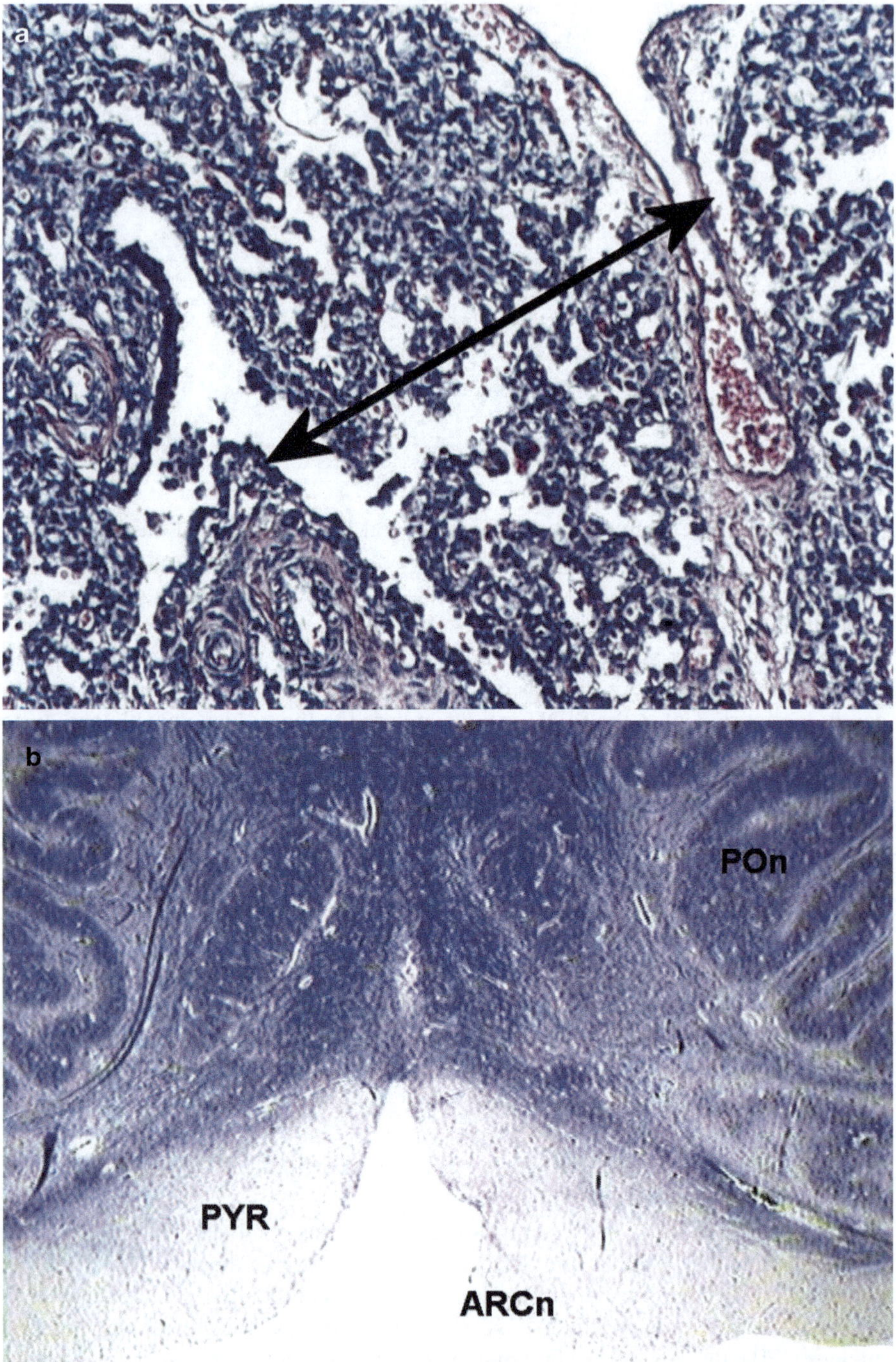

Fig. 3.27 (**a**, **b**) Combined pulmonary and arcuate nucleus hypoplasia in a SIUD fetus at 39 weeks of gestation. (**a**) Hypoplastic lung. The *black line* illustrates the method for determining the radial alveolar count (*RAC*) (H&E, ×100). (**b**) Medulla oblongata with severe hypoplasia of the arcuate nucleus (*ARCn*) (*PYR* pyramid, *POn* principal inferior olivary nucleus; Klüver-Barrera, ×25)

3.3.3.2 Lateral Parabrachial Nucleus

In transverse sections this nucleus is located between the lateral surface of the superior cerebellar peduncles (SCP) and the lateral lemniscus. It extends rostrocaudally from the level of the pons–mesencephalon junction (cranial pole) to the level where the lateral nucleus lemniscus is clearly visible (caudal pole). The section marking the passage from the pons to the mesencephalon is recognizable because the SCP forms a continuous line with their decussation. In the more caudal sections, the lPB is reduced because the distance between the lateral lemniscus and the SCP is very short. The neurons are round or tapering, with a light, often central nucleus, a prominent nucleolus, and scarce cytoplasm. Many neurons are dorsoventrally oriented, parallel to the axis of the SCP [13, 17].

3.3.3.3 Medial Parabrachial Nucleus

This nucleus lies medial to the SCP in transverse sections, running between the motor nucleus of the trigeminal nerves and the locus coeruleus up to the ventral termination of the SCP. Longitudinally, its size does not change from the rostral pole (pons–mesencephalon junction) to the caudal pole (where the lateral nucleus lemniscus is clearly visible). It contains numerous oval and polygonal neurons, which are usually larger than the lPB neurons and have a darker and more evident cytoplasm [13, 17].

3.3.3.4 Kölliker-Fuse Nucleus

This extends from the caudal pole of the parabrachial nuclei in the rostral pons along the whole of the lower portion of the mesencephalon, up to the level where the caudal pole of the red nucleus is visible.

In transverse pontine sections, it appears as a group of large neurons, located ventral to the lPB, between the medial limit of the SCP and the medial lemniscus. The neurons, which are noticeably larger than those of the PB nuclei, have a large, distinct, eccentric nucleus with a very evident nucleolus, abundant cytoplasm with Nissl substance located at the cell periphery.

On the basis of the neuronal disposition, it is possible at all levels to define two KF subnuclei: the subnucleus compactus, made up of a cluster of a few neurons, whose outline is sometimes indistinct, and the subnucleus dissipatus, adjacent to the compactus. In more rostral sections, in the caudal mesencephalon, the KF, located between the lateral limit of the SCP decussation and the medial lemniscus, shows similar cytological features and neuronal distribution [13, 17].

3.3.3.5 Morphometric Analysis of the Parabrachial/Kölliker-Fuse Complex

All the morphometric parameters were very similar in SIUD and SIDS victims to those in the respective control groups, as shown by the absence of statistically significant differences between the fetus and infant groups.

The transverse areas and volumes of the PB and KF nuclei in the unexplained stillbirth and control groups were very frequently lower than those of the SIDS and infant controls; instead, the number of neuronal cells and the cell body areas in fetuses were on the whole larger than in infants, but the differences were not significant.

The coronal size of the lPB decreased from the cranial (total mean area in the four groups $11.29 \pm 0.20\ mm^2$) to the caudal pole (total mean area $2.15 \pm 0.28\ mm^2$). In contrast, the transverse sectional areas of both mPB and KF were similar at the lower and upper extremities (mPB, total mean rostral area $9.28 \pm 0.26\ mm^2$, total mean caudal area $8.55 \pm 0.35\ mm^2$; KF, total mean rostral area $1.75 \pm 0.47\ mm^2$, total mean caudal area $1.88 \pm 0.25\ mm^2$).

Comparing the sectional areas of the body of the three PB/KF nuclei, it was evident that the mPB neurons were larger than the lPB neurons (total mean areas 310.58 ± 0.28 and $268.70 \pm 0.36\ \mu m^2$, respectively) and that the neuronal areas of the KF were significantly larger, being more than twice those of the PB neurons (mean $878 \pm 0.40\ \mu m^2$) [13].

In an infant born by cesarian section at 41 weeks of gestation with severe signs of asphyxia and dead 20 h after delivery, rare and immature neurons were observed in the brainstem areas of both lateral and medial PB nuclei together with a total absence of the characteristic neurons of the KF nucleus [18].

3.3.4 c-Fos Expression in Brainstem

The immunohistochemical labeling of the c-fos protein in the control group was overall negative or very low. In the medulla oblongata of SIDS victims there was a substantial and significant increase in c-fos expression, limited to the dorsal motor vagal nucleus. Indeed, in 60% of SIDS infants we observed positive neurons with strong cytoplasmic staining distributed in the dorsal motor nucleus of the vagal nerve bilaterally (score from ++ to +++). The c-fos-positive cells were consistently found throughout the rostral-intermediate extent of this nucleus. In contrast, in the caudal sections of the dorsal vagal motor nucleus, the immunohistochemical staining was negative or limited.

A non-significant scattered distribution of a few c-fos-stained neurons was also present in some cases, irrespective of the positivity of the dorsal vagal motor nucleus, in the inferior olive. Other nuclei of the medulla oblongata examined for c-fos immunoreactivity were negative [12].

3.3.5 En-2 Expression in Neurons

In fetuses, from 17 to 22 gw, the immunohistochemical study of the En-2 protein expression showed an intense positivity in all the neurons in the ArcN, in the inferior olivary nucleus and in the cerebellar granule cell layers equally in sudden death and control groups. The En-2 expression decreases up to the first days after birth and disappears in the newborn. A negative En-2 expression was registered in 29% of SIUD cases and in no control cases [19, 21].

3.3.6 Somatostatin Expression in Brainstem

The immunohistochemical study for somatostatin (SS) showed a prevalent SS expression in the nuclei of the brainstem involved in respiratory activity with a variable distribution. In particular, in fetuses, an intense positivity was constantly seen in the cell bodies and fibres of the tractus solitarii nucleus, dorsal vagus motor nucleus, ambiguus nucleus and the reticular formation in the medulla oblongata, and of the PB/KF complex, the locus coeruleus in the pons.

In all the postnatal death cases, an abrupt reduction of SS-positivity was detected. Even in the first day, a moderate number of positive cell bodies limited to two subnuclei of the tractus solitarii nu cleus (ventrolateral and ventral subnuclei) and in some cases also to the dorsal vagus motor nucleus and locus coeruleus were observed.

In 33% of SIUD and in 17% of controls the neurons of the hypoglossus nucleus were not immunostained for SS. The observation of a SS-negative hypoglossus nucleus is more frequent in SIUD versus fetal deaths of known causes. On the contrary, the frequency of SS-positivity of the hypoglossus nucleus is significantly higher in SIDS than in infants dead of other causes [15, 16, 19].

3.3.7 Tyrosine Hydroxilase Expression in Brainstem

In the medulla oblongata the tyrosine hydroxilase (TH) immunohistochemistry showed immunoreactive neurons in the dorsal motor vagal nucleus, in the tractus solitarius nucleus and in the ventrolateral reticular formation. The number and intensivity of positive neurons did not differ significantly between the sudden unexplained death and the control victims. On the contrary, in the pons, a variable expression of the TH, limited to the locus coeruleus was detected. In 57% of SIUD cases and in only 17% of victims of known diseases, the TH was not expressed in the locus coeruleus [19].

3.3.8 Combined Cardiac Conduction and Brainstem Findings

In SIDS infants with ARCn hypoplasia, Mahaim fibers were observed in 50% of those with severe bilateral hypoplasia (Fig. 3.28) and in 71% of those with monolateral hypoplasia. Thus, Mahaim fibers were significantly more frequent in SIDS infants with ARCn hypoplasia than in those with a well-developed ARCn (control and other SIDS infants; $p < 0.005$). The resorptive degeneration, cartilaginous metahyperplasia, and dispersion of the bundle of His bundle were statistically unrelated to the presence of ARCn hypoplasia [35].

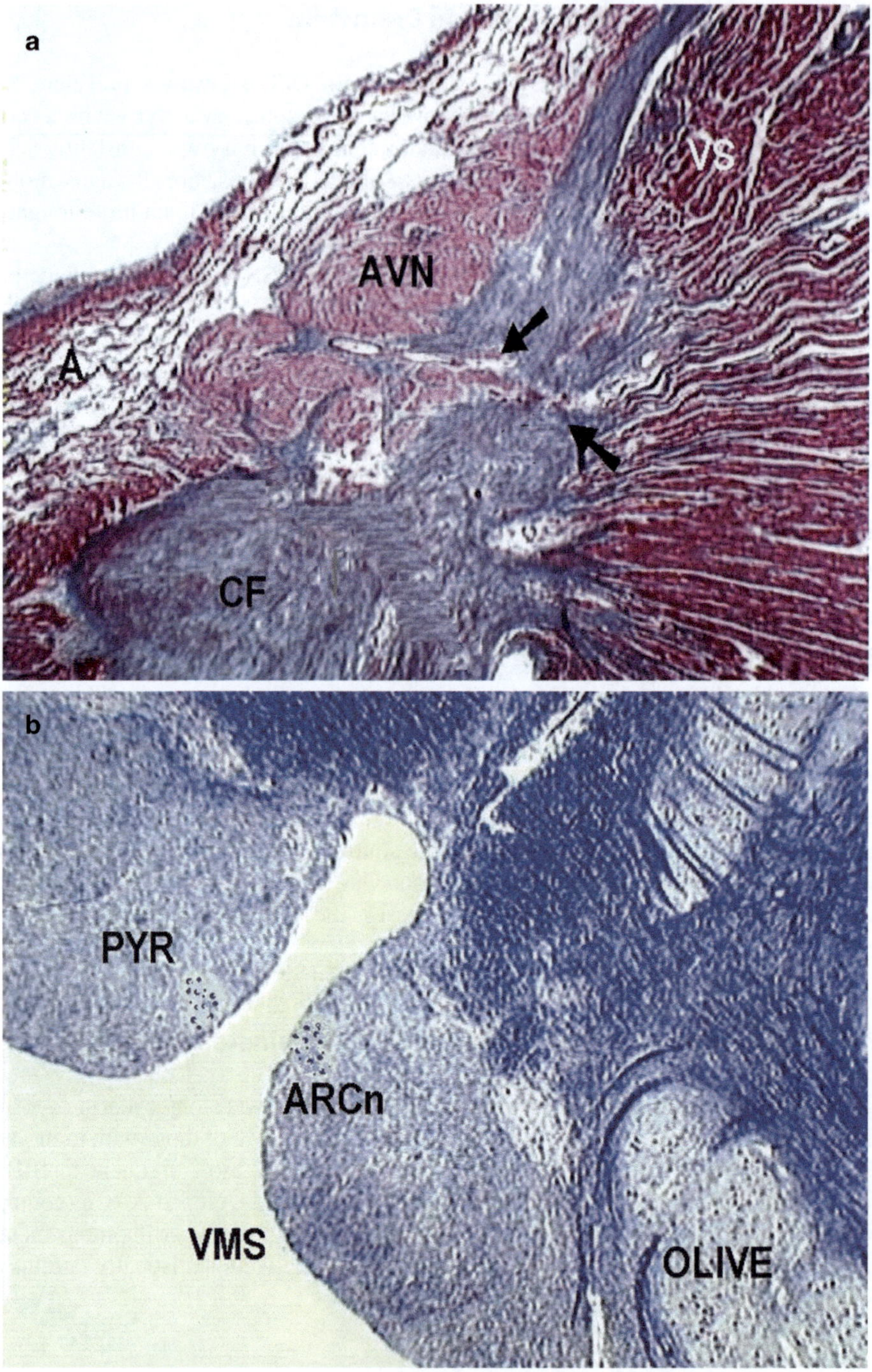

Fig. 3.28 (**a**, **b**) Simultaneous presence of Mahaim fiber and arcuate nucleus hypoplasia in a SIDS infant. (**a**) Accessory Mahaim fiber (*arrows*) bridge the atrioventricular node (*AVN*) and the ventricular septum (*VS*) (*A* right atrium, *CF* central fibrous body; trichromic Heidenhain, ×25). (**b**) Severe hypoplasia of the arcuate nucleus (*ARCn*) (*VMS* ventral medullary surface, *PYR* pyramid; Klüver-Barrera, ×25)

3.3.9 SIDS "Grey-Zone"/Borderline Findings

As described above, a total of 7% of SIDS and 11% of unexplained perinatal death victims were classified as grey zone/borderline cases. Below, some examples of SIDS grey zone cases classified in the basis of the brainstem findings are described.

- Case 1: In a SIDS case, the brainstem analysis on serial sections showed a discrete T-lymphocytic leptomeningitis of the ventral medullary surface, with involvement of the ARCn [29].
- Case 2: In a SIDS case, the brainstem analysis on serial sections showed toxoplasma encephalitis involving the ambiguus nucleus [56].
- Case 3: In a SIDS case, the brainstem analysis on serial sections showed degeneration with a necrotic focus with breaking of nerve fibers into the nucleus of the solitary tract, of unknown cause, perhaps viral in origin [56].
- Case 4: In a SIDS case, the brainstem analysis on serial sections showed a benign hemangioendothelioma arising bilaterally from the area postrema invading the medulla oblongata [30].
- Case 5: In a SIUD case, presenting with chorioamnionitis and vasculitis of the amino-chorial plate, the brainstem analysis on serial section disclosed a bilateral hypoplasia of the arcuate nucleus [62].

3.4 Peripheral Autonomic Nervous System Findings

Among the SIDS victims, immature neurons in both the upper cervical ganglia, associated with poorly developed capsular cells and neurons with interneuronal argentaffin elements (small intensely fluorescent – SIF cells) were detected in 9% of cases. Hyperplasia of the mediastinal paraganglia was detected in 25% of cases. An intracapsular glomus in the left stellate ganglion was detected in 2% of cases, and inflammatory foci in the right stellate ganglion was detected in 5% of cases [11].

3.4.1 Paraganglionic Hyperplasia

Hyperplasia of the aorticopulmonary paraganglia (APP) was detected in 25% of SIDS infants. It was not so marked in intercarotid glomera as in the mediastinal glomera [46, 63]. A few, small, discrete lobules showed great enlargement with irregular and elongated profiles. The enlargement of the APP was due in small part to this increase in size of lobules. The cell clusters and cell diameters were not significantly different from those in age-matched controls. Thus, enlargement of the APP involved an increase in the number rather than size of cells, favoring hyperplasia rather than hypertrophy [63–65]. The prominence of dark cells may be superimposed on the histological features of APP hyperplasia. These were distributed diffusely throughout the glomic tissue, exhibiting a compact basophilic cytoplasm, often in strap-like cytoplasmic extensions with an eccentric hyperchromatic nucleus [65]. The APP of the control group were greater in number and size at birth and decreased dramatically during the first year of life [63].

3.4.2 Stellate Ganglion Alterations

In 2% of SIDS infants an intracapsular glomus in the left stellate ganglion was found. In 5% of SIDS cases inflammatory foci in the right stellate ganglion have been detected. Alterations in the stellate ganglia may lead to asynchronism of the vagal parasympathetic bradycardic activity with a prevalence of left sympathetic tachycardic activity, and a consequent prolongation of the QT time, i.e., long QT syndrome [71, 72].

3.5 Cerebellar Findings

At 17–18th gw, the cerebellar cortex shows high, diffuse cellularity. Only the external granular layer is outlined, whereas the molecular layer, Purkinje cell layer, and internal granular layer are scarcely or not identifiable.

From the 20th–22nd gw, besides a well-defined 10–12 cells thick pluristratified external granular layer, a dense row of small cells appears in the Purkinje cell layer.

After the 30th gw, a four-layered structure of the cerebellar cortex is recognizable. The external granular layer is formed by 6–8 rows of densely packed small round cells. In this layer, several mitoses can be detected. The molecular layer contains numerous cells resembling cells of the external granular layer, in the migratory phase. The Purkinje cells form an ordered five to six cells thick layer of round immature larger neurons located between the molecular layer and the internal granular layer. This morphological pattern remains stable until the first days of life.

At the 1st month after birth the external granular layer presents a superficial zone of small round cells and a substrate of horizontal bipolar neurons, sometimes oriented centripetally toward the molecular layer.

From the 2nd month after birth the external granular layer becomes progressively thinner, while the molecular layer increases in thickness and shows lower cell density. The Purkinje cell layer is composed by numerous large cells with immature dendritic trees aligned in a single layer. Clusters of Purkinje cells are detectable in only a few tracts. The internal granular layer is increased in thickness and neuronal density.

At the 5–7th months of life the external granular layer is composed by three to four rows of prevalently elongated bipolar neurons and Purkinje cells show large mature somata, frequently polygonal in shape, with an evident axon and dendrites. They are now much more widely spaced and reduced in number. At the 10th month the external granular layer is a discontinuous single layer. In many areas the molecular layer represents the external surface.

At the 1st year of age the external granular layer is totally absent. The cerebellar cortex shows the three-layered definitive structure (molecular layer, Purkinje cell layer, and internal granular layer).

The average neuronal density and the number of reactive astrocytes in the inferior olivary nucleus and the dentate nucleus were decreased in sudden unexplained death victims as compared with explained perinatal and infant deaths. From the comparative histologic observations of both inferior olive and dentate nuclei, significant differences were observed between sudden unexplained perinatal and infant death groups and perinatal and infant control groups related to the morphometric data (one-way ANOVA, $p=0.001$) and biologic markers in both the olivary and dentate nuclei (Fisher's exact test, $p=0.05$). In the sudden death groups, there was an increased number of reactive astrocytes and of c-fos and apoptotic positive neurons as compared with the control groups [24].

3.5.1 PCNA Immunohistochemistry

In fetuses, PCNA immunoreactivity was observed throughout the cerebellar cortex thickness from the 20th gw. Successively, positive cells are mainly localized in the external granular layer, being far less represented in the molecular layer and internal granular layer and absent in the Purkinje cell layer. Within the internal granular layer, positive nuclei are mostly located at the boundaries of the Purkinje cell layer. This pattern of immunopositivity is observed up to birth and declines thereafter. At the 2nd month of life, rare PCNA-immunoreactive cells are detectable and only in the upper portiona of the external granular layer [23].

3.5.2 Apoptosis Immunohistochemistry

In prenatal life and up to the 1st postnatal month the immunostaining for apoptotic cells reveals only sporadic positive nuclei in the external granular layer.

At the 2nd–4th months, the apoptosis is positive as the number of dying cells increases and is confined to the outer part of the external granular layer. This process becomes more marked during external granular layer regression, affecting the vast majority of its cells. Apoptotic neurons display intense staining with margination of highly condensed chromatin, various nuclear fragmentation stage and apoptotic bodies [23].

High percentages of apoptotic neurons have been observed in the inferior olive and the dentate nuclei of 36% of sudden unexplained perinatal deaths, 50% of SIDS victims and in 25% of the control group [24].

3.5.3 c-Fos Immunohistochemistry

From the 17–25th gw, the vast majority of cells in the cerebellar cortex is c-fos labeled. Then the positivity decreases and at 35 gw only rare c-fos positive cells are visible, scattered in the external granular layer. By the last fetal period and in postnatal life c-fos expression is fully negative [23].

In 36% of sudden death victims, more than 80% of the neurons of both the inferior olive and the dentate nuclei were intensely c-fos-labeled. In the control cases, the c-fos expression was entirely negative [24].

In the cerebellar cortex, abnormal patterns of maturation were observed in about 50% of cases of sudden unexplained perinatal or infant death and in 5% of controls, i.e., an immature structure of the external granular layer which resulted to be constituted exclusively by small round cells, without any bipolar neurons in the inner rows; an external granular layer negative for apoptosis; positivity for apoptosis in the internal granular layer and in the Purkinje cells [22, 23, 25].

In the cerebellar nuclei, overall, high glial indices and biologic alterations of the dentate-olivary system were present in 64% of sudden unexplained infant and perinatal and only in 10% of the explained death victims (Fisher's exact test, $p = 0.05$) [24].

The cerebellar alterations were significantly related to maternal smoking [22, 24].

3.6 Review Questions

This test, composed of 10 multiple-choice questions, is designed to measure knowledge about the contents of this chapter on Pathological and related Epidemiological Findings in Sudden Infant and Perinatal Death. Questions have only one correct answer and cover the major content areas of this chapter. Check the correct responses and score your test using the answer keys on page 136.

31. At which age does SIDS most frequently occur?
    - □ A. Infants 10–12 month-old
    - □ B. Infants 8–10 month-old
    - □ C. Infants 6–8 month-old
    - □ D. Infants 4–6 month-old
    - □ E. Infants 2–4 month-old
32. In which season does SIDS more frequently occur?
    - □ A. Spring
    - □ B. Summer
    - □ C. Winter
    - □ D. Fall
    - □ E. SIDS incidence is not related to season
33. In about which percentage of SIDS and sudden unexplained perinatal deaths are the parents cigarette smokers?
    - □ A. 95% of cases
    - □ B. 55% of cases
    - □ C. 25% of cases
    - □ D. 15% of cases
    - □ E. 5% of cases
34. Which one of the following is the most important preventable risk factor for SIDS, related to morphological and/or functional alterations of brainstem centers?
    - □ A. Maternal cigarette smoking
    - □ B. Position in the crib
    - □ C. Prematurity
    - □ D. Maternal alcohol abuse
    - □ E. Maternal drug abuse

35. Which of the following accessory pathways are more frequently detected in the cardiac conduction system of SIDS cases?
   - □ A. Kent fibers, detected in 10% of SIDS cases
   - □ B. James fibers, detected in 23% of SIDS cases
   - □ C. Mahaim fibers, detected in 40% of SIDS cases
   - □ D. Mahaim fibers, detected in 23% of SIDS cases
   - □ E. James fibers, detected in 60% of SIDS cases
36. A previously healthy 3-month-old male infant is brought to the ER by his mother, who found early in the morning the child in the crib unarousable for feeding. The child is determined to be dead after resuscitative efforts. An autopsy is requested.

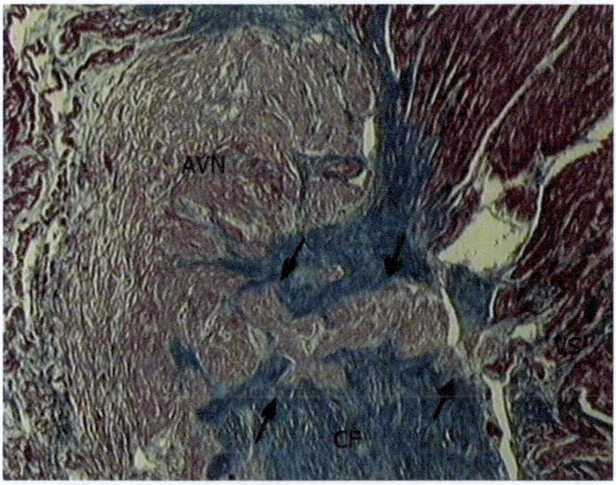

   What is detected at the histopathological exam of the cardiac conduction system?
   - □ A. Myocardial infarction
   - □ B. James fiber
   - □ C. Split atrio-ventricular node
   - □ D. Cartilagineous metaplasia
   - □ E. Mahaim fiber
37. When do the preatherosclerotic lesions in coronary arteries start to be detectable?
   - □ A. in fetuses
   - □ B. in newborns
   - □ C. in infants
   - □ D. in children
   - □ E. in adults
38. A 3-month old baby boy is found dead in his crib suddenly and unexpectedly. A hypertrophic cardiomyopathy is diagnosed at autopsy. How is this case classified?
   - □ A. SIDS
   - □ B. SIDS grey zone
   - □ C. Explained death
   - □ D. Sudden unexplained perinatal death
   - □ E. SIUD

39. An hypoplasia of the arcuate nucleus has been detected in which approximate percentage of SIDS and sudden unexplained perinatal cases?
    - □ A. 100% of cases
    - □ B. 50% of cases
    - □ C. 30% of cases
    - □ D. 15% of cases
    - □ E. 0% of cases
40. Which of the following cerebellar alterations have been detected in SIDS?
    - □ A. Immaturity of the external granular layer, apoptosis of the Purkinje cells, and apoptosis of the inner granular layer of the cerebellar cortex, detected in about 50% of SIDS cases
    - □ B. Immaturity of the external granular layer, apoptosis of the Purkinje cells, and apoptosis of the inner granular layer of the cerebellar cortex, detected in about 20% of SIDS cases
    - □ C. Immaturity of the external granular layer, apoptosis of the Purkinje cells, and apoptosis of the inner granular layer of the cerebellar cortex, detected in about 70% of SIDS cases
    - □ D. Immaturity of the internal granular layer, apoptosis of the external granular layer of the cerebellar cortex, detected in about 50% of SIDS cases
    - □ E. Immaturity of the internal granular layer, apoptosis of the external granular layer of the cerebellar cortex, detected in about 30% of SIDS cases

3.7 Answer Keys

Block 3 (Questions 21–30)

31. E
32. C
33. B
34. A
35. D
36. E
37. A
38. C
39. B.
40. A

References

1. Bharati S, Krongrad E, Lev M (1985) Study of the conduction system in a population of patients with sudden infant death syndrome. Pediatr Cardiol 6:29–40.
2. Eisenberg MS, Mengert TJ (2000) Cardiac resuscitation. N Engl J Med 343:1206–1209.

3. Gerlis LM (1996) Covert congenital cardiovascular malformations discovered in an autopsy series of nearly 5000 cases. Cardiovasc Pathol 5:11–19.
4. James TN (1961) Morphology of the human atrioventricular node, with remarks pertinent to its electrophysiology. Am Heart J 62:756–777.
5. James TN (1968) Sudden death in babies: new observation in the heart. Am J Cardiol 22:479–506.
6. James TN (1983) The Mikamo lecture. Structure and function of AV junction. Jpn Circ J 47:1–47.
7. James TN (1994) Normal and abnormal consequences of apoptosis in the human heart. From postnatal morphogenesis to paroxysmal arrhythmias. Circulation 90:556–573.
8. James TN (2001) The internodal pathways of the human heart. Prog Cardiovasc Dis 43:495–535.
9. James TN, Marshall TK (1976) De Subitaneis Mortibus XVIII. Persistent fetal dispersion of the atrioventricular node and His bundle within the central fibrous body. Circulation 6:1026–1034.
10. Kent AFS (1893) Researches on the structure and function of the mammalian heart. J Physiol 14:233–254.
11. Lavezzi AM, Matturri L, Ballabio G, Ottaviani G, Rossi L (2002) Study of the cytoarchitecture of the parabrachial/Kölliker-Fuse complex in SIDS and fetal late stillbirth. In: Proceedings of the 7th International Conference on SIDS, Florence, p 132.
12. Lavezzi AM, Ottaviani G, Matturri L (2003) Identification of neurons responding to hypoxia in sudden infant death syndrome (SIDS). Pathol Int 53:769–774.
13. Lavezzi AM, Ottaviani G, Ballabio G, Rossi L, Matturri L (2004) Preliminary study on the cytoarchitecture of the human parabrachial/Kölliker-Fuse complex, with reference to sudden infant death syndrome and sudden intrauterine unexplained death. Pediatr Dev Pathol 7:171–179.
14. Lavezzi AM, Ottaviani G, Mauri M, Matturri L (2004) Hypoplasia of the arcuate nucleus and maternal smoking during pregnancy, in perinatal and infant sudden unexpected death. Neuropathology 24:284–289.
15. Lavezzi AM, Ottaviani G, Matturri L (2004) Involvement of somatostatin in breathing control before and after birth, and in perinatal and infant sudden unexplained death. Folia Neuropathol 42:59–65.
16. Lavezzi AM, Ottaviani G, Matturri L (2004) Role of somatostatin and apoptosis in breathing control in sudden perinatal and infant unexplained death. Clin Neuropathol 23:304–310.
17. Lavezzi AM, Ottaviani G, Rossi L, Matturri L (2004) Cytoarchitectural organization of the Parabrachial/Kölliker-Fuse complex in man. Brain Dev 26:316–320.
18. Lavezzi AM, Ottaviani G, Rossi L, Matturri L (2004) Hypoplasia of the parabrachial/Kölliker-Fuse complex in perinatal death. Biol Neonate 86:92–97.
19. Lavezzi AM, Ottaviani G, Matturri L (2005) Adverse effects of prenatal tobacco smoke exposure on biological parameters of the developing brainstem. Neurobiol Dis 20:601–607.
20. Lavezzi AM, Ottaviani G, Matturri L (2005) Biology of the smooth muscle cells in human atherosclerosis. APMIS 113:112–121.
21. Lavezzi AM, Ottaviani G, Mauri M, Terni L, Matturri L (2005) Involvement of the EN-2 gene in normal and abnormal development of the human arcuate nucleus. Int J Exp Pathol 86:25–31.
22. Lavezzi AM, Ottaviani G, Mauri M, Matturri L (2006) Alterations of biological features of the cerebellum in sudden perinatal and infant death. Curr Mol Med 6:429–435.
23. Lavezzi AM, Ottaviani G, Terni L, Matturri L (2006) Histological and biological developmental characterization of the human cerebellar cortex. Int J Dev Neurosci 24:365–371.
24. Lavezzi AM, Ottaviani G, Mauri M, Matturri L (2007) Biopathology of the dentate-olivary complex in sudden unexplained perinatal death and sudden infant death syndrome related to maternal cigarette smoking. Neurol Res 19:525–532.
25. Lavezzi AM, Ottaviani G, Matturri L (2007) Ontogenesis of human cerebellar cortex and biopathological characterization in sudden unexplained fetal and infant death. Virchows Arch 450:31–40.

26. Mahaim I, Benatt A (1938) Nouvelles recherches sur les connexions superiors de la branche gauche du faisceau de His-Tawara avec cloison interventriculaire. Cardiologia 1:61–120.
27. Massing GK, James TN (1976) Anatomical configuration of the His bundle and bundle branches in the human heart. Circulation 53:609–621.
28. Matturri L, Nappo A, Varesi C, Martini I, Rossi L (1997) Dualismo del nodo atrioventricolare per la presenza del nodo del seno coronarico di Zahn in un caso di morte improvvisa del lattante (SIDS). Riv Ital Pediatr 23:130–133.
29. Matturri L, Ottaviani G, Biondo B, Ramos SG, Rossi L (1998) Discrete T-lymphocytic leptomeningitis of the ventral medullary surface in a case of sudden unexpected infant death. Adv Clin Path 2:313–316.
30. Matturri L, Ottaviani G, Rossi L (1999) Sudden and unexpected infant death due to an hemangioendothelioma located in the medulla oblongata. Adv Clin Path 3:29–33.
31. Matturri L, Ottaviani G, Ramos SG, Rossi L (2000) Sudden infant death syndrome (SIDS). A study of cardiac conduction system. Cardiovasc Pathol 9:137–145.
32. Matturri L, Ottaviani G, Lavezzi AM, Turconi P, Cazzullo A, Rossi L (2001) Expression of apoptosis and proliferating cell nuclear antigen (PCNA) in the cardiac conduction system of crib death (SIDS). Adv Clin Path 5:79–86.
33. Matturri L, Minoli I, Lavezzi AM, Cappellini A, Ramos S, Rossi L (2002) Hypoplasia of medullary arcuate nucleus in unexpected late fetal death (stillborn infants): a pathological study. Pediatrics 109:E43.
34. Matturri L, Ottaviani G, Ballabio G, Lavezzi AM (2002) Medullary arcuate nucleus' cellular differentiation in SIDS and unexpected late fetal stillbirth cases. In: Proceedings of the 7th SIDS International Conference, Florence, p 135.
35. Matturri L, Ottaviani G, Biondo B, Rossi L (2002) Sudden infant death syndrome (SIDS): associated alterations of the cardiac conduction system and brainstem. In: Proceedings of the 7th International Conference on SIDS, Florence, p 133.
36. Matturri L, Ottaviani G, Rossi L (2002) Should overdone external cardiac massage in infants dying of SIDS be discouraged? In: Proceedings of the 7th International Conference on SIDS, Florence, p 136.
37. Matturri L, Lavezzi AM, Minoli I, Ottaviani G, Cappellini A, Rubino B, Rossi L (2003) Association between pulmonary hypoplasia and hypoplasia of arcuate nucleus in stillbirth. J Perinatol 23:328–332.
38. Matturri L, Lavezzi AM, Ottaviani G, Rossi L (2003) Intimal preatherosclerotic thickening of the coronary arteries in human fetuses of smoker mothers. J Thromb Haemost 1:2234–2238.
39. Matturri L, Ottaviani G, Rossi L (2003) External cardiac massage in infants. Intensive Care Med 29:1199–1200.
40. Matturri L, Ottaviani G, Alfonsi G, Crippa M, Rossi L, Lavezzi AM (2004) Study of the brainstem, particularly the arcuate nucleus, in sudden infant death syndrome (SIDS) and sudden intrauterine unexplained death (SIUD). Am J Forensic Med Pathol 25:44–48.
41. Matturri L, Ottaviani G, Corti G, Lavezzi AM (2004) Pathogenesis of early atherosclerotic lesions in infants. Pathol Res Pract 200:403–410.
42. Matturri L, Ottaviani G, Lavezzi AM, Rossi L (2004) Early atherosclerotic lesions of the cardiac conduction system arteries in infants. Cardiovasc Pathol 13:276–281.
43. Matturri L, Ottaviani G, Lavezzi AM (2005) Early atherosclerotic lesions in infancy: role of parental cigarette smoking. Virchows Arch 447:74–80.
44. Matturri L, Ottaviani G, Lavezzi AM (2005) Techniques and criteria in pathologic and forensic-medical diagnostics in sudden unexpected infant and perinatal death. Am J Clin Pathol 124:259–268.
45. Matturri L, Ottaviani G, Lavezzi AM (2005) Unexpected sudden death related to medullary brain lesions. Acta Neuropathol (Berl) 109:554–555.
46. Matturri L, Ottaviani G, Lavezzi AM, Ramos SG (2005) Peripheral chemoreceptors and sudden infant death syndrome: a wide open problem. Curr Cardiol Rev 1:65–70.

47. Matturri L, Ottaviani G, Lavezzi AM (2006) Maternal smoking and sudden infant death syndrome: epidemiological study related to pathology. Virchows Arch 449:697–706.
48. Morpurgo CV, Lavezzi AM, Ottaviani G, Rossi L (2004) Bulbo-spinal pathology and sudden respiratory infant death syndrome. Eur J Anaesthesiol 21:589–593.
49. Ottaviani G, Ramos SG, Matturri L (1997) Defective "resorptive degeneration" of the heart's conduction system and sudden infant death syndrome. Ann Españ Pediatr 92(Suppl):53.
50. Ottaviani G, Goisis M, Ramos SG, Matturri L (1998) Dispersione del tessuto giunzionale e sue conseguenze in un caso di morte improvvisa del lattante. Cardiologia 43:737–739.
51. Ottaviani G, Rossi L, Bondurri A, Ramos SG, Matturri L (1998) Morte improvvisa del lattante: un caso di sdoppiamento del nodo atrio-ventricolare. Riv Ital Pediatr 24:1165–1167.
52. Ottaviani G, Rossi L, Ramos SG, Matturri L (1999) Pathology of the heart and conduction system in a case of sudden death due to a cardiac fibroma in a 6-month-old child. Cardiovasc Pathol 8:109–112.
53. Ottaviani G, Matturri L, Lavezzi AM, Rossi L, James TN (2002) Postnatal apoptosis of the cardiac conduction system in crib death: preliminary results. In: Proceedings of the 7th SIDS International Conference, Florence, p 132.
54. Ottaviani G, Matturri L, Rossi L, James TN (2003) Crib death: further support for the concept of fatal cardiac electrical instability as the final common pathway. Int J Cardiol 92:17–26.
55. Ottaviani G, Matturri L, Rossi L, Lavezzi AM, James TN (2004) Multifocal cardiac Purkinje cell tumor in infancy. Europace 6:138–141.
56. Ottaviani G, Matturri L, Bruni B, Lavezzi AM (2005) Sudden infant death syndrome "gray zone" disclosed only by a study of the brain stem on serial sections. J Perinat Med 33:165–169.
57. Ottaviani G, Rossi L, Matturri L (2005) Myocardial injury attributable to external cardiac massage in infants. Cardiology 1:25–29.
58. Ottaviani G, Matturri L, Mingrone R, Lavezzi AM (2006) Hypoplasia and neuronal immaturity of the hypoglossal nucleus in sudden infant death. J Clin Pathol 59:497–500.
59. Ottaviani G (2006) Studio istopatologico del sistema di conduzione cardiaco nella morte improvvisa del lattante e perinatale. In: Proceedings of the Convegno "Morte improvvisa del lattante e morte inaspettata del feto. La rilevanza giuridica e medico-sociale della ricerca scientifica: la legge n. 31 del 2006", Gargnano, pp 63–74.
60. Ottaviani G, Matturri L (2008) Histopathology of the cardiac conduction system in sudden intrauterine unexplained death. Cardiovasc Pathol 17:146–155.
61. Ottaviani G, Mingrone R, Lavezzi AM, Matturri L (2009) Infant and perinatal pulmonary hypoplasia frequently associated with brainstem hypodevelopment. Virchows Arch 454:451–456.
62. Ottaviani G (2008) Sudden intrauterine unexplained death (SIUD) «gray zone» or borderline. Neurosci Imaging 2:127–133.
63. Ramos SG, Matturri L, Biondo B, Ottaviani G, Rossi L (1998) Hyperplasia of the aorticopulmonary paraganglia: a new insight into the pathogenesis of sudden infant death syndrome? Cardiologia 43:953–958.
64. Ramos SG, Matturri L, Ottaviani G, Rossi L (1998) Maternal smoking and aorticopulmonary paraganglia in sudden infant death syndrome. In: Proceedings of the 5th SIDS International Conference, Rouen, p 169.
65. Ramos SG, Ottaviani G, Biondo B, Rossi L, Matturri L (1999) Hyperplasia of the aorticopulmonary paraganglia in infants dying of SIDS: further supports for the cardio-respiratory hypothesis. In: Proceedings of the International Symposium on SIDS and Lombardy Region project for the reduction of the risk for sudden infant death and unexplained intrauterine death, Milan, pp 117–128.
66. Rossi L (1969) Histopathologic features of cardiac arrhythmias. Casa Editrice Ambrosiana, Milan.
67. Rossi L (1978) Intramural ramification of the left bundle branch. Am Heart J 96:271–272.
68. Rossi L, Matturri L (1988) His bundle haematoma and external cardiac massage: histopathological findings. Br Heart J 59:586–587.

69. Rossi L, Matturri L (1990) Clinicopathological approach to cardiac arrhythmias. A color atlas. Centro Scientifico Torinese, Turin.
70. Rossi L, Matturri L (1995) Anatomo-histological features of the heart's conduction system and innervation in SIDS. In: Rognum TO (ed) Sudden infant death syndrome: new trends in the nineties. Scandinavian University Press, Oslo, pp 207–212.
71. Rossi L, Matturri L (1995) Cardiac conduction and nervous system in health disease and sudden death: an anatomoclinical overview. Osp Maggiore 89:239–257.
72. Rossi L, Thiene G (1983) Arrhythmologic pathology of sudden cardiac death. Casa Editrice Ambrosiana, Milan.
73. Rossi L, Knippel M, Taccardi B (1975) Histological findings. His bundle recordings and body-surface potential mappings in a case of Wolff-Parkinson-White syndrome. An anatomoclinical comparison. Cardiology 60:265–279.
74. Rossi L, Thiene G, Knippel M (1978) A case of surgically corrected Wolff-Parkinson-White syndrome: clinical and histological data. Br Heart J 40:581–585.
75. Suàrez-Mier MP, Gamallo C (1998) Atrioventricular node fetal dispersion and His fragmentation of the cardiac conduction system in sudden cardiac death. J Am Coll Cardiol 32:1885–1890.
76. Waldo AL, James TN (1973) A retrospective look at A-V nodal rhythms (A Zahn). Circulation 47:222–224.
77. Wolff GS, Han J, Curran G (1978) Wolff-Parkinson-White syndrome in the neonate. Am J Cardiol 41:559–563.
78. Wolff L, Parkinson J, White PD (1930) Bundle-branch block with short P-R interval in healthy young people prone to paroxysmal tachycardia. Am Heart J 5:685–704.
79. Zahn A (1912) Experimentelle untersuchungen über die reizbildung im atrioventrikularnoten und sinus coronarius. Zentralbl Physiol 26:495.

Moving Forward the Discussion on Sudden Infant and Perinatal Unexplained Death

4

Sudden infant death syndrome (SIDS) or crib death and sudden perinatal unexplained death (SPUD) represent facets of a multifactorial problem that has not yet found an unified approach on the clinical plane, and therefore the only field of study that allows for the possibility of scientific progress is anatomic pathology.

In today's medicine SIDS remains one of the major social health problems still lacking a solution. It is defined as the sudden death of an infant under one year of age which remains unexplained after a thorough case investigation, including performance of a complete autopsy, examination of the death scene, and a review of the clinical history [213]. It strikes one infant in every 1,700–2,000 live births, and is the most frequent form of demise within the first year of life [16].

Sudden intrauterine unexplained death (SIUD) or unexplained stillbirth is up to ten-fold more frequent than SIDS, representing about one-half of perinatal deaths, with a prevalence of 5–12 per 1,000 births [16, 21, 47]. This tragic form of death is still frequent. Despite the advances in maternal and fetal care that have produced a significant reduction in perinatal mortality, the prevalence of SIUD has not significantly changed [16, 96].

Many cases of sudden neonatal death remain unexplained after the usual gross and microscopic examination, and are referable to similar histopathological mechanisms underlying equally SIDS, sudden neonatal unexplained death (SNUD) and SIUD [128, 157, 161], so the term sudden unexplained perinatal death (SPUD) [156] has been used to indicate both sudden fetal and neonatal unexplained deaths. SPUD is therefore herein defined as the sudden unexpected death of a fetus from the 22nd gw or of a newborn since birth to the completion of the 1st month of postnatal life that remains unexplained after a thorough investigation of the case, including the review of the clinical history and the performance of a complete *post mortem* examination.

The emotional consequences of infants and fetus loss among families are devastating and the cost of adaptation therapies is remarkable [15]. As these tragic events are so frequent, a better knowledge of SIDS and sudden unexplained perinatal death aims also to limit the subsequent environmental damage due to the loss of many potentially productive individuals. The scientific and financial advantages theoretically deriving from a better understanding of SIDS and unexplained perinatal death are certainly significant.

G. Ottaviani, *Crib Death - Sudden Infant Death Syndrome (SIDS): Sudden Infant and Perinatal Unexplained Death: The Pathologist's Viewpoint*,
DOI 10.1007/978-3-319-08347-6_4

The need to submit the young victims to necropsy procedures is unanimously recognized and the chance of preventing SIDS and unexplained perinatal death relies mainly on a better knowledge of the underlying histopathological alterations and etiopathogenetic mechanisms. An accurate examination of the circumstances and environment where the death occurred is also mandatory.

Frequent alterations of the autonomic nervous system, both central and peripheral, in SIDS and unexplained perinatal death victims have been described. These structural alterations are mainly of a congenital nature, representing a common morphological substrate in both fetal and infant sudden death. The functional consequences consist of severe disturbances of the neuroreceptorial activities, including the synthesis of tyrosine hydroxylase, somatostatin, substance P, etc., that contribute to cause marked alterations of the nuclei and/or structures presiding over the vital cardio-respiratory, arousal, upper digestive tract activities [82, 83, 86, 92]. In addition to congenital anomalies, in SIDS "grey zone", acquired alterations of an inflammatory nature have been observed to be localized in these vital centers [103, 125, 150].

The congenital anomalies of the brainstem and cerebellum, seem to be factors on the development of the fetal lungs, as pulmonary hypoplasia has been found in the victims of sudden unexplained perinatal death and SIDS [88–90, 112, 161].

Malignant arrhythmias are known to be another substrate of infant and fetal sudden death, mostly caused by accessory atrio-ventricular pathways [105, 147, 162]. Therefore, an accurate examination of the cardiac conduction system, again under the control of the nervous system, is also indispensable.

In view of these results, the need to make an in-depth study of the cardiac conduction system and of the autonomic nervous system, according to *ad hoc* guidelines [115, 120, 124, 131], is self evident. The diagnostic protocol consists of an anatomo-pathologic examination of all the organs, including the thymus. In fetuses, in particular, the adnexa, i.e., placenta, umbilical cord and membranes, must be examined according to the usual procedure.

4.1 Advances in Cardiac Conduction Pathology

SIDS infants do not show any abnormality of the ordinary myocardium, while the core of the heart, where the cardiac rhythm arises and spreads, represents an insight into the solution to the problem. The involvement of conducting tissue in the cardiac pathology of crib death has been a controversial issue for years [3]. A pathologist may not consider very small lesions in the general myocardium to have any functional significance and, without experience of looking at the cardiac conduction system, may fail to understand how crucially important a lesion with maximal dimensions of one mm could be in the cardiac conduction system [147].

In the 1970s several authors focused the study of crib death on the conducting tissue [5, 32, 33, 52, 53, 94]. The most common finding discussed was the "resorptive degeneration" first defined by James [51] as a process of postnatal morphogenesis consisting of areas of degeneration, cell death mainly by apoptosis, and replacement fibrosis, beginning about 1 or 2 weeks after birth [59, 62, 63], and being usually completed in the first year of life. James' concept has been confirmed by Ferris [32], Marino and Kane [98], and Rossi and Matturri [180–182], but the validity of his findings has been questioned by other investigators; since this finding was also present in the control group, the studies were considered inconclusive by some authors and thus abandoned [4, 94, 205, 207]. Despite that cardiac hypothesis of crib death was controversial [3], the concept that crib death may be related to lethal cardiac arrhythmias or heart block due to structural abnormalities has been the focus of renewed interest [39, 105, 139–142, 146, 147, 162]. There also continues to be interest in the relationship between crib death and the occurrence of fetal and infant junctional tachycardia [204, 216].

The morphological *post mortem* study of the conducting tissue in all cases of suspected SIDS is based on the cardiac theory, which postulates that SIDS-SPUD could be due to lethal cardiac electrical instability [147, 162]. The cardiac theory of crib death was introduced by James [51–54] who described postnatal morphological changes described in infants dying in the crib who had no morphological abnormalities other then in the cardiac conduction system. The cardiac theory of SIDS is based on what James [51] first referred to as "resorptive degeneration", as a developmental process of molding and shaping of the atrioventricular (AV) node and bundle of His (HB), mediated by apoptosis [61, 62].

4.1.1 Resorptive Degeneration

During human fetal development, the entire cardiac conduction system is essentially in place and almost completed by the end of the first trimester of gestation. Teleologically, one can reason that this becomes a necessity as a fetus grows and distribution of blood within its body can be facilitated by assisting the circulation provided through the maternal placenta. Once this conduction system has been formed and is in place, there are relatively few morphological changes in it until birth. What happens then is a remarkable transformation and, although the general organization remains, the cytological and histological changes are rather dramatic [52, 64, 65].

The AV node and HB undergo a remarkable postnatal morphogenesis, defined by James [51] in 1968 as "resorptive degeneration", consisting of degeneration, cell death and replacement in an orderly programmed way [51–59, 139, 147]. This term indicates a tidying-up process in which loose strands of surplus conducting tissue are gradually reabsorbed to change the AV node and HB into their more smooth adult configuration [51, 52, 55, 59]. The areas of resorptive degeneration have been described as clusters of young fibroblasts depositing collagen caught in the central fibrous body, sometimes isolated from the "overdeveloped" specialized structures, sometimes adjacent to them, without association of inflammation or massive necrosis or hemorrhage [51, 182].

The resorptive degeneration is a process not claimed to be unique to crib death that itself must be considered a normal postnatal morphological process [51, 56, 59,

147]. This postnatal morphogenesis is mediated by apoptotic death of myocytes in both the sinus node and the AV junctional tissue [62, 106]. Since there is no associated inflammation or other indicators of necrosis, some authors have considered such changes as normal or harmless. A misunderstanding of this interpretation has come from two directions: first, those who conclude that a normal process could not be seen as pathological; and, second, those who are seeking a single or unique abnormality to blame for crib death. The problem here is that it is not correct to say that the resorptive degeneration, itself something normal, is not necessarily dangerous. The resorptive degeneration, itself a normal process occurring up to the completion of the first year of postnatal life, being a process of molding and shaping, represents a period of physiological electrical instability of the infant's heart.

Since we do not all die during these ubiquitous changes, the changes usually are harmless. We all survive the risk of crib death because no additional other stressful events encountered in a baby's life, such as fever, vomiting or diarrhea, electrolytic imbalance or neurovegetative influence, coincided with the period of postnatal morphogenesis [56–59, 147]. Thus, both resorptive degeneration and otherwise innocuous events are harmless if they occur alone. On the other hand, the resorptive degeneration, itself physiological, can become pathological. It is defective if fails to reabsorb redundant conduction tissue leaving in place accessory pathways or islands of conducting tissue, or is exaggerated if the reabsorption is so extensive to cause hypoplasia of the cardiac conduction system structures [61, 69, 70, 139, 177].

Areas of resorptive degeneration were observed in 97% of SIDS infants and in 75% of controls (Fig. 3.6). Statistical analysis showed a significant difference between the two infant groups ($p<0.05$). In the SPUD victims, areas of resorptive degeneration were observed in 55% of cases and in 47% of the age-matched controls, without statistically significant differences [155, 157].

In these resorptive degeneration areas clusters of young fibroblasts depositing collagen caught in the central fibrous body were observed, sometimes isolated from the overdeveloped specialized structures, sometimes adjacent to them. In these areas there was no associated inflammation nor any massive necrosis or hemorrhage. Macrophages were sometimes present adjacent to the small foci of degeneration, acting eventually as scavenger cells [51, 59, 105, 138] (Figs. 3.7 and 3.8).

As described by James [51], resorptive degeneration was detected in both SIDS and control infants, but it was significantly more frequent in the former ($p<0.05$).

James [56] stated that there is no clear correlation between the extent or presence of degeneration and the age at death in infants. Similarly, we found that the presence of resorptive degeneration was not significantly different among age-related SIDS subgroups ($p>0.05$). James, in his original work [51], emphasized that the process is ubiquitous in the infancy period, being a normal phenomenon rather than a pathological one, but that ubiquity cannot be read as synonymous with safety or stability [59, 66]. In fact, it seems that this normal orderly process, if exaggerated, could provoke blocking disruption of the pathway itself [69, 70], and if defective could leave in place some accessory communications between the AV pathway and the adjacent ordinary myocardium [39, 105, 141, 181]. Over the years, James' studies have been confirmed by some authors [98, 139–141, 180–182, 200, 201], but have been considered inconclusive by others [3–5, 205, 207]. Davies et al. [24] pointed out that there is no association between resorptive degeneration and sudden infant death, the process being present equally in SIDS and control infants. Valdés-Dapena et al. [207], Anderson et al. [4] and Lie et al. [94] described fetal dispersion of the AV node without evidence of cell death, phagocytosis or replacement fibrosis. Thiene [203] concluded that the search needs to be continued for a better definition of what is normal and what is abnormal in the conduction system of the infant heart. Resorptive degeneration remains a contentious issue and in a commentary on a cardiac conduction study in a large series of SIDS cases [105], Anderson [3] questioned the definition of "resorptive degeneration" itself.

James [52–59] first introduced the concept of resorptive degeneration as a process of postnatal molding occurring in infants. Being resorptive degeneration found also in perinatal cases [155–157, 162], it is instead to be consider both a peri- and post-natal process that, if defective can leave in place accessory pathways, and if exaggerated can cause hypoplasia of the conduction system, as morphological substrates for both infant and perinatal sudden and unexpected death.

4.1.2 Atrioventricular Node and Bundle of His Dispersion/ Septation

The dispersion or septation of the AV node and/or HB is characterized by fragmentation of the main node/bundle within the central fibrous body [66, 105, 182, 201]. The consequences of this alteration should be intrahissian slowing of the conduction rate producing reentrants, increased automaticity, and paroxysmal block due to fractionation of transmission of the impulse, ventricular arrhythmias and sudden death [64–66, 174].

Dispersion or septation of the HB has been observed in 33% of SIDS infants and in 17% of control infants, without a statistically significant difference ($p > 0.05$) (Fig. 3.8). Being present in both groups, therefore, the HB dispersion cannot be implicated as an unequivocal cause of crib death. Ho and Anderson [44] found HB dispersion and molding in a higher proportion of hearts from controls than from infants dying suddenly and unexpectedly.

AVN dispersion/septation [105, 147] has been detected in 7% of SIDS infants, while has been not detected in control infants. Dispersion or septation of the AV junction was observed in 64.5% of SPUD victims and in 53% of the control cases, with no statistically significant difference [155, 157].

As for the septate/dispersed HB, the consequences of this alteration could be a deceleration of the conduction speed with the phenomenon of reentry, increased automaticity, blocking due to the splitting of the transmission of the impulse, ventricular arrhythmias, and sudden death [9, 147].

4.1.3 Persistent Fetal Dispersion

The islands of conduction tissue in the central fibrous body, designated as persistent fetal dispersion, have been described as islands of the conduction system separated from the AV node and HB, dispersed in the central fibrous body, resembling the normal fetal pattern [55, 66].

Islands of conduction tissue in the fibrous body were found in 25% of SIDS and in 17% of control infants, and in 80% of SIUD and in 73% of age-matched controls. These islands of conduction system were separated from the AVN and HB, dispersed in the central fibrous body, resembling the normal fetal pattern [55, 66, 146] (Fig. 3.8). No statistically significant difference was observed between the SIDS/SIUD and control groups ($p > 0.05$).

Davies et al. [24] and Suàrez-Mier and Gamallo [201] postulated that fetal dispersion and HB fragmentation may be a normal variation present for many years in life, and must not be considered the anatomic substrate for arrhythmias and sudden death without electrocardiographic abnormalities.

According to James [57, 64, 65], the persistent fetal dispersion would represent a suitable anatomic substrate for reentrant pathways, dissociation of the conduction impulse and paroxysmal tachycardias. If the dispersed fragments of conducting tissue are separated from the AV node or HB but remain attached to the crest of the interventricular septum, their cytological content and anatomic location would serve as parasystolic foci with either spontaneous or triggered automatic rhythms, and thus they would serve as abnormal foci of automaticity [57, 58].

4.1.4 Accessory Pathways

Frequent alterations in the cardiac conduction system are represented by accessory pathways, the Mahaim (Fig. 3.9), Kent, and James fibers. These fibers, under particular conditions and under autonomic neural stimulation, may underlie potentially lethal arrhythmias. These arrhythmias are generally junctional reentrant in nature, and are actually the most frequent in fetuses and infants [52, 105, 181, 204, 216, 217].

The accessory AV pathways can play an important role as the pathogenetic background to a significant number of cardioarrhythmogenic SIDS victims [105, 147, 154–157]. The uncommonly numerous group of SIDS and SPUD victims studied exhibited, as unique histopathological evidence, accessory AV communications, which, however, were "silent" at the clinical level, since they lacked ECG-confirmed tachyarrhythmias [105, 191]. Most of the high-risk tachyarrhythmias in term fetuses and early infancy show the typical ECG of a junctional reentry, together with the inherent implications of a potential or actual degeneration into ventricular fibrillation [191, 216, 217].

4.1.4.1 Mahaim Fibers

The Mahaim fibers, first described in 1938 by Mahaim et al. [97], are specialized accessory pathways connecting the AV junction and the upper ventricular septum. The Mahaim fibers are subdivided into superior (nodo-ventricular), middle (fascicular-ventricular) and inferior (bifurcation-ventricular), depending if the accessory pathway connects to the ventricle the AVN, bundle of His or bifurcation respectively. They are associated with forms of pre-excitation syndrome [144, 177, 180–183].

It seems that whenever the physiological process of resorptive degeneration fails or slows down, some peripheral bundles of the conduction system remain connected to the common myocardial tissue of the ventricular septum, configuring the Mahaim fibers [139, 144, 180, 182]. These fibers, under particular conditions and/or neuro-vegetative stimuli, may cause potentially malignant junctional arrhythmias [147, 182, 183, 189], described in cases of sudden infant and perinatal death [19, 39, 138, 154–157, 162, 178, 180–182].

Suàrez-Mier and Aguilera [200] found Mahaim fibers in 16% of SIDS cases and in none of the control infants. Mahaim fibers have been detected in 23% of SIDS and in 8% of control infants and in 20% of SIUD victims, while they were absent in the age-matched control cases [157] (Fig. 3.9). When there is a working accessory AV connection, the whole AV system or its junctional tract, can become part of a classic circuit of a tachycardic macroloop. The preexcitation depends on the presence of AV accessory pathways where the impulse can diffuse in an antegrade direction, and thus this type of accessory pathway may be responsible for death in SIDS and SPUD victims.

4.1.4.2 James Fibers

The James fibers were described in 1961 by James [50], whose name is the eponym now used to describe them. They are atriofascicular accessory pathways connecting the atrium with the AVN or the bundle of His. James fibers have been observed in 2% of SIDS infants and in none of the SPUD victims nor of the age-matched controls. The pathogenetic significance of the mediate bundles of James type is unclear, but together with the Mahaim fibers, they are considered to be related to the Lown-Ganong-Levine (LGL) syndrome [95, 185, 188].

4.1.4.3 Kent Fibers

A defective resorptive degeneration that may rarely result in accessory pathways between the atrial and ventricular myocardium [180, 182], the Kent fibers representing the anatomical substrate for the pre-excitation syndrome originally described by Wolff, Parkinson and White [215], detected in 2% of SIDS infants, but not found in any of the SPUD victims nor in age-matched control cases.

The Kent fibers, first described in 1893 by Kent [74], are accessory pathways that have an arrhythmogenic action, since they provide direct communication between the atrium and the ventricle, bypassing the classic conduction system pathway. This Kent bundle allows the passage of a faster impulse than that continuing in the normal conduction system pathway, since the deceleration of the AVN has been bypassed. This could result in serious tachyarrhythmias, i.e., a ventricular tachycardic preexcitement and atrial retrograde excitement through the Kent bundle. The presence of this bundle does not mean that it necessarily conducts an impulse bypassing the AVN to prematurely excite the HB, since the AVN and HB can conduct the impulse only in a retrograde and/or intermittent way [180, 186, 189]. Moreover, a more rapid conduction in the bypass would produce excitement in the HB before the impulse could reach the ventricle through the AVN; in such a case, a simultaneous diffusion of the impulse both toward the HB, or toward the AVN, could result in fusion of the ventricular complex (delta wave) [175, 186, 187, 214].

4.1.5 Cartilaginous Meta/Hyperplasia

A cartilaginous metahyperplasia of the central fibrous body [147, 182] was detected in 6% of SIDS infants and in 4% of control infants, in 20% of SPUD victims and in 18% of age-matched controls, without a statistically significant difference ($p > 0.05$) between the sudden infant/perinatal death and control groups (Fig. 3.10).

The central fibrous body in adult humans is a structure composed by dense collagen, while in fetuses and infants is soft and gelatinous in consistency [55, 174]. Since the AV node lies directly upon the central fibrous body and the HB courses through it, they both seem to be in some jeopardy because of their proximity when an alteration of the central fibrous body is present [53, 55]. In particular, a central fibrous body presenting with cartilaginous metahyperplasia could potentially have provoked compression of the HB and the conduction system in many cases of SIDS [105, 147, 178] as well as in SPUD victims [155–157].

The fibroblasts of the central fibrous body seem to have a pluripotential nature, although the functional meaning of this is still unknown [55, 105]. In normal circumstances they produce dense collagen, but there are examples of cartilage or sometimes even bone present in the central fibrous body [34, 66]. It is reasonable that the fibroblasts of the fibrous body, essential to complete the morphogenesis of the adjoining AV node and HB, may sometimes work improperly, becoming both hyperactive and inactive. If they are able to produce media different from collagen, they could also show metaplastic transformation. What could induce such metaplasia is unknown, although it could logically be suspected that it is a consequence of physical stress, ischemia or other unknown factors [33, 147], considering that the synthesis of the DNA of the cartilaginous cells is stimulated by oscillating electric fields [170].

Ferris and Aherne [34] described two infants dying unexpectedly with the *post mortem* findings of nodules of fibrocartilage within the central fibrous body adjacent to the HB and AV node. James [57] reported that cartilaginous or bony metaplasia in infants suffering sudden and unexpected death originates from the pluripotential fibroblasts of the fibrous body, but their role in causing death is not yet entirely understood.

4.1.6 Hemorrhage of the Cardiac Conduction System

Hemorrhage of the conducting tissue characterized by red blood cells seen in the intercellular spaces [4, 179] was detected in 16% of SIDS infants, in 7% of SPUD victims and in 9% of age-matched controls [105, 147, 155, 157]. In some cases the red cells were widely dispersed over an area of specialized myocardium, in others discrete clumps of red cells were present enclosing several working as well as specialized myocardial fibers. Since an emergency resuscitation effort was made in most of the analyzed infants, Rossi et al. [179] considered that the hemorrhage occurred after death, due to injury caused by the attempted resuscitation efforts, but the hemorrhage of the conducting tissue was also detected in fetuses who died *in utero* [155, 157], clearly without undergoing resuscitation maneuvers. Other investigators [4, 71, 94, 200], found hemorrhagic lesions in SIDS infants, but they did not analyze perinatal cases. Hemorrhages of the conduction system caused by injury during external cardiac massage have been reported in the literature underlying the danger of this resuscitative maneuver if it is carried out in an overly vigorous fashion [111, 114, 151].

4.1.7 Intramural Right Bundle Branch

An intramural right bundle branch was present, respectively, in 20% and 25% of SIDS and control infants, in 6.5% and in 5% of SPUD and age-matched controls, and the differences were not significant ($p>0.05$). In SIDS infants dying from 3 to 60 days an intramural right bundle was more frequent than in those dying from 61 to 120 days ($p=0.01$). James [57] reported the intramural right bundle as a normal variation in the location of the right bundle branch. An intramural right bundle, like an intramural left bundle branch [176], might be vulnerable to an impaired blood supply by the nutrient arteries [157].

4.1.8 Left-Sided Bundle of His

A left-sided HB was present in 20% of SIDS infants and in 8% of explained death infants [105], without a statistically significant difference. In 2% of SIDS infants the HB was left-sided and intramural (Fig. 3.12). A left-sided bundle of His was detected in 7% of SPUD cases and in none of the age-matched controls [157]. Bharati et al. [12] observed a left-sided HB significantly more commonly in crib death infants (53%) than in explained death infants (25%), suggesting that this may be a factor promoting crib death. A left-sided HB has been described in association with sudden death in previously healthy individuals [9, 12] and in young asthmatics [10]. Massing and James [101] found a left-sided HB in 62.5% of normal human hearts of various ages.

4.1.9 Intramural Left Bundle Branch

An intramural left bundle [176] was observed in 2% of SIDS infants and in none of the control infants (Figs. 3.6 and 3.12). Rossi [176] reported that an intramural left bundle branch is comparatively more vulnerable to an impaired blood supply through the nutrient arteries.

4.1.10 Septation of the Bifurcation

Septation of the bifurcation, also known as anomalous bifurcation, characterized by interposition of fibrous tissue of the central fibrous body in the His bundle bifurcation [105, 182], was detected in 13% of SIDS infants and was not found in control infants (Fig. 3.13). These changes might be responsible for death in SIDS infants due to the fractionation of the cardiac impulse transmission within the His bundle bifurcation, resulting in conduction decrease, reentrants, increased automaticity, paroxysmal block, and sudden death.

4.1.11 Hypoplasia of the Cardiac Conduction System

A SAN hypoplasia [12, 182] was found in 6% of SIDS infants (Fig. 3.6) and in 3% of SPUD victims, but was not found in explained death controls [105, 155]. Studies of the cardiac conduction system in crib death are usually directed towards the AV node and HB, but clearly alterations of the SAN may also be involved. Ho et al. [45] described three perinatal infants with a hypoplastic sinus node and cardiac arrhythmia immediately before death. They considered the hypoplasia of the sinus node as due to an arrest or defect in development rather than due to an active degenerative process. Kozakewich et al. [77], examining the sinus node of 30 crib death and 18 explained death infants, found no difference in size between the two groups, but found intimal lesions of the sinus node intranodal artery in three crib death infants.

Hypoplasia of the HB was detected in 5% of SIDS infants and in none of the control infants (Fig. 3.6) [105].

Hypoplasia of the central fibrous body [155, 157] was detected in 7% of the SPUD victims while it was absent in age-matched controls. This abnormality seems to be a defective development rather than an active processes caused by an exaggerated processes of resorptive degeneration. Daliento et al. [23] reported two siblings presenting with an hypoplasia of the central fibrous body associated with accessory pathways and suggested these hypoplasias were part of a malformative complex.

4.1.12 Atrioventricular Node/Bundle of His Dualism

The AV node and/or the HB show a dualism when they appear stratified into two portions by interposition of a fibrous diaphragm, so configuring the morphological basis of dual AV pathways [105, 142, 147].

An AVN dualism or split AVN was present in 3% of our SIDS infants (Fig. 3.14), all in the SIDS subgroup who died at between 3 and 120 days of life, and in none of the explained death infants (Fig. 3.6).

A HB dualism or split HB was present in 3% of SIDS infants and in 4% of the control infants.

Bharati et al. [11] described a distinct AV node-like structure on the parietal wall of the right atrium in a patient with a history of paroxysmal supraventricular tachycardia.

4.1.13 Zahn Node

The Zahn node, whose name refers to Zahn's original studies in 1912 [210, 219] is also known as the coronary sinus node because it is situated near the myocardium of the coronary sinus outlet [102, 174]. In 1957, Doerr [26] presented a large illustration of a Zahn node represented as a Y-shaped bundle of loosely arranged myocardial fibers embracing a neurovegetative ganglion and protruding from an "atrial tail" of the AV node, close to the coronary sinus. Doerr and Schiebler [27] recognized that it is difficult to decide whether a coronary sinus node can be considered as a separate entity of the conducting system or only as the dorsal atrial part of the AV node.

A Zahn node was present in 3% of the SIDS infants but in none of the control infants (Fig. 3.6). In these infants, close to the major axis of the AVN, a formation of small myocytes, lengthened or stellate in shape, arranged with a muscular network was observed, morphologically definable as a small AVN. A typical feature of a Zahn node is a posterosuperior prolongation with a pseudohissian fascicle. Matturri et al. [102] reported a SIDS case in which a Zahn node has a plausible substrate for reentry tachyarrhythmias in SIDS.

4.1.14 Apoptosis Expression in the Conducting Tissue

The programmed cell death called apoptosis is of particular interest for its occurrence in the cardiac conduction system that plays a role in the pathogenesis of crib death [20, 59, 61–63, 106, 145, 147], as well as in SPUD [155, 157].

The apoptotic indices (AI) in the cardiac conduction system of SIDS infants (range 0.80–4.50, mean ± SEM 2.45 ± 0.44) and of controls (range 2.79–3.00, mean ± SEM 2.89 ± 0.05) were found to show no statistically significant difference ($p > 0.05$, Student's *t* test), while in the resorptive degeneration areas the AI was higher in the controls than in the SIDS infants ($p < 0.05$, Student's *t* test), but not in SIUD cases. The SAN in both groups showed an AI similar to that of the common myocardium. The AI was higher in the AVN, HB and the initial tract of the bundle branches than in the common myocardium ($p < 0.05$, Student's *t* test) [106, 147]. In almost all cases, TUNEL labeling was detected in the peripheral region of the AVN, close to the atrial myocardium (Fig. 3.16). This is in agreement with the observations of James [54] who reported that the AV node, during postnatal morphogenesis, becomes smaller towards its adult configuration, being reabsorbed mainly at its periphery and almost always along its left margin, and that apoptosis is a major and possibly the main mechanism by which cell death occurs during the postnatal morphogenesis of the cardiac conduction system [59].

The postnatal morphogenesis of the sinus node by apoptosis also occurs generally in the same time period, the first year of life, as the postnatal morphogenesis of the AV node and HB. This involves multifocal cell death by apoptosis and could serve to distort further the normal rhythm of the baby's heart. While the changes in the AV node and HB are mainly smoothing of the margins of these two structures, eliminating surplus tissue that may be dangerous if not removed, the changes in the sinus node are quite different, amounting more or less to a total restructuring of the interior of the sinus node itself. The fetus and the infant have sinus nodes composed primarily of P cells, whereas the sinus node of the adult human always contains a mixture of slender cells and P cells. The changes occur either by transformation of some of the P cells to slender cells or by the death of P cells to be replaced by slender cells, perhaps migrating in from the margins of the sinus node [59, 62]. Cardiac arrhythmias, such as atrial fibrillation or atrial flutter, as well as distortions in sinus rhythm, including episodes of sinus arrest or tachycardia or ectopic beading, are facilitated by impaired activity of the sinus node during this molding process of the conducting tissue that occurs mostly in the first year of postnatal life, creating an electrically instable heart.

In both infants and fetuses the apoptosis of the cardiac conduction system of the developing heart could be a process favoring electrical instability in two opposite ways: deficit and exaggeration. On one hand, a defective apoptosis could leave in place some accessory communication between the AV pathway and the adjacent ordinary myocardium, and would leave the sinus node in its fetal configuration, eliminating the beneficial evolution into an appropriate mixture and distribution of P cells among slender cells [59, 139, 147]. On the other hand, an exaggerated apoptosis, could provoke blocking disruption of the pathway itself, and disfigure the sinus node structure or even completely destroy it [59, 69, 70, 182]. Kajstura et al. [73], in their study in rats on programmed cell death found that myocyte death is absent in the fetal heart but affects the myocardium postnatally, particularly the right ventricle but they did not study the cardiac conduction system.

4.1.15 PCNA Expression in the Conducting Tissue

Although for years many experimental cell kinetic studies have demonstrated that the number of proliferating myocytes in the mammalian heart is high during embryogenesis, but gradually decreases becoming similar to a "non-dividing" tissue [7, 99], the several studies [6, 143, 193] show that, in some pathological conditions, myocardial cells are able to express PCNA and nuclear mitotic division, especially in fetuses and infants. This prompted to hypothesize that, during the pre- and postnatal cardiac process of molding/resorptive degeneration, cell death could be accompanied by cell proliferation. However, in both the SIDS and the control groups there were no findings of positive PCNA immunoreactivity either in the conducting system or in the common myocardium [106]. Kajstura et al. [73] found that in rats the DNA synthesis in myocytes decreases postnatally.

4.1.16 ECG Findings

One or more electrocardiograms were available in 15% of SIDS infants. A careful clinicopathological and electrocardiographic correlation is particularly important and always should to be done. Schwartz et al. [196], in their prospective study, performed follow-up ECG in an unselected population of 33,034 infants. They found that prolongation of the QT interval in the first week of life is strongly associated with SIDS. However, Schwartz et al. [196] did not consider the *post mortem* histopathological findings in the SIDS cases, whose diagnosis relies on autopsy which is also obviously considered of great importance long QT (LQT) syndrome [11, 60, 68, 184]. In particular, James [60] studied in detail the pathophysiological significance of the conduction morphological abnormalities in LQT syndrome. According to the most recent expert consensus statement on inherited primary arrhythmias syndromes [165], the diagnoses of LQT, Brugada syndrome, catecholaminergic polymorphic ventricular tachycardia, short QT syndrome, early relarization, progressive cardiac conduction disease, and unexplained cardiac arrest are all based on ECG recordings, even in absence of a pathogenic mutation found with genetic tests.

4.1.17 Coronary and Cardiac Conduction Arteries

The histopathological examination of the serially sectioned coronary arteries and cardiac conduction arteries from infants and fetuses who died suddenly and unexpectedly revealed the frequent presence of preatherosclerotic lesions, indicating the atherogenic effect of cigarette smoke (Fig. 3.19) [116, 117, 121, 133].

Both intrauterine and postnatal exposure to cigarette smoke appear to increase the risk of sudden death in infancy [86, 136]. Nicotine seems to interact directly with the endogenous nicotinic and muscarinic cholinergic receptors present in the brainstem regions involved in cardio-respiratory activity, jeopardizing their normal function in vulnerable subjects.

The consequences of formula feeding are also significant. The coronary and cardiac conduction system artery lesions were larger and more diffuse in formulated infants whose parents both smoked. The combination of both risk factors seems to increase the early atherogenic effect of each noxa [116].

Early and severe atherogenic action of both baby formula and cigarette smoke was demonstrable in the cardiac conduction system arteries as well as in the coronary walls of infants. The association of the two atherogenic noxae results in a cumulative effect [117]. On the other hand, according to the American Academy of Pediatrics' policy statement, maternal smoking, while it should be strongly discouraged, is not an absolute contraindication to breastfeeding [1].

Fibromuscular hyperplasia or dysplasia [58] of the sinus node and/or AV node arteries has been described as a cause of death in young people and adults [66, 67]. Anderson and Hill [2], analyzing 40 victims of crib death, found five infants (12.5%) with increased thickness of the AV artery and one infant with reduced thickness of the sinus node artery. The authors hypothesized that this thickness may explain ischemia of the conducting tissue with consequent cardiac arrhythmias and/or heart block.

Early preatherosclerotic lesions of the SAN and/or AVN arteries were detected in 21% of infants (Fig. 3.15). This percentage is much higher than that found by Suàrez-Mier and Aguilera (1.8%) [200] and more similar to that found by Anderson and Hill (12.5%) [2].

It has been suggested that these lesions should be regarded as "initial preatherosclerotic lesions" instead of "fibromuscular hyperplasia" or "dysplasia" of the cardiac conduction system arteries [117].

In the cardiac conduction system arteries, the early atherosclerotic lesions are already detectable in fetuses and early infancy and might have a significant role in determining sudden unexpected death. These results suggest the importance of studying suitable strategies for eliminating the risk factors, i.e. parents smoking and lack of breast feeding in infants, thus preventing the development and progression of early atherosclerotic lesions [116, 117].

4.1.17.1 Infants

The histological examination of serially sectioned coronary arteries revealed the frequent presence, in 61% of SIDS infants, of initial atherosclerotic lesions, indicating the atherogenic effect of passive cigarette smoke.

The severity of the lesions ranged from initial preatherosclerotic alterations, mainly affecting the anterior descending branch of the left coronary artery, observed in 30.5% of infants, to juvenile soft plaques, which can be so extensive as to reduce the arterial lumen by up to 30–40%. These soft plaques were observed in all the coronary walls of 30.5% of infants.

The morphological appearance of the preatherosclerotic lesions varies in relation to the type of atherogenic noxa. In infants in whom the atherogenic factor is related exclusively to cigarette smoke, particularly if the mother smoked before becoming pregnant, the lesions can usually be detected very early, within the first few months of life. Another notable feature is the structural disorder of the tunica media, which appears to be fragmented and is also the site of intense proliferation. The myointimal thickening consists predominantly of smooth muscle cell (SMC) infiltrates, rare monocytes and B lymphocytes. The deposits of amorphous material, which contribute to the myointimal thickening, are made up of acid mucopolysaccharides (Fig. 3.19) [113].

Both intrauterine and postnatal exposure to cigarette smoke increase the risk of SIDS [93, 113]. Nicotine seems to interact directly with the endogenous nicotinic and muscarinic cholinergic receptors present in the brainstem regions involved in cardio-respiratory activity, jeopardizing their normal function in vulnerable subjects [76].

The consequences of formula feeding may also be significant. Recently, the AAP [1] reaffirmed its recommendation of exclusive breast feeding for at least the first 6 months of life, to avoid the serious damage caused by formula feeding. Maternal milk contains long-chain polyunsaturated fatty acids (LCPUFAs) which are necessary for the normal development of many tissues [49]. The positive effects of breast feeding have also been demonstrated with regard to SIDS, whose incidence is lowered by 36% in breastfed infants [48].

The coronary lesions were larger and more diffuse in formula-fed infants whose parents both smoked. The combination of both risk factors seems to increase the atherogenic effect of each noxa. The association of the two atherogenic noxae appears to have a cumulative effect and leads to the early development of typical atherosclerotic plaques [116].

4.1.17.2 Fetuses

The morphological pattern of preatherosclerotic coronary artery lesions in human fetuses and the possible atherogenic role of maternal cigarette smoking before and during pregnancy have been reported [113].

In the literature, the few studies carried out on fetal coronary arteries have predominantly been performed in experimental animals. Bolande et al. [14] observed that proliferative modifications of the coronary arteries are present in 100% of piglet fetuses and regress after birth, and they conclude that such lesions represent a physiological developmental process and therefore cannot be related to coronary atherogenesis in the adult.

The rare studies of the coronary arteries of human fetuses in the literature yield controversial findings and date back over 50 years. In 1957, Moon [134] did not observe any pathological process, while a few years later, Robertson [171] reported an altered architecture of the coronary walls only in fetuses at term.

The results of our histopathological study performed on the major epicardial coronary arteries, serially sectioned, from a considerable number of late stillborns, have demonstrated the incidence and characteristics of intimal preatherosclerotic lesions of proliferative appearance and the possible role of maternal cigarette smoking. In particular, in the early atherosclerotic process, the intima at first appears to be infiltrated by SMCs which, due to loss of polarity, seem to be arranged in a column perpendicular to the main axis of the media. The longitudinally oriented SMCs probably originate from the media but they are intimal structures. Only later the intimal thickening contains acid mucopolysaccharide deposits, probably synthesized by SMCs, that give an edematous appearance to the subendothelial connective tissue. Few monocytes are present [113] (Fig. 3.20). Intimal preatherosclerotic lesions of proliferative appearance were observed in 55% of stillborns, 83% of which had mothers who smoked.

In 9% of fetuses and in 4% of infants of non-smoking parents, but living in highly industrialized areas the lesions were similar to those detected in fetuses and infants of smoker mothers. Noteworthy is also the possible atherogenic effects of air pollution [123].

Molecular biology analyses have made it possible to clarify the biological nature of the observed coronary wall alterations. These studies revealed intense activation of the protooncogene c-fos in the smooth muscle cells of the media, and in some of these, positivity for apoptosis was observed, suggesting that c-fos overexpression may promote proliferation, as evidenced by PCNA-positive cells [87, 133].

The c-fos gene belongs to the family of immediate early genes, so defined for their ability to be rapidly activated in many tissues in response to various injuries, because they do not require protein synthesis. Therefore, c-fos positivity in fetal coronary lesions represents the first biological reaction in response to the gaseous products of nicotine combustion. By crossing the cellular membrane, particularly of the SMCs, the nicotine products can directly modify the expression of the c-fos gene, interacting with nuclear receptors [87].

It has been demonstrated that very early preatherosclerotic alterations of the coronary arteries are already detectable in the prenatal period and are significantly associated with maternal cigarette smoking even before the beginning of pregnancy [113].

The studies on the passive cigarette smoke effects already detectable in fetuses have allowed description of the features of the initial coronary atherosclerotic lesions and their progression in infancy if the passive smoke exposure persists. Alterations ranged from focal areas with mild myointimal thickening in prenatal life to early soft parietal plaques in infants. The fetus represents the ideal model for the evaluation of the passive cigarette smoke effects, and also to re-exame the actual concept on the natural history of the atherosclerotic process [118, 119, 133].

4.1.18 Other Cardiac Findings

In some cases submitted to the *post mortem* investigation with the clinical suspicion of SIDS, an explained cardiac cause of death was identified, such as cardiac fibroma, or hypertrophic cardiomyopathy, complicated with ischemia, or myocardial infarction (Figs. 3.23 and 3.24).

Valdés-Dapena and Gilbert-Barness [206] have pointed out that cardiac causes for sudden infant death include viral myocarditis, congenital heart disease particularly congenital aortic stenosis, endocardial fibroelastosis, and anomalous origin of the left coronary artery from the pulmonary artery. Other cardiac conditions that may result in sudden death include rhabdomyomas of the heart in tuberous sclerosis and conduction system disorders. Frequent conduction system disorders resulting in sudden death include histiocytoid cardiomyopathy, congenital heart block that may be associated with maternal lupus erythematosus, arrhythmogenic right ventricular dysplasia, and the long QT syndrome.

4.1.19 Long QT Syndrome

The long QT (LQT) syndrome is mostly a familiar disease that affects one every 2,000 individuals and is characterized by a prolonged QT interval on ECG, usually longer than 440 ms for males and 460 ms for females. The LQT syndrome is a potentially fatal condition, with increased risk for serious arrhythmias, i.e., ventricular tachycardias and torsade de pointes, which may degenerate into ventricular fibrillation, torsadogenic-mediated syncope, and sudden death [37].

The hereditary LQT syndrome is mostly an autosomic dominant genetic disorder, the so-called Romano-Ward syndrome (R-W), but can also be transmitted as autosomal recessive, denominated Jervell and Lange-Nielsen syndrome (J-LN), characterized by the coexistence of congenital QT prolongation and deafness [164]. The LQT syndrome has marked incomplete penetrance and variable expressivity and is predominantly caused by mutations in at least 12 known genes involved in the function of ion channels in the heart. There are seven known types of inherited LQT syndrome, types 1 through 7. The most common types are LQT1, LQT2, and LQT3. Three major susceptibility genes account for about 75% of cases of LQT syndrome: *KCNQ1/LQT1* in 30–35% of cases; *KCNH2/LQT2* in 25–30% of cases, and *SCN5A/LQT3* in 5–10% of cases [37, 173, 202].

A notable example of multifocal apoptotic degeneration of the sinus node occurs in victims dying of the LQT syndrome, a clinical entity characterized by sinus bradycardia [60, 68]. Sudden unexpected death is one of the clinical characteristics of the LQT syndrome and has often been found to be mediated by lethal ventricular arrhythmias. According to James [69], it can be anticipated that the normal occurrence of apoptotic cell death during postnatal morphogenesis of the sinus node will periodically distort or suppress the normal sinus rhythm. Furthermore, in the LQT syndrome apoptotic destruction involves not only the myocytes of the sinus node but also many local nerves and ganglia [60, 68].

The QT prolongation could be dangerous in infants [41, 164, 198] and fetuses [21, 22] and a possible cause of their fatal arrhythmia.

In 1957, Jervell and Lange-Nielsen [72] described four children suffering from prolonged QT interval, hearing deficits and sudden cardiac death with an autosomal recessive inheritance, later called the Jervell and Lange-Nielsen syndrome.

In 1963, Romano et al. [172] and in 1964 Ward [211] separately described the more common variant of LQT syndrome with normal hearing and autosomal dominant inheritance, later called the Romano-Ward syndrome.

In 1976, Maron et al. [100] and Schwartz et al. [195] first introduced the hypothesis that the QT prolongation could be responsible for some SIDS cases.

In 1998, Schwartz et al. [196], in a 19-year prospective study, performed follow-up electrocardiography in an unselected population of over 33,000 infants, and concluded that congenital prolongation of the QT interval accounts for a proportion of SIDS cases. Their results underline the potential value of neonatal electrocardiographic screening for an early identification of a prolonged long QT interval and consequent preventive treatment of the affected infants. However, Schwartz et al. [196, 197] admitted that the LQT syndrome may account for only a fraction of the crib death cases, and precise quantification of this fraction remains difficult despite the data obtained from their large epidemiological study. Guntheroth and Spiers [40] stated that submitting all infants and newborns to electrocardiographic screening would be ineffective and a waste of medical resources, and it would cruelly alarm thousands of parents.

Further close clinicopathogenetic analogies with arrhythmogenic lethal late repolarization, attended by fetal developmental impairments of the conduction system, often resulting in accessory AV pathways, in SIDS and SPUD have been documented to be consistent with junctional tachycardia [190, 191]. An important report, in this connection, is that of Kuo et al. [78] who emphasize the possible role of the conduction system among the ontogenetic substrates of the Ito abnormalities. This genetic clinicopathological suggestion is further substantiated by studies on the life-threatening potential of WPW syndrome, whose common accessory AV pathway substrate was proven occasionally to have a genetic association [8, 38].

Since 2000, Viskin et al. [209] recommended genetic screening in every case of probable LQT syndrome, and stated that a positive result will confirm the diagnosis but that no mutations are found in many patients with a definite diagnosis of LQT syndrome, so a negative result is not very helpful. In any case, genetic testing might take months.

Sudden unexpected perinatal death can occur more frequently in fetuses and infants of mothers suffering positive for anti-SSA/anti-Ro or anticardiolipin antibodies, due to AV blocks and severe autoimmune reaction of the AV junction tissue [18, 148, 192]. Despite the emphasis given to the possibly lethal association of maternal autoantibodies and QT prolongation, once again no conclusions can be reached if the postmortem examination does not included the study of the cardiac conduction system and the brainstem on serial sections.

In 2013, Cuneo et al. [22] reported that an arrhythmia phenotype during fetal life suggests an LQT syndrome genotype. Thus, prenatal arrhythmia phenotype suggests prenatal and neonatal management while awaiting the results of genetic testing.

4.2 Advances in Neuropathology

Among the most important pathogenetic theories of SIDS (respiratory, cardiac, and visceral dyskinetic), the congenital and acquired abnormalities of the central nervous system, particularly of the brainstem have been attracting the greatest interest.

4.2.1 Hypoplasia and Agenesis of the Arcuate Nucleus

In SIDS mono- or bilateral hypoplasia or even agenesis of the arcuate nucleus (ARCn) was found to be particularly frequent, as it occurs in about 50% of the SIDS and SPUD victims (Figs. 3.25 and 3.26) [81, 109, 112, 120, 127].

The ARCn is a bulbar chemosensitive nucleus which takes part in the regulation of cardio-respiratory activity [35, 75, 81, 107, 109]. This anatomic site, relevant to the central cardiopulmonary hypothesis in SIDS and SPUD, is located near the surface of the ventrolateral, ventral, and ventromedial medulla oblongata [137]. This region is an integrative site for autonomic function, ventilation, and chemosensitivity. It contains sympathetic premotor pressor and depressor zones which regulate blood pressure, cardiac rate and rhythm, and hemodynamic aspects of temperature regulation, as well as neurons which integrate "defense" responses [35].

A high frequency of hypoplasia of the ARCn occurs in fetuses who died *sine causa* (SIUD) in a similar manner to that observed in SIDS, as well as in newborns (SNUD) who died suddenly and unexpectedly [81, 88, 109, 112, 116, 135].

The study of ARCn cellular maturation suggests that in some SIDS infants even an architecturally well-developed ARCn could have a pattern of anomalous neuronal differentiation. Such a maturation defect may be related to developmental disorders of the ARCn chemoreceptor function and consequently to respiratory regulation impairment [110].

Cigarette smoking is significantly associated with structural alterations of the ARCn, i.e., bilateral hypoplasia, monolateral hypoplasia, partial hypoplasia, delayed neuronal maturation, decreased neuronal density [81].

4.2.2 Combined Pulmonary and Brainstem Hypodevelopment

Using specific macro- and microscopic criteria, the presence of pulmonary hypoplasia in 65% of unexplained stillbirths has been reported. In 31% of fetuses lung hypoplasia was associated with hypoplasia of the medullary ARCn (Fig. 3.27) [112]. Pulmonary hypoplasia was detected in 85% of SIDS cases and was significantly more frequent in the SIDS group compared to the control group.

About 20% of cases presenting with both brainstem and pulmonary hypodevelopment have been exposed to passive cigarette smoke [159].

The presence of a combined ARCn and lung hypoplasia suggests that in these cases the hypoplasia of the ARCn exerts a negative effect on respiratory movements *in utero* and therefore on lung development. In fetuses in which pulmonary hypoplasia is not accompanied by hypodevelopment of this nucleus, the explanation could be a wrong physiological mechanism, more precisely a failure to block the inhibitory action on the Kölliker-Fuse nucleus exerted by the gigantocellular nucleus.

Fetal respiration appears to be a feature of mammalian development, even though it has been studied in detail only in sheep. In 1972, Dawes et al. [25] described in the fetal lamb rapid and irregular breathing movements alternating with apneic pauses of varying duration, very long in the early stages of gestation and reducing gradually thereafter in relation to pulmonary development, irrespective of the gas profile of the blood.

In 1995, experimental physiological studies by Blanco et al. [13] have shown that the predominant absence of ventilation *in utero* is determined by the inhibitory effect exerted mainly by the Kölliker-Fuse nucleus. In the fetus there is periodic disinhibition of the Kölliker-Fuse nucleus to allow breathing movements which favor pulmonary development. This interruption of inhibitory activity seems to be determined by a nucleus located in the caudal portion of the pons, the gigantocellular nucleus, which after birth has the task of intervening rhythmically to interrupt the inhibitory effect on inspiration normally exerted by the Kölliker-Fuse nucleus, and enabling expiration to start [31, 112].

Developments in magnetic resonance imaging have led to the possibility of analyzing the development of fetal lungs [163] and brainstem [29] *in utero* and therefore to the ability to diagnose both ARCn and lung hypoplasia prenatally [112]. This correlation of ARCn and lung hypoplasia has provided potentially clinically useful applications, suggesting close prenatal and postnatal monitoring in order to prevent sudden perinatal or infant death.

4.2.3 Cytoarchitectural Organization and Hypoplasia of the Parabrachial/Kölliker-Fuse Complex

In the rostral pons and caudal mesencephalon of 35% of perinatal unexplained deaths, particularly intra-partum deaths, hypoplasia with neuronal immaturity or agenesis of the parabrachial/Kölliker–Fuse (PB/KF) complex were observed [132].

The PB/KF complex has been defined in different animal species as lying in the dorsolateral part of the pontine tegmentum and is subdivided into three well-defined regions: the medial parabrachial (mPB) nucleus, the lateral parabrachial (lPB) nucleus, and the Kölliker-Fuse (KF) nucleus. Experimental studies have demonstrated that the PB/KF complex is involved in a variety of functional activities and plays an important role in respiratory activity. In humans, the impossibility of using experimental approaches makes it difficult to characterize the cytoarchitecture and the pathophysiology of these structures. Only a few studies have provided morphological data regarding the human PB complex [17, 43, 80, 84].

The *post mortem* brainstem findings confirm the hypothesis that functional or structural alterations of components of the vegetative nervous system which modulate fetal breathing may lead to disturbances in the development of the respiratory apparatus, in particular to pulmonary hypoplasia in unexplained stillbirth [108, 112]. Although irrelevant to fetal life, the chemoreceptors become of vital importance in the intrapartum and postpartum periods; therefore, when they are impaired in development, they may underlie cardioventilatory abnormalities critical to SIDS and unexplained perinatal death [82–85, 108, 112].

A relevant question concerns how this congenital anomaly may cause respiratory disturbances immediately after birth, as suggested by the examination of a well documented intrapartum case [85]. In this newborn, an anomalous position of the umbilical cord could have enhanced a chemoreceptor dysfunction and this may have been an important predisposing or contributing lethal factor. Respiratory insufficiency was seen immediately at birth, a fact that seems to indicate that the pathogenetic mechanism of respiratory death involves two factors: (1) vulnerability due to hypoplasia of the parabrachial/Kölliker-Fuse complex, and (2) an exogenous stress manifested and triggered by the trauma of birth.

The parabrachial/Kölliker-Fuse complex is a ill-understood reflex-blocking center, exerting in the fetus the life-preserving inhibitory action upon respiration. This brainstem area, in the near-term fetus accounts for the strong inhibitory action of chemoreflexogenesis that prevents potentially lethal active respiratory motions in the fetus. During a still-indefinite phase of partum, the Kölliker-Fuse nucleus quickly reverses to an active respiration-facilitating function, and it is then actually regrouped among the respiratory centers in postnatal physiology [108]. Not only may abnormalities of the respiratory chemoreceptors underlie sudden unexpected perinatal or infant death by defective regulation, but anomalous persistence of post-partum blockade or disfacilitation of respiratory fetal chemoreflexes may also play a part in the respiratory, life-threatening mechanisms of the SPUD-SIDS complex itself.

4.2.4 Brainstem Neurons Responding to Hypoxia (c-Fos-Positive)

Immunohistochemistry of c-fos applied to the medulla oblongata of SIDS victims has shown that in 60% of SIDS infants there is a high density of labeled neurons in the dorsal motor vagal nucleus [79]. The cellular changes induced by increased Fos protein in the dorsal motor vagal nucleus neurons are still unclear. According to Dony and Gruss [28], in many proliferative processes, particularly during embryonic development and in some types of tumors, the rapid activation of the c-fos gene in the presence of different noxae causes activation of other genes related to DNA synthesis. This mitogenic effect does not occur in the nerve cells. The increased Fos expression in the dorsal motor vagal nucleus neurons observed in SIDS victims could enhance the production of catecholamines, indispensable for the breathing stimuli [79]. Although the functioning of the c-fos gene remains poorly understood, the increase in fos immunoreactivity observed in SIDS infants suggests that the neurons of the dorsal motor nucleus of the vagal nerve involved in breathing regulation may yield an intense, immediate ventilatory response to hypoxia.

4.2.5 Significance of Paraganglia Hyperplasia

Paraganglia hyperplasia was detected in 25% of SIDS infants and it has been considered to be caused by prolonged hypoxia. This abnormality is not so marked in intercarotid as in mediastinal glomera. In fact, the mediastinal glomera are a part of the cardiac nerve plexus and are functionally more pertinent to the cardiocirculatory regulation [126, 166–168]. Enlargement of the aorticopulmonary paraganglia (APP) in infants dying of SIDS was confirmed by the use of morphometric techniques. Hyperplasia of the APP can be readily observed from sections under the low power objective of the microscope, but an unequivocal proof of glomic cell proliferation can only be confirmed by morphometric measurement [166].

Previous reports describe a more extensive and prominent distribution of paraganglia cells in human fetuses and infants than in adults [42]. Our results confirm this aspect: the APP of control infants were greater in number and size at birth and decreased dramatically during the first year of life. The mechanism underlying this morphological variation is not yet known. Programmed cell death may play a role in the process [42, 166]. Interactions of the ARCn with the peripheral chemoreceptors have been postulated [166]. The paraganglia hyperplasia observed in some SIDS infants could be compensatory, beginning from alterations in the central chemoreceptor mechanisms [166, 169].

Stephan-Blanchard et al. [199] measured the peripheral chemoreceptor activity at thermoneutrality in preterm neonates born to nonsmoking and smoking mothers, performing a hyperoxic test during active and quiet sleep. They reported that prenatal smoking exposure in neonates has a negative impact on peripheral chemoreceptor tonic activity, hypothesizing the presence of preexisting damage in the brainstem and cardiac conduction. The common physiopathology of sudden unexplained infant and perinatal death is attributed to impaired developmental processes in the peripheral chemoreceptors, i.e., in the carotid and aortic bodies and the aorticopulmonary paraganglia. At the functional level, a sudden death implies a defective resetting, slow or incomplete, of the sensitivity to hypoxia and hypercapnia and/or a defective processing of signals in the brainstem cardio-respiratory centers. A normal infant's nervous system receives prompt information on a progressive hypercapnia and hypoxia event, and triggers respiration or arousal. In fetuses and infants with peripheral or central chemoreception defects, these protective reflexes are not released, and prolonged apnea can develop which may be fatal and lead to sudden death. In this scenario, smoke exposure *in utero* acts as a triggering phenomenon in fetuses and infants with brainstem or cardiac conduction developmental abnormalities [160].

4.3 "Grey Zone"/ Borderline SIDS and SPUD

A case is classified as SIDS or SPUD "grey zone" or borderline when the infant or fetus dies suddenly and unexpectedly following a concomitant pathological event, itself not deadly – such as a mild leptomeningitis, a bronchus-pneumonic infection or a chorionamnionitis – that acts as a triggering phenomenon in particularly vulnerable individuals, i.e., suffering from undetected preexisting nervous autonomic or cardiac conduction alterations, such as an hypoplasia of the ARCn or a Mahaim fiber [129, 150, 158, 162].

About of 7% of SIDS and 11% of SPUD victims are classified as grey zone or borderline cases. In these borderline SIDS or SPUD victims whose microscopic examination showed specific lesions interacting with the conduction system or with the brainstem.

A multifocal Purkinje tumor near the AV node (Fig. 3.22) makes a SIDS case a grey zone or a borderline if the combination of a multifocal nodular Purkinje tumor of the heart is associated with a bilateral hypoplasia of the arcuate nucleus (ARCn). The Purkinje cell tumor alone may have or may not have accounted for the sudden death, but could have played a triggering role in this baby suffering from a hypoplastic ARCn [149].

Accessory fibers, under particular conditions and under autonomic neural stimulation, may underlie potentially lethal arrhythmias. These arrhythmias are generally junctional reentrant in nature, being actually the most frequent in the fetus and newborn [215]. Severe oxygen-consuming tachycardias can underlie, in hypoxic infants, the risk of myocardial infarction.

Inflammatory brainstem lesions, sometimes of suspected viral origin, are significant in SIDS and SPUD cases. The observation of a 4-month-old infant with a

T-lymphocytic leptomeningitis affecting the ventral medullary surface and the outer layer of a hypoplastic ARCn [103] illustrates the etiopathogenetic importance of a combined lesion of the central chemosensitive field.

Focal degeneration and necrosis of the solitary nucleus or a hypoplastic hypoglossus nucleus were observed in infants dying suddenly and unexpectedly. The impairment of the nucleus hypoglossus caused recurrent aspiration pneumonia [150, 152, 153] could be a clinically ignored infection that might have simultaneously compromised respiratory and cardiac activity, together with the kinesis of the tongue, glottis, esophagus and/or stomach. In particular, a lingual/glottic kinetic problem might have compromised the tone of the tongue, with the risk of high respiratory obstruction in the supine position, besides provoking glottic spasm and/or inspiration of gastroesophageal reflux.

Studies on the pathophysiology of SIDS have focused on the cardio-respiratory brainstem of infants, with important results pointing to a reflexogenic lethal mechanism [122, 194]. In a 4-month-old male, who suffered from deglutition and respiratory disorders the *post mortem* investigation disclosed a hemangioendothelioma located in the area postrema, which widely infiltrated the posterior–middle brainstem bilaterally, sparing only the dorsal vagal nucleus, while diffusely compromising, even cancelling, the neuronal circuitries of the hypoglossus, solitary tract, ambiguous nucleus, and the reticular formation [104]. It was evident that the baby survived 4 months because of preservation of the chemosensitive respiratory ventral medullary surface areas together with the ARCn, and the dorsal visceromotor nucleus.

The inflammatory and neoplastic infiltrates, in the cases discussed above, alone would probably not account for sudden death, but could have played a triggering role. All these observations confirm the pathological evidence and the inherent clinical implications, focused upon the cardiac conduction system and the brainstem cardiovascular and respiratory centers, whose derangement can trigger a sudden unexpected infant or perinatal death. These borderline cases seem in part consistent with the triple-risk model of SIDS [36], a hypothesis that invokes underlying biological vulnerability to exogenous stressors or triggering factors in a critical developmental period. The cases presented here seem to usefully contribute to the orientation of research in the field of sudden infant and perinatal unexplained death. Further studies on triggering factors and related mechanisms will lead to a better understanding of the complex interactions involved in the SIDS and SPUD pathophysiology.

4.4 Genetics of SIDS and SPUD

The investigation of sudden unexplained infant and perinatal death should always focus on genetic analyses, but only as a completion to the in-depth histopathology study of the brainstem and cardiac conduction system which remains mandatory.

In 1970, Weinberg et al. [212] published the first report of genetic autopsy, performing karyotype analyses in 12 SIDS cases. Only in one of these cases had a normal karyotype; the anomalous karyotypes of the other cases consisted of deletions, chromatid breaks, abnormal chromosomal association and telemeric association of unknown significance.

Only in 2003, new gene tests could disclose that cases of repeated sudden infant death within a family, initially judged to be murders, were instead proven to be cases of familial SIDS [30].

In 2013, the expert consensus recommendations [165] stated that for sudden unexplained infant death an expert cardiac pathologist "may be considered" at autopsy assessment to rule out the presence of microscopic indicators of structural heart disease. An expert cardiac pathologist assessment should instead "be mandatory" for autopsy assessment! Who else can identify or rule out the structural heart disease underlying the sudden unexplained death of infants and fetuses? Netherless it should be stressed that no conclusions on inherited primary arrhythmia syndromes can ever be drawn without an accurate *post mortem* investigation of the cardiac conduction system carried out by an expert cardiovascular pathologist.

At least five categories of genes are involved in the pathogenesis of SIDS:

1. Genes for ion channel proteins involved in cardiac channelopathies. Mutations in cardiac ion channel genes underlie many cases of inherited arrhythmia syndromes, mainly the LQT syndrome. Several mutated genes have been reported, mainly the sodium channel gene (*SCN5A*), potassium channel genes (*KCNQ1*, *KCNH12*, *KCNE2*), the RyR2-encoded caveolin-3 gene, the sodium channel beta-4 subunit gene (*SCN4B*), the glycerol-3-phosphate dehydrogenase 1-like genr (GPD1-L) [37, 46].
2. Genes for serotonin (5-hydrxytryptamine, 5-HT) transporter based on decreased serotonergic receptor binding in brainstems. The promoter long (L) allele of the serotonin transporter (5-HTT) gene was detected in 75% of SIDS compared to 30% of controls cases [130]. The presence of the L allele represents a predisposing factor for sudden perinatal and infant unexplained death in association with morphologic developmental defects of the raphé nuclei and cigarette smoke exposure [91].
3. Genes pertinent to the autonomic nervous system (ANS) development. The *EN-2* gene is a genetic marker for rhombic lip-derived structures, such as the arcuate nucleus. Its expression is very high in the arcuate nucleus neurons from the 17th to the 22nd gestational week, then decreases up to the first days after birth and later disappears [87]. Mutational or functional alterations of the *EN-2* gene have been reported in the hypoplasia of the arcuate nucleus [81].
4. Genes regulating inflammation and infections, including polymorphisms in complement C4, interleukin (IL)-6, IL-10, and vascular endothelial growth factor (VEGF) [46].
5. Genes regulating energy production, hypoglycemia, and thermal regulation. In any case of suspected SIDS or SPUD, according to Yang et al. [218], analysis of the medium-chain acyl CoA dehydrogenase (MCAD) genes is necessary to diagnose the deficiency of fatty acids β-oxidation. As suggested by Van Norstrand

et al. [208], although the MCAD deficiency can result in a sudden death in the first year of life, it is unlikely that this death will be given a diagnosis of SIDS rather than of MCAD deficiency-associated death.

In conclusion, increasing attention to the genetic studies should be addressed to identify the involvement of abnormal genes in developmental defects in the brainstem and cardiac conduction system underlying both SIDS and SPUD.

4.5 Review Questions

This test, composed of 10 multiple-choice questions, is designed to measure knowledge about the contents of this chapter on Moving Forward the Discussion on Sudden Infant and Perinatal Unexplained Death. Questions have only one correct answer and cover the major content areas of this chapter. Check the correct responses and score your test using the answer keys on page 169.

41. What is the sudden perinatal unexplained death (SPUD)?
    - □ A. Sudden perinatal unexplained death (SPUD) is the sudden unexpected death of a fetus from the 22nd gw or of a newborn since birth to the completion of the 1st month of postnatal life that remains unexplained after a thorough investigation of the case, including the review of the clinical history and the performance of a complete post mortem examination.
    - □ B. Sudden perinatal unexplained death (SPUD) is the sudden unexpected death of a term fetus from the 32nd gw or of a newborn in the first two weeks of postnatal life that remains unexplained after a thorough investigation of the case, including the review of the clinical history and the performance of a complete *post mortem* examination.
    - □ C. Sudden perinatal unexplained death (SPUD) is the sudden unexpected death of a term fetus from the 22nd gw or of a newborn since birth to the completion of the 1st month of postnatal life.
    - □ D. Sudden perinatal unexplained death (SPUD) is defined as the sudden unexpected death of a term fetus from the 22nd gw or of an infant under one year of age that remains unexplained after a thorough investigation of the case, including the review of the clinical history and the performance of a complete *post mortem* examination.
    - □ E. Sudden perinatal unexplained death (SPUD) is defined as the sudden unexpected death of a term fetus from the 22nd gw or of an infant since birth to the completion of the 1st year of postnatal life.
42. Which of the following statements on the anomalies detected in the cardiac conduction system of sudden infant statements and perinatal unexplained death is correct?
    - □ A. The anomalies of the cardiac conduction system have been detected in a similar manner both in sudden death and in control groups.
    - □ B. Some abnormalities of the cardiac conduction system, such as the sinoatrial node hypoplasia, Mahaim, James and Kent fibers, Zahn node have

been detected only in the SIDS-SPUD groups and not in the age-matched controls.

- □ C. Resorptive degeneration has been detected only in SIDS cases and ins absent in age-matched controls.
- □ D. Mahaim fibers has been detected exclusively in SIDS cases and are absent in age-matched controls.
- □ E. Resorptive degeneration has been detected exclusively in SIDS and in SPUD cases and is absent in age-matched controls.

43. What is the resorptive degeneration and what is its possible role in SIDS-SPUD?
    - □ A. Resorptive degeneration is itself a pathological process that has been detected only in SIDS and SPUD cases and has been absent in age-matched controls.
    - □ B. Resorptive degeneration is itself a pathological process, detected in cases of SIDS or SPUD and always responsible for sudden death, as it can account for peripheral bundles of the conduction system that remain connected to the common myocardial tissue of the ventricular septum, the so-called Mahaim fibers.
    - □ C. Resorptive degeneration is itself a physiological process that can become pathological if it is defective, lacking to reabsorb redundant conduction tissue leaving in place accessory pathways or islands of conducting tissue, or exaggerated if the reabsorption is so extensive to cause hypoplasia of the cardiac conduction system structures.
    - □ D. Resorptive degeneration is itself a pathological process of postnatal morphogenesis mediated by apoptotic death of myocytes in both the sinus node and the AV junctional tissue unique to SIDS.
    - □ E. Resorptive degeneration is always a physiological harmless process of cardiac conduction system molding and shaping toward the its adult configuration occurring up to the completion of the first year of postnatal life.
44. What are the Mahaim fibers and what is their possible role in SIDS-SPUD?
    - □ A. Mahaim fibers are accessory pathways connecting the AV junction and the upper ventricular septum, detected in SIDS and SPUD cases and absent in age-matched control cases.
    - □ B. Mahaim fibers are accessory pathways that have an arrhythmogenic action, since they provide direct communication between the atrium and the ventricle, bypassing the classic conduction system pathway, resulting in serious tachyarrhythmias, i.e., a ventricular tachycardic preexcitement and atrial retrograde excitement through the accessory fibers, detected in SIDS cases and absent in age-matched control cases.
    - □ C. Mahaim fibers are accessory pathways that have an arrhythmogenic action, since they provide direct communication between the atrium and the ventricle, bypassing the classic conduction system pathway, resulting in serious tachyarrhythmias, i.e., a ventricular tachycardic preexcitement and atrial retrograde excitement through the accessory fibers detected in both SIDS and SPUD cases.

- □ D. Mahaim fibers are accessory pathways connecting the AV junction and the upper ventricular septum, associated with pre-excitation, junctional, supraventricular arrhythmias in SIDS and SPUD cases.
- □ E. Mahaim fibers are atriofascicular accessory pathways connecting the atrium with the AVN or the bundle of His that may be may be responsible for Lown-Ganong-Levine syndrome and SIDS.

45. What are the James fibers and what is their possible role in SIDS?
    - □ A. James fibers are accessory pathways connecting the AV junction and the upper ventricular septum, detected in SIDS and SPUD cases and absent in age-matched control cases.
    - □ B. James fibers are accessory pathways that have an arrhythmogenic action, since they provide direct communication between the atrium and the ventricle, bypassing the classic conduction system pathway, resulting in serious tachyarrhythmias, i.e., a ventricular tachycardic preexcitement and atrial retrograde excitement through the accessory fibers, detected in SIDS cases and absent in age-matched control cases.
    - □ C. James fibers are accessory pathways that have an arrhythmogenic action, since they provide direct communication between the atrium and the ventricle, bypassing the classic conduction system pathway, resulting in serious tachyarrhythmias, i.e., a ventricular tachycardic preexcitement and atrial retrograde excitement through the accessory fibers, detected in both SIDS and SPUD cases.
    - □ D. James fibers are accessory pathways connecting the AV junction and the upper ventricular septum, associated with pre-excitation, junctional, supraventricular arrhythmias in SIDS and SPUD cases.
    - □ E. James fibers are atriofascicular accessory pathways connecting the atrium with the AVN or the bundle of His that may be responsible for Lown-Ganong-Levine syndrome and SIDS.
46. What are the Kent fibers and what is their possible role in SIDS?
    - □ A. Kent fibers are accessory pathways connecting the AV junction and the upper ventricular septum, detected in SIDS and SPUD cases and absent in age-matched control cases.
    - □ B. Kent fibers are accessory pathways that have an arrhythmogenic action, since they provide direct communication between the atrium and the ventricle, bypassing the classic conduction system pathway, resulting in serious tachyarrhythmias, i.e., a ventricular tachycardic preexcitement and atrial retrograde excitement through the accessory fibers, detected in SIDS cases and absent in age-matched control cases.
    - □ C. Kent fibers are accessory pathways that have an arrhythmogenic action, since they provide direct communication between the atrium and the ventricle, bypassing the classic conduction system pathway, resulting in serious tachyarrhythmias, i.e., a ventricular tachycardic preexcitement and atrial retrograde excitement through the accessory fibers, detected in both SIDS and SPUD cases.
    - □ D. Kent fibers are accessory pathways connecting the AV junction and the upper ventricular septum, associated with pre-excitation, junctional, supraventricular arrhythmias in SIDS and SPUD cases.

□ E. Kent fibers are atriofascicular accessory pathways connecting the atrium with the AVN or the bundle of His that may be responsible for Lown-Ganong-Levine syndrome and SIDS.

47. Which of the following statements concerning the initial preatherosclerotic process is correct?
 □ A. The histopathological examinations of the serially sectioned coronary arteries and cardiac conduction arteries from infants and fetuses that died suddenly and unexpectedly revealed the frequent presence of preatherosclerotic lesions, indicating the atherogenic effect of cigarette smoke.
 □ B. The initial phases of the atherosclerotic process does not affect the arteries of the sino-atrial node and of the atrio-ventricular node in perinatal age.
 □ C. The coronary arteries should be carefully inspected and sampled, as initial pre-atherosclerotic reversible lesions have been reported to start in young adults.
 □ D. The initial pre-atherosclerotic lesions detected in perinatal age should be analyzed post mortem in coronary and cardiac conduction system arteries cut on a single section.
 □ E. The coronary arteries should be carefully inspected and sampled, as initial pre-atherosclerotic reversible lesions have been reported to start in elderly.

48. Which of the following statements concerning the arcuate nucleus is correct?
 □ A. The arcuate nucleus is located in the pons. It is an important integrative site for autonomic function that has been found to be hypoplastic in about 30% of SIDS and SPUD cases.
 □ B. The arcuate nucleus is located in the mesencephalon. It has been found to be hypoplastic in about 70% of SIDS and SPUD cases.
 □ C. The arcuate nucleus, relevant to the central cardiopulmonary hypothesis in SIDS and SPUD, being found hypoplastic in about 50% of cases, is located near the surface of the ventrolateral, ventral, and ventromedial medulla oblongata. This region is an integrative site for autonomic function, ventilation, and chemosensitivity.
 □ D. The arcuate nucleus, relevant to the central cardiopulmonary hypothesis in SIDS and SPUD, being found hypoplastic in about 50% of cases, is located in the pons. This region is an integrative site for autonomic function, ventilation, and chemosensitivity.
 □ E. The arcuate nucleus, relevant to the central cardiopulmonary hypothesis in SIDS and SPUD, being found hypoplastic in about 50% of cases, is located in the mesencephalon.

49. Which of the following statements concerning pulmonary hypoplasia is correct?
 □ A. Pulmonary hypoplasia has been detected in 30% of SIDS infants.
 □ B. Pulmonary hypoplasia has been detected in both SIDS-SPUD and age-matched controls, without significant differences.
 □ C. Pulmonary hypoplasia in SIDS-SPUD is rarely associated with brainstem hypodevelopment.

- □ D. Pulmonary hypoplasia has been detected in 65% of unexplained stillbirth.
- □ E. Pulmonary hypoplasia has been detected in 20% of unexplained stillbirth.

50. Which genes are involved in the congenital long QT syndrome?
- □ A. KCNQ1/LQT1 in 5–10% of cases; KCNH2/LQT2 in 25–30% of cases, and SCN5A/LQT3 in 30–35% of cases
- □ B. KCNQ1/LQT1 in 25–30% of cases; KCNH2/LQT2 in 5–10% of cases, and SCN5A/LQT3 in 30–35% of cases
- □ C. KCNQ1/LQT1 in 40–50% of cases and KCNH2/LQT2 in 30–40% of cases
- □ D. KCNQ1/LQT1 in 80–90% of cases
- □ E. KCNQ1/LQT1 in 30–35% of cases; KCNH2/LQT2 in 25–30% of cases, and S*CN5A*/LQT3 in 5–10% of cases

4.6 Answer Keys

Block 4 (Questions 41–50)

41. A
42. B
43. C
44. D
45. E
46. B
47. A
48. C
49. D
50. E

References

1. American Academy of Pediatrics (2012) Policy statement. Breastfeeding and the use of human milk. Pediatrics 129:e827–e841.
2. Anderson KR, Hill RW (1982) Occlusive lesions of cardiac conducting tissue arteries in sudden infant death syndrome. Pediatrics 69:50–52.
3. Anderson RH (2000) Sudden and unexpected death in infancy and the conduction system of the heart. Cardiovasc Pathol 9:147–148.
4. Anderson RH, Bouton J, Burrow CT, Smith A (1974) Sudden death in infancy: a study of cardiac specialized tissue. Br Med J 2:135–139.
5. Anderson WR, Edland JF, Schenk EA (1970) Conducting system changes in the sudden infant death syndrome. Am J Pathol 59:35a.
6. Arbustini E, Diegoli M, Grasso M, Fasani R, D'Armini A, Martinelli L, Goggi C, Campana C, Gavazzi A, Vigano M (1993) Expression of proliferating cell markers in normal and diseased human hearts. Am J Cardiol 72:608–614.

7. Barton JR, Boheler KR, Brand NJ, Thomas PS (1995) Molecular biology of cardiac development and growth. Springer, Berlin/Heidelberg/New York.
8. Basso C, Corrado D, Rossi L, Thiene G (2001) Ventricular preexcitation in children and young adults: atrial myocarditis as a possible trigger of sudden death. Circulation 103:269–275.
9. Bharati S, Lev M (1986) Congenital abnormalities in the conduction system in sudden death in young adults. J Am Coll Cardiol 8:1096–1104.
10. Bharati S, Lev M (1994) Conduction system findings in sudden death in young adults with a history of bronchial asthma. J Am Coll Cardiol 23:741–746.
11. Bharati S, Dreifus L, Bucheleres G, Molthan M, Covitz W, Isenberg HS, Lev M (1985) The conduction system in patients with a prolonged QT interval. J Am Coll Cardiol 6:1110–1119.
12. Bharati S, Krongrad E, Lev M (1985) Study of the conduction system in a population of patients with sudden infant death syndrome. Pediatr Cardiol 6:29–40.
13. Blanco CE, Hanson MA, Kumar P (1995) Breathing and sleep states in the fetus and at birth. In: Loughlin GM, Carrol JL, Marcus CL (eds) Sleep and breathing in children. A developmental approach. Marcel Dekker, Inc, New York, pp 161–179.
14. Bolande RP, Leistikow EA, Wartman F, Louis T (1996) The development of preatherosclerotic coronary artery lesions in perinatal piglets. Biol Neonate 69:109–118.
15. Cacciatore J (2013) Psychological effects of stillbirth. Semin Fetal Neonatal Med 18:76–82.
16. Centers for Disease Control and Prevention (CDC) (2014) Linked birth/infant death records, 2007–2010 results. http://wonder.cdc.gov/lbd-current.html. Accessed July 26, 2014.
17. Chamberlin NL, Saper CB (1994) Topographic organization of respiratory responses to glutamate microstimulation of the parabrachial nucleus in the rat. J Neurosci 414:6500–6510.
18. Cimaz R, Stramba-Badiale M, Brucato A, Catelli L, Panzeri P, Meroni PL (2000) QT interval prolongation in asymptomatic anti-SSA/Ro-positive infants without congenital heart block. Arthritis Rheum 43:1049–1053.
19. Cohle SD, Lie JT (1991) Pathologic changes of the cardiac conduction tissue in sudden unexpected death. A review. Pathol Annu 26(Pt 2):33–57.
20. Colombo B, Ottaviani G, Ramos SG, Matturri L (1998) Apoptosis in cardiac conduction system in sudden infant death syndrome (SIDS): preliminary results. In: Proceedings of the 5th SIDS International Conference, Rouen, p 157.
21. Crotti L, Tester DJ, White WM, Bartos DC, Insolia R, Besana A, Kunic JD, Will ML, Velasco EJ, Bair JJ, Ghidoni A, Cetin I, Van Dyke DL, Wick MJ, Brost B, Delisle BP, Facchinetti F, George AL, Schwartz PJ, Ackerman MJ (2013) Long QT syndrome-associated mutations in intrauterine fetal death. JAMA 309:1473–1482.
22. Cuneo BF, Etheridge SP, Horigome H, Sallee D, Moon-Grady A, Weng HY, Ackerman MJ, Benson DW (2013) Arrhythmia phenotype during fetal life suggests long-QT syndrome genotype: risk stratification of perinatal long-QT syndrome. Circ Arrhythm Electrophysiol 6:946–951.
23. Daliento L, Nava A, Fasoli G, Mazzucco A, Thiene G (1984) Dysplasia of the atrioventricular valves associated with conduction system anomalies. Br Heart J 51:243–251.
24. Davies MJ, Anderson RH, Becker AE (1983) The conduction system of the heart. Butterworth, London.
25. Dawes GS, Fox HE, Leduc BM, Liggins GC, Richards RT (1972) Respiratory movements and rapid eye movement sleep in the fetal lamb. J Physiol 220:119–143.
26. Doerr W (1957) Die morphologie des reizleitungssystemes ihre orthologie und pathologie. In: Spang K (ed) Rhythmusstörungen des herzens. Thieme, Stuttgart, pp 11–16.
27. Doerr W, Schiebler TH (1963) Pathologische anatomie des reizleitungssystems. In: Bargmann W, Doerr W (eds) Das Herz des Menschen. Thieme, Stuttgart.
28. Dony C, Gruss P (1987) Proto-oncogene c-fos expression in growth regions of fetal bone and mesodermal tissue. Nature 299:711–714.
29. Drobyshevsky A, Derrick M, Luo K, Zhang LQ, Wu YN, Takada SH, Yu L, Tan S (2012) Near-term fetal hypoxia-ischemia in rabbits: MRI can predict muscle tone abnormalities and deep brain injury. Stroke 43:2757–2763.
30. Eastman Q (2003) Genetics. Crib death exoneration could usher in new gene tests. Science 300:1858.

31. Euler C (1986) Brainstem mechanisms for generation and control of breathing pattern. In: Cherniack NS, Waddicombe JG (eds) Handbook of physiology, Section 3. Respiration, vol 2: Control of breathing. American Psychological Society, Bethesda, pp 1–67.
32. Ferris JA (1972) Cot death – why not the heart? Med Sci Law 12:173–177.
33. Ferris JA (1973) Hypoxic changes in conducting tissue of the heart in sudden death in infancy syndrome. Br Med J 2:23–25.
34. Ferris JA, Aherne WA (1971) Cartilage in relation to the conducting tissue of the heart in sudden death. Lancet 1:64–66.
35. Filiano JJ, Kinney HC (1992) Arcuate nucleus hypoplasia in the sudden infant death syndrome. J Neuropathol Exp Neurol 51:394–403.
36. Filiano JJ, Kinney HC (1994) A perspective on neuropathologic findings in victims of sudden infant death syndrome: the triple risk model. Biol Neonate 65:194–197.
37. Giudicessi JR, Ackerman MJ (2013) Arrhythmia risk in long QT syndrome: beyond the disease-causative mutation. Circ Cardiovasc Genet 6:313–316.
38. Gollob MH, Green MS, Tang AS-L, Gollob T, Karibe A, Hassa A, Ahmad F, Lozado R, Shah G, Fananapazir L, Bachinski L, Roberts R (2001) Identification of a gene responsible for familial Wolff-Parkinson-White syndrome. N Engl J Med 344:1823–1831.
39. Guareschi M, Ottaviani G, Ramos SG, Matturri L (1998) Morte improvvisa del lattante (SIDS): un caso con vie accessorie e resorptive degeneration. Pathologica 90:294–297.
40. Guntheroth WG, Spiers PS (1996) Are bedding and rebreathing suffocation a cause of SIDS? Pediatr Pulmonol 22:335–341.
41. Guntheroth WG, Spiers PS (1999) Prolongation of the QT interval and the sudden infant death syndrome. Pediatrics 10:813–814.
42. Hervonen A, Vaalasti A, Partanen M, Kanerva L, Vaalasti T (1976) The paraganglia, a persisting endocrine system in man. Am J Anat 146:207–210.
43. Hirano T, Simbulan D, Kumayawa T (1994) Effects of kainic acid in the parabrachial region for ongoing respiratory activity and reflexive respiratory suppression. Brain Res 665:54–62.
44. Ho SY, Anderson RH (1988) Conduction tissue and SIDS. Ann N Y Acad Sci 533:176–190.
45. Ho SY, Mortimer G, Anderson RH, Pomerance A, Keelings JW (1985) Conduction system defects in three perinatal patients with arrhythmia. Br Heart J 53:158–163.
46. Hunt CE, Hauck FR (2010) Sudden infant death syndrome: gene-environment interactions. In: Brugada R (ed) Clinical approach to sudden cardiac death syndromes. Springer, London, pp 7–21
47. Iams JD, Lynch CD (2011) Stillbirth and lessons for pregnancy care. JAMA 306:2506–2507.
48. Ip S, Chung M, Raman G, Trikalinos TA, Lau J (2009) A summary of the agency for healthcare research and quality's evidence report on breastfeeding in developed countries. Breastfeed Med 1(Suppl):S17–S30.
49. Iranpour R, Kelishadi R, Babaie S, Khosravi-Darani K, Farajian S (2013) Comparison of long chain polyunsaturated fatty acid content in human milk in preterm and term deliveries and its correlation with mothers' diet. J Res Med Sci 18:1–5.
50. James TN (1961) Morphology of the human atrioventricular node, with remarks pertinent to its electrophysiology. Am Heart J 62:756–777.
51. James TN (1968) Sudden death in babies: new observation in the heart. Am J Cardiol 22:479–506.
52. James TN (1970) Cardiac conduction system: fetal and postnatal development. Am J Cardiol 25:213–226.
53. James TN (1976) Sudden death of babies. Circulation 53:1–2.
54. James TN (1983) Change and sudden death. J Am Coll Cardiol 1:164–183.
55. James TN (1983) The Mikamo lecture. Structure and function of AV junction. Jpn Circ J 47:1–47.
56. James TN (1985) Crib death. J Am Coll Cardiol 5:1185–1187.
57. James TN (1985) Normal variations and pathologic changes in structure of the cardiac conduction system and their functional significance. J Am Coll Cardiol 5:71B–78B.
58. James TN (1993) Congenital disorders of cardiac rhythm and conduction. J Cardiovasc Electrophysiol 4:702–718.

59. James TN (1994) Normal and abnormal consequences of apoptosis in the human heart. From postnatal morphogenesis to paroxysmal arrhythmias. Circulation 90:556–573.
60. James TN (1996) Long reflections on the QT interval: the sixth annual Gordon K. Moe lecture. J Cardiovasc Electrophysiol 7:738–759.
61. James TN (1997) Apoptosis in congenital heart disease. Coron Artery Dis 8:599–616.
62. James TN (1998) Normal and abnormal consequences of apoptosis in the human heart. Annu Rev Physiol 60:309–325.
63. James TN (1999) Apoptosis in cardiac disease. Am J Med 107:606–620.
64. James TN (2002) Structure and function of the sinus node, AV node and His bundle of the human heart: part I – structure. Prog Cardiovasc Dis 45:235–267.
65. James TN (2003) Structure and function of the sinus node, AV node and His bundle of the human heart: part II – function. Prog Cardiovasc Dis 45:327–360.
66. James TN, Marshall TK (1976) De Subitaneis Mortibus XVIII. Persistent fetal dispersion of the atrioventricular node and His bundle within the central fibrous body. Circulation 6:1026–1034.
67. James TN, Froggatt P, Marshall TK (1967) Sudden death in young athletes. Ann Intern Med 67:1013–1021.
68. James TN, Froggatt P, Atkinson WJ Jr, Lurie PR, McNamara DG, Miller WW, Schloss GT, Carroll JF, North RL (1978) De subitaneis mortibus XXX. Observations on the pathophysiology of the QT syndromes with special reference to the neuropathology of the heart. Circulation 57:1221–1231.
69. James TN, Nichols MM, Sapire DW, Di Patre PL, Lopez SM (1996) Complete heart block and fatal right ventricular failure in an infant. Circulation 93:1588–1600.
70. James TN, St. Martin E, Willis PW 3rd, Lohr TO (1996) Apoptosis as a possible cause of gradual development of complete heart block and fatal arrhythmias associated with absence of the AV node, sinus node and internodal pathways. Circulation 93:1424–1438.
71. Jankus A (1976) The cardiac conduction system in sudden infant death syndrome: a report on three cases. Pathology 8:275–280.
72. Jervell A, Lange-Nielsen F (1957) Congenital deaf-mutism, functional heart disease with prolongation of the QT interval and sudden death. Am Heart J 54:59–68.
73. Kajstura J, Mansukhani M, Cheng W, Reiss K, Krajewski S, Reed JC, Quaini F, Sonnenblick EH, Anversa P (1995) Programmed cell death and expression of the protooncogene bcl-2 in myocytes during postnatal maturation of the heart. Exp Cell Res 219:110–121.
74. Kent AFS (1893) Researches on the structure and function of the mammalian heart. J Physiol 14:233–254.
75. Kinney HC, Filiano JJ, Harper RM (1992) The neuropathology of the sudden infant death syndrome. A review. J Neuropathol Exp Neurol 51:115–126.
76. Kinney HC, O'Donnel TJ, Kriger P, White WF (1993) Early developmental changes in H3-nicotine binding in the human brainstem. Neuroscience 55:1127–1138.
77. Kozakewich HPW, McManus BM, Vawter G (1982) The sinus node in sudden infant death syndrome. Circulation 65:1242–1246.
78. Kuo HC, Cheng CF, Clark RB, Lin JJ, Lin JL, Gu Y, Ikeda Y, Chu PH, Ross J Jr, Giles WR, Chien KR (2001) A defect in the Kv channel-interacting protein 2 (KchIP2) gene leads to a complete loss of Ito and confers susceptibility to ventricular tachycardia. Cell 107:801–812.
79. Lavezzi AM, Ottaviani G, Matturri L (2003) Identification of neurons responding to hypoxia in sudden infant death syndrome (SIDS). Pathol Int 53:769–774.
80. Lavezzi AM, Ottaviani G, Ballabio G, Rossi L, Matturri L (2004) Preliminary study on the cytoarchitecture of the human parabrachial/Kölliker-Fuse complex, with reference to sudden infant death syndrome and sudden intrauterine unexplained death. Pediatr Dev Pathol 7:171–179.
81. Lavezzi AM, Ottaviani G, Mauri M, Matturri L (2004) Hypoplasia of the arcuate nucleus and maternal smoking during pregnancy, in perinatal and infant sudden unexpected death. Neuropathology 24:284–289.
82. Lavezzi AM, Ottaviani G, Matturri L (2004) Involvement of somatostatin in breathing control before and after birth, and in perinatal and infant sudden unexplained death. Folia Neuropathol 42:59–65.

83. Lavezzi AM, Ottaviani G, Matturri L (2004) Role of somatostatin and apoptosis in breathing control in sudden perinatal and infant unexplained death. Clin Neuropathol 23:304–310.
84. Lavezzi AM, Ottaviani G, Rossi L, Matturri L (2004) Cytoarchitectural organization of the Parabrachial/Kölliker-Fuse complex in man. Brain Dev 26:316–320.
85. Lavezzi AM, Ottaviani G, Rossi L, Matturri L (2004) Hypoplasia of the parabrachial/ Kölliker-Fuse complex in perinatal death. Biol Neonate 86:92–97.
86. Lavezzi AM, Ottaviani G, Matturri L (2005) Adverse effects of prenatal tobacco smoke exposure on biological parameters of the developing brainstem. Neurobiol Dis 20:601–607.
87. Lavezzi AM, Ottaviani G, Matturri L (2005) Biology of the smooth muscle cells in human atherosclerosis. APMIS 113:112–121.
88. Lavezzi AM, Ottaviani G, Mauri M, Terni L, Matturri L (2005) Involvement of the EN-2 gene in normal and abnormal development of the human arcuate nucleus. Int J Exp Pathol 86:25–31.
89. Lavezzi AM, Ottaviani G, Mauri M, Matturri L (2006) Alterations of biological features of the cerebellum in sudden perinatal and infant death. Curr Mol Med 6:429–435.
90. Lavezzi AM, Ottaviani G, Terni L, Matturri L (2006) Histological and biological developmental characterization of the human cerebellar cortex. Int J Dev Neurosci 24:365–371.
91. Lavezzi AM, Casale V, Oneda R, Weese-Mayer DE, Matturri L (2009) Sudden infant death syndrome and sudden intrauterine unexplained death: correlation between hypoplasia of raphé nuclei and serotonin transporter gene promoter polymorphism. Pediatr Res 66:22–27.
92. Lavezzi AM, Mehboob R, Matturri L (2011) Developmental alterations of the spinal trigeminal nucleus disclosed by substance P immunohistochemistry in fetal and infant sudden unexplained deaths. Neuropathology 31:405–413.
93. Liebrechts-Akkerman G, Lao O, Liu F, van Sleuwen BE, Engelberts AC, L'hoir MP, Tiemeier HW, Kayser M (2011) Postnatal parental smoking: an important risk factor for SIDS. Eur J Pediatr 170:1281–1291.
94. Lie JT, Rosenberg HS, Erickson EE (1976) Histopathology of the conduction system in the sudden infant death syndrome. Circulation 53:3–8.
95. Lown B, Ganong WF, Levine SA (1952) The syndrome of short P-R interval, normal QRS complex and paroxysmal rapid heart action. Circulation 5:693–706.
96. MacDorman MF, Kirmeyer SE, Wilson EC (2012) Fetal and perinatal mortality, United States, 2006. Natl Vital Stat Rep 60:1–23. www.cdc.gov/nchs/data/nvsr/nvsr60/nvsr60_08.pdf. Accessed July 26, 2014.
97. Mahaim I, Benatt A (1938) Nouvelles recherches sur les connexions superiors de la branche gauche du faisceau de His-Tawara avec cloison interventriculaire. Cardiologia 1:61–120.
98. Marino TA, Kane BM (1985) Cardiac atrioventricular junctional tissues in hearts from infants who died suddenly. J Am Coll Cardiol 5:1178–1184.
99. Marino TA, Haldar S, Williamson EC, Beaverson K, Walter RA, Marino DR, Beatty C, Lipson KE (1991) Proliferating cell nuclear antigen in developing and adult rat cardiac muscle cells. Circ Res 69:1353–1360.
100. Maron BJ, Clark CE, Goldstein RE, Epstein SE (1976) Potential role of QT interval prolongation in sudden infant death syndrome. Circulation 54:423–430.
101. Massing GK, James TN (1976) Anatomical configuration of the His bundle and bundle branches in the human heart. Circulation 53:609–621.
102. Matturri L, Nappo A, Varesi C, Martini I, Rossi L (1997) Dualismo del nodo atrioventricolare per la presenza del nodo del seno coronarico di Zahn in un caso di morte improvvisa del lattante (SIDS). Riv Ital Pediatr 23:130–133.
103. Matturri L, Ottaviani G, Biondo B, Ramos SG, Rossi L (1998) Discrete T-lymphocytic leptomeningitis of the ventral medullary surface in a case of sudden unexpected infant death. Adv Clin Path 2:313–316.
104. Matturri L, Ottaviani G, Rossi L (1999) Sudden and unexpected infant death due to an hemangioendothelioma located in the medulla oblongata. Adv Clin Path 3:29–33.
105. Matturri L, Ottaviani G, Ramos SG, Rossi L (2000) Sudden infant death syndrome (SIDS). A study of cardiac conduction system. Cardiovasc Pathol 9:137–145.

106. Matturri L, Ottaviani G, Lavezzi AM, Turconi P, Cazzullo A, Rossi L (2001) Expression of apoptosis and proliferating cell nuclear antigen (PCNA) in the cardiac conduction system of crib death (SIDS). Adv Clin Path 5:79–86.
107. Matturri L, Biondo B, Suàrez-Mier MP, Rossi L (2002) Brain stem lesions in the sudden infant death syndrome: variability in the hypoplasia of the arcuate nucleus. Acta Neuropathol (Berl) 194:12–20.
108. Matturri L, Lavezzi AM, Ottaviani G, Rossi L (2002) Anatomia patologica della sindrome della morte improvvisa del lattante (SIDS) e della morte inaspettata del feto. In: Proceedings of the National Symposium "Sudden Infant Death Syndrome (SIDS) and Sudden Unexplained Intrauterine Death", Milan, pp 13–23.
109. Matturri L, Minoli I, Lavezzi AM, Cappellini A, Ramos S, Rossi L (2002) Hypoplasia of medullary arcuate nucleus in unexpected late fetal death (stillborn infants): a pathological study. Pediatrics 109:E43.
110. Matturri L, Ottaviani G, Ballabio G, Lavezzi AM (2002) Medullary arcuate nucleus' cellular differentiation in SIDS and unexpected late fetal stillbirth cases. In: Proceedings of the 7th SIDS International Conference, Florence, p 135.
111. Matturri L, Ottaviani G, Rossi L (2002) Should overdone external cardiac massage in infants dying of SIDS be discouraged? In: Proceedings of the 7th International Conference on SIDS, Florence, p 136.
112. Matturri L, Lavezzi AM, Minoli I, Ottaviani G, Cappellini A, Rubino B, Rossi L (2003) Association between pulmonary hypoplasia and hypoplasia of arcuate nucleus in stillbirth. J Perinatol 23:328–332.
113. Matturri L, Lavezzi AM, Ottaviani G, Rossi L (2003) Intimal preatherosclerotic thickening of the coronary arteries in human fetuses of smoker mothers. J Thromb Haemost 1:2234–2238.
114. Matturri L, Ottaviani G, Rossi L (2003) External cardiac massage in infants. Intensive Care Med 29:1199–1200.
115. Matturri L, Ottaviani G, Alfonsi G, Crippa M, Rossi L, Lavezzi AM (2004) Study of the brainstem, particularly the arcuate nucleus, in sudden infant death syndrome (SIDS) and sudden intrauterine unexplained death (SIUD). Am J Forensic Med Pathol 25:44–48.
116. Matturri L, Ottaviani G, Corti G, Lavezzi AM (2004) Pathogenesis of early atherosclerotic lesions in infants. Pathol Res Pract 200:403–410.
117. Matturri L, Ottaviani G, Lavezzi AM, Rossi L (2004) Early atherosclerotic lesions of the cardiac conduction system arteries in infants. Cardiovasc Pathol 13:276–281.
118. Matturri L, Ottaviani G, Lavezzi AM, Grana DR, Milei J (2005) Natural history of perinatal and infant coronary atherosclerosis due to maternal cigarette smoking. In: Proceedings of the "4th World Congress of Pediatric Cardiology and Cardiac Surgery" Buenos Aires, p 31.
119. Matturri L, Ottaviani G, Lavezzi AM, Grana DR, Milei J (2005) Perinatal and infant early atherosclerotic coronary lesions related to maternal smoking. In: Proceedings of the "4th World Congress of Pediatric Cardiology and Cardiac Surgery", Buenos Aires, p 48.
120. Matturri L, Ottaviani G, Benedetti G, Agosta E, Lavezzi AM (2005) Unexpected perinatal death and sudden infant death syndrome (SIDS): anatomopathologic and legal aspects. Am J Forensic Med Pathol 26:155–160.
121. Matturri L, Ottaviani G, Lavezzi AM (2005) Early atherosclerotic lesions in infancy: role of parental cigarette smoking. Virchows Arch 447:74–80.
122. Matturri L, Ottaviani G, Lavezzi AM (2005) Sudden infant death triggered by dive reflex. J Clin Pathol 58:77–80.
123. Matturri L, Ottaviani G, Lavezzi AM (2005) Perinatal and infant atherosclerotic coronary lesions related to maternal smoking. In: Proceedings of the "6th International Congress on Coronary Artery Disease: from Prevention to Intervention", Istanbul, p 66.
124. Matturri L, Ottaviani G, Lavezzi AM (2005) Techniques and criteria in pathologic and forensic-medical diagnostics in sudden unexpected infant and perinatal death. Am J Clin Pathol 124:259–268.

125. Matturri L, Ottaviani G, Lavezzi AM (2005) Unexpected sudden death related to medullary brain lesions. Acta Neuropathol (Berl) 109:554–555.
126. Matturri L, Ottaviani G, Lavezzi AM, Ramos SG (2005) Peripheral chemoreceptors and sudden infant death syndrome: a wide open problem. Curr Cardiol Rev 1:65–70.
127. Matturri L, Ottaviani G, Lavezzi AM (2006) Maternal smoking and sudden infant death syndrome: epidemiological study related to pathology. Virchows Arch 449:697–706.
128. Matturri L, Ottaviani G, Minoli I, Mauri M, Lavezzi AM (2007) Neonatal pulmonary hypoplasia frequently associated with brainstem hypodevelopment. 8th World Congress of Perinatal Medicine. Florence, Italy. J Perinat Med 35(Suppl):209.
129. Matturri L, Ottaviani G, Mingrone R, Lavezzi AM, Fulcheri E (2007) Sudden intrauterine unexplained death (SIUD) «gray zone» or borderline. 8th World Congress of Perinatal Medicine. Florence, Italy. J Perinat Med 35(Suppl):210.
130. Matturri L, Ottaviani G, Nonnis Marzano F, Lavezzi AM (2006) Stillbirth versus SIDS. Pathology of the autonomic nervous system and DNA polymorphisms in SIUD and SIDS. In: Proceedings of the 9th SIDS International Conference, Yokohama, pp 105–106.
131. Matturri L, Ottaviani G, Lavezzi AM (2008) Guidelines for neuropathologic diagnostics of perinatal unexpected loss and sudden infant death syndrome (SIDS) – a technical protocol. Virchows Arch 452:19–25.
132. Matturri L, Lavezzi AM (2011) Unexplained stillbirth versus SIDS: common congenital diseases of the autonomic nervous system–pathology and nosology. Early Hum Dev 87:209–215.
133. Milei J, Ottaviani G, Lavezzi AM, Grana DR, Stella I, Matturri L (2008) Perinatal and infant early atherosclerotic coronary lesions. Can J Cardiol 24:137–141.
134. Moon HD (1957) Coronary arteries in fetuses, infants and juveniles. Circulation 16:263–267.
135. Morpurgo CV, Lavezzi AM, Ottaviani G, Rossi L (2004) Bulbo-spinal pathology and sudden respiratory infant death syndrome. Eur J Anaesthesiol 21:589–593.
136. Nachmanoff DB, Panigrahy A, Filiano JJ, Sieeper LA, Valdes-Dapena M, Krous HF, White WF, Kinney HC (1998) Brainstem H3-nicotine receptor binding in the sudden infant death syndrome. J Neuropathol Exp Neurol 57:1018–1025.
137. Olszewski J, Baxter D (1982) Cytoarchitecture of the human brain stem. Karger, Basel.
138. Ottaviani G (2006) Histological observation of the cardiac conduction system in the diagnostics of sudden infant death syndrome (SIDS). "SIDS e ALTE Aggiornamento 2005. Primo Corso Teorico Pratico di Anatomia-Patologica in casi di Sospetta SIDS e di morte inaspettata fetale", Parma, Italy. Acta Biomed Ateneo Parmense 77:52.
139. Ottaviani G, Ramos SG, Matturri L (1997) Defective "resorptive degeneration" of the heart's conduction system and sudden infant death syndrome. Ann Españ Pediatr 92(Suppl):53.
140. Ottaviani G, Goisis M, Ramos SG, Matturri L (1998) Dispersione del tessuto giunzionale e sue conseguenze in un caso di morte improvvisa del lattante. Cardiologia 43:737–739.
141. Ottaviani G, Matturri L, Ramos SG, Rossi L (1998) Resorptive degeneration of the heart's conduction system and sudden infant death syndrome: preliminary results. In: Proceedings of the 5th SIDS International Conference, Rouen, p 156.
142. Ottaviani G, Rossi L, Bondurri A, Ramos SG, Matturri L (1998) Morte improvvisa del lattante: un caso di sdoppiamento del nodo atrio-ventricolare. Riv Ital Pediatr 24:1165–1167.
143. Ottaviani G, Lavezzi AM, Rossi L, Matturri L (1999) Proliferating cell nuclear antigen (PCNA) and apoptosis in hyperacute and acute myocardial infarction. Eur J Histochem 43:7–14.
144. Ottaviani G, James TN, Rossi L, Matturri L (2002) Significance of Mahaim fibers in crib death. In: Proceedings of the 7th SIDS International Conference, Florence, p 136.
145. Ottaviani G, Matturri L, Lavezzi AM, Rossi L, James TN (2002) Postnatal apoptosis of the cardiac conduction system in crib death: preliminary results. In: Proceedings of the 7th SIDS International Conference, Florence, p 132.
146. Ottaviani G, Matturri L, Rossi L, James TN (2002) Crib death: further support for the concept of fatal cardiac electrical instability as the final common pathway. In: Proceedings of the 7th SIDS International Conference, Florence, p 66.

147. Ottaviani G, Matturri L, Rossi L, James TN (2003) Crib death: further support for the concept of fatal cardiac electrical instability as the final common pathway. Int J Cardiol 92:17–26.
148. Ottaviani G, Lavezzi AM, Rossi L, Matturri L (2004) Sudden unexpected death of a term fetus in a anticardiolipin positive mother. Am J Perinatol 21:31–35.
149. Ottaviani G, Matturri L, Rossi L, Lavezzi AM, James TN (2004) Multifocal cardiac Purkinje cell tumor in infancy. Europace 6:138–141.
150. Ottaviani G, Matturri L, Bruni B, Lavezzi AM (2005) Sudden infant death syndrome "gray zone" disclosed only by a study of the brain stem on serial sections. J Perinat Med 33:165–169.
151. Ottaviani G, Rossi L, Matturri L (2005) Myocardial injury attributable to external cardiac massage in infants. Cardiology 1:25–29.
152. Ottaviani G, Matturri L, Mingrone R, Lavezzi AM (2006) Hypoplasia and neuronal immaturity of the hypoglossal nucleus in sudden infant death. J Clin Pathol 59:497–500.
153. Ottaviani G (2006) A case of respiratory unexpected death. "SIDS e ALTE Aggiornamento 2005. Primo Corso Teorico Pratico di Anatomia-Patologica in casi di sospetta SIDS e di morte inaspettata fetale". Parma, Italy. Acta Biomed Ateneo Parmense 77:45.
154. Ottaviani G (2006) Morte improvvisa inaspettata perinatale e del lattante (SIDS): studio istopatologico del sistema di conduzione cardiaco. In: Proceedings of the Conference "Morte improvvisa del lattante (SIDS) e morte inaspettata del feto: La rilevanza medico-sociale e formativa della ricerca scientifica: la legge 31 del 2006". Corso di .alta formazione continua: "Tecniche e criteri anatomo-patologici e medico-legali nella diagnostica della morte inaspettata del feto versus SIDS", Milan, pp 73–78.
155. Ottaviani G (2006) Studio istopatologico del sistema di conduzione cardiaco nella morte improvvisa del lattante e perinatale. In: Proceedings of the Convegno "Morte improvvisa del lattante e morte inaspettata del feto. La rilevanza giuridica e medico-sociale della ricerca scientifica: la legge n. 31 del 2006", Gargnano, pp 63–74.
156. Ottaviani G, Matturri L (2007) Cardiovascular pathology of sudden perinatal unexpected death (SPUD) and sudden infant death syndrome (SIDS). 8th World Congress of Perinatal Medicine, Florence, Italy. J Perinat Med 35(Suppl):229–230.
157. Ottaviani G, Matturri L (2008) Histopathology of the cardiac conduction system in sudden intrauterine unexplained death. Cardiovasc Pathol 17:146–155.
158. Ottaviani G, Bergui G (2009) Sudden unexpected death in infancy (SUDI): A new anatomo-clinical approach. Europace 11:395.
159. Ottaviani G, Mingrone R, Lavezzi AM, Matturri L (2009) Infant and perinatal pulmonary hypoplasia frequently associated with brainstem hypodevelopment. Virchows Arch 454:451–456.
160. Ottaviani G (2010) In utero exposure to smoking and peripheral chemoreceptor function. Pediatrics [E-letter]. http://pediatrics.aappublications.org/content/125/3/e592/reply. Accessed July 26, 2014.
161. Ottaviani G (2011) Sudden deaths in term infants within 24 hours of birth. Pediatrics. http://pediatrics.aappublications.org/content/127/4/e869/reply. Accessed July 26, 2014.
162. Ottaviani G (2011) Sudden infant and perinatal unexplained death: are we moving forward yet? Cardiovasc Pathol 10:302–306.
163. Pacharn P, Kline-Fath B, Calvo-Garcia M, Linam LE, Rubio EI, Salisbury S, Brody AS (2013) Congenital lung lesions: prenatal MRI and postnatal findings. Pediatr Radiol 43:1136–1143
164. Priori SG, Bloise R, Crotti L (2001) The long QT syndrome. Europace 3:16–27.
165. Priori SG, Wilde AA, Horie M, Cho Y, Behr ER, Berul C, Blom N, Brugada J, Chiang CE, Huikuri H, Kannankeril P, Krahn A, Leenhardt A, Moss A, Schwartz PJ, Shimizu W, Tomaselli G, Tracy C, Document Reviewers, Ackerman M, Belhassen B, Estes NA 3rd, Fatkin D, Kalman J, Kaufman E, Kirchhof P, Schulze-Bahr E, Wolpert C, Vohra J, Refaat M, Etheridge SP, Campbell RM, Martin ET, Quek SC (2013) Executive summary: HRS/EHRA/APHRS expert consensus statement on the diagnosis and management of patients with inherited primary arrhythmia syndromes. Europace 15:1389–1406.
166. Ramos SG, Matturri L, Biondo B, Ottaviani G, Rossi L (1998) Hyperplasia of the aorticopulmonary paraganglia: a new insight into the pathogenesis of sudden infant death syndrome? Cardiologia 43:953–958.

167. Ramos SG, Matturri L, Ottaviani G, Rossi L (1998) Maternal smoking and aorticopulmonary paraganglia in sudden infant death syndrome. In: Proceedings of the 5th SIDS International Conference, Rouen, p 169.
168. Ramos SG, Matturri L, Ottaviani G, Rossi L, Rossi MA (1999) Lesions of aorticopulmonary paraganglia related to sudden death: histopathologic considerations. J Heart Dis 1:141.
169. Ramos SG, Ottaviani G, Biondo B, Rossi L, Matturri L (1999) Hyperplasia of the aortico-pulmonary paraganglia in infants dying of SIDS: further supports for the cardio-respiratory hypothesis. In: Proceedings of the International Symposium on SIDS and Lombardy Region project for the reduction of the risk for sudden infant death and unexplained intrauterine death, Milan, pp 117–128.
170. Rodan GA, Bourret LA, Norton LA (1978) DNA synthesis in cartilage cells is stimulated by oscillating electric fields. Science 199:690–692.
171. Robertson JH (1960) The significance of intimal thickening in the arteries of the newborn. Arch Dis Child 35:588–590.
172. Romano C, Gemme G, Pongiglione R (1963) Rare cardiac arrythmias of the pediatric age. II. Syncopal attacks due to paroxysmal ventricular fibrillation. Presentation of the 1st case in Italian literature. Clin Pediatr (Bologna) 45:656–683.
173. Rossenbacker T, Priori SG (2007) Clinical diagnosis of long QT syndrome: back to the caliper. Eur Heart J 28:527–528.
174. Rossi L (1969) Histopathologic features of cardiac arrhythmias. Casa Editrice Ambrosiana, Milan.
175. Rossi L (1975) A histological survey of pre-excitation syndrome and related arrhythmias. G Ital Cardiol 5:816–828.
176. Rossi L (1978) Intramural ramification of the left bundle branch. Am Heart J 96:271–272.
177. Rossi L (1983) The pathologic basis of cardiac arrhythmias. Cardiol Clin 1:13–17.
178. Rossi L (1998) Histopathology of the cardiac conduction system in the problem of arrhythmogenic SIDS. In: Proceedings of the 18th International Symposium on Neonatal Intensive Care, Milan, p 75.
179. Rossi L, Matturri L (1988) His bundle haematoma and external cardiac massage: histopathological findings. Br Heart J 59:586–587.
180. Rossi L, Matturri L (1990) Clinicopathological approach to cardiac arrhythmias. A color atlas. Centro Scientifico Torinese, Turin.
181. Rossi L, Matturri L (1991) Anatomohistological features of sudden infant death. New Trends Arrhyt 6:135–142.
182. Rossi L, Matturri L (1995) Anatomo-histological features of the heart's conduction system and innervation in SIDS. In: Rognum TO (ed) Sudden infant death syndrome: new trends in the nineties. Scandinavian University Press, Oslo, pp 207–212.
183. Rossi L, Matturri L (1995) Cardiac conduction and nervous system in health disease and sudden death: an anatomoclinical overview. Osp Maggiore 89:239–257.
184. Rossi L, Matturri L (1998) Neuronal degeneration localized in the thoracic spinal cord sympathetic center in a case with prolonged QT interval. G Ital Cardiol 28(Suppl):535–537.
185. Rossi L, Thiene G (1983) Arrhythmologic pathology of sudden cardiac death. Casa Editrice Ambrosiana, Milan.
186. Rossi L, Knippel M, Taccardi B (1975) Histological findings. His bundle recordings and bodysurface potential mappings in a case of Wolff-Parkinson-White syndrome. An anatomo-clinical comparison. Cardiology 60:265–279.
187. Rossi L, Thiene G, Knippel M (1978) A case of surgically corrected Wolff-Parkinson-White syndrome: clinical and histological data. Br Heart J 40:581–585.
188. Rossi L, Piffer R, Turolla E, Frigerio B, Coumel P, James TN (1985) Multifocal purkinje-like tumor of the heart. Occurrence with other anatomic abnormalities in the atrioventricular junction of an infant with junctional tachycardia, Lown-Ganong-Levine syndrome, and sudden death. Chest 87:340–345.
189. Rossi L, Matturri L, Lotto A (1988) Cardiac conduction blocks and pacemaking. An anatomoclinical color atlas. Clas International, Brescia.

190. Rossi L, Pozzato R, Matturri L (1991) L'anatomia patologica della morte cardiaca oggi. Riv Ital Med Leg 13:93–110.
191. Rossi L, Matturri L, Ottaviani G (2002) Arrhythmogenic sudden death in the modern setting SIDS. An overview. In: Proceedings of the 7th International Conference on SIDS, Florence, p 153.
192. Rossi L, Matturri L, Ottaviani G (2002) Sudden unexpected death of a term fetus with maternal infant anti-cardiolipin antibodies. A case report. In: Proceedings of the 7th International Conference on SIDS, Florence, p 137.
193. Rumyantsev PP (1977) Interrelations of the proliferation and differentiation processes during cardiac myogenesis and regeneration. Int Rev Cytol 51:187–273.
194. Schaller B, Cornelius JF, Sandu N, Ottaviani G, Perez-Pinzon MA (2009) Oxygen-conserving reflexes of the brain: the current molecular knowledge. J Cell Mol Med 13:644–647.
195. Schwartz PJ (1976) Cardiac sympathetic innervation and the sudden infant death syndrome. A possible pathogenetic link. Am J Med 60:167–172.
196. Schwartz PJ, Stramba-Badiale M, Segantini A, Austoni P, Bosi G, Giorgetti RR, Grancini F, Marini ED, Perticone F, Rositi D, Salice P (1998) Prolongation of the QT interval and the sudden infant death syndrome. N Engl J Med 338:1709–1714.
197. Schwartz PJ, Priori SG, Dumaine R, Napolitano C, Antzelevitch C, Stramba-Badiale M, Richard TA, Berti MR, Bloise R (2000) A molecular link between the sudden infant death syndrome and the long-QT syndrome. N Engl J Med 343:262–267.
198. Southall DP, Arrowsmith WA, Stebbins V, Alexander JR (1986) QT interval measurements before sudden infant death syndrome. Arch Dis Child 61:327–333.
199. Stéphan-Blanchard E, Chardon K, Léké A, Delanaud S, Djeddi D, Libert JP, Bach V, Telliez F (2010) In utero exposure to smoking and peripheral chemoreceptor function in preterm neonates. Pediatrics 125:e592–e599.
200. Suàrez-Mier MP, Aguilera B (1998) Histopathology of the conduction system in sudden infant death. Forensic Sci Int 93:143–154.
201. Suàrez-Mier MP, Gamallo C (1998) Atrioventricular node fetal dispersion and His fragmentation of the cardiac conduction system in sudden cardiac death. J Am Coll Cardiol 32:1885–1890.
202. Tester DJ, Ackerman MJ (2009) Cardiomyopathic and channelopathic causes of sudden unexplained death in infants and children. Annu Rev Med 60:69–84.
203. Thiene G (1988) Problems in the interpretation of cardiac pathology in reference to SIDS. Ann N Y Acad Sci 533:191–199.
204. Turner CJ, Wren C (2013) The epidemiology of arrhythmia in infants: a population-based study. J Paediatr Child Health 49:278–281.
205. Valdès-Dapena M (1985) Are some crib deaths sudden cardiac deaths? J Am Coll Cardiol 5(6 Suppl):113B–117B.
206. Valdés-Dapena M, Gilbert-Barness E (2002) Cardiovascular causes for sudden infant death. Pediatr Pathol Mol Med 21:195–211.
207. Valdés-Dapena MA, Greene M, Basavanand N, Catherman R, Truex RC (1973) The myocardial conduction system in sudden death in infancy. N Engl J Med 289:1179–1180.
208. Van Norstrand DW, Ackerman MJ (2010) Genomic risk factors in sudden infant death syndrome. Genome Med 2:86.
209. Viskin S, Fish R, Roth A, Schwartz PJ, Belhassen B (2000) QT or not QT? N Engl J Med 343:352–356.
210. Waldo AL, James TN (1973) A retrospective look at A-V nodal rhythms (A Zahn). Circulation 47:222–224.
211. Ward OC (1964) A new familial cardiac syndrome in children. J Ir Med Assoc 54:103–106.
212. Weinberg SB, Purdy BA (1970) Postmortem leukocyte culture studies in sudden infant death. Nature 226:1264–1265.
213. Willinger M, Hoffman HJ, Hartford RB (1994) Infant sleep position and risk for sudden infant death syndrome: report of meeting held January 13 and 14, 1994, National Institutes of Health, Bethesda, MD. Pediatrics 93:814–819.

214. Wolff GS, Han J, Curran G (1978) Wolff-Parkinson-White syndrome in the neonate. Am J Cardiol 41:559–563.
215. Wolff L, Parkinson J, White PD (1930) Bundle-branch block with short P-R interval in healthy young people prone to paroxysmal tachycardia. Am Heart J 5:685–704.
216. Wren C (1998) Mechanism of fetal tachycardia. Heart 79:536–539.
217. Wren C, Vogel M, Lord S, Abrams D, Bourke J, Rees P, Rosenthal E (2012) Accuracy of algorithms to predict accessory pathway location in children with Wolff-Parkinson-White syndrome. Heart 98:202–206.
218. Yang Z, Lantz PE, Ibdah JA (2007) Post-mortem analysis for two prevalent beta-oxidation mutations in sudden infant death. Pediatr Int 49:883–887.
219. Zahn A (1912) Experimentelle untersuchungen über die reizbildung im atrioventrikularnoten und sinus coronarius. Zentralbl Physiol 26:495.

5 Concluding Remarks on Sudden Infant and Perinatal Unexplained Death

Sudden infant death syndrome (SIDS), or crib death, is defined as the sudden death of an infant under one year of age which remains unexplained after a thorough investigation of the case, including the performance of a complete autopsy, examination of the death scene, and a review of the clinical history [81]. SIDS is the most frequent death-causing syndrome occurring during the first year of life, at a death rate of 0.47 per 1,000 births striking one baby in every 1,700–2,000 in the USA [1]. Despite a wide spectrum of proposed theories, its etiology remains uncertain. Since it is a particularly tragic event for a healthy vigorous infant to die suddenly and unexpectedly, it is not surprising that the subject is of great medical and public interest and concern.

SIDS is a syndrome which represents a tragedy, scientifically and humanly not understandable. However, the initial definition of SIDS as "unexplained after thorough postmortem examination" should be revised. In fact, while it is believed to reduce the age of the subject in question less than a month, histopathological findings, entrusted to experienced observers, highlight some objective morphological alterations. From the literature data SIDS merges as a multifactorial problem, whose pathogenetic aspects cannot be traced to a single cause. Indeed, the definition of syndrome – as the "run together" of various different morbid conditions – should consider the extension and the variety of the microscopic features, warning risk factors, and clinical signals.

Many risk factors are considered to be related to SIDS. They can be arbitrarily subdivided into non-amenable to prevention, such as gender, ethnicity, age and amenable to prevention, such as parental cigarette smoking, prone position in the crib, and bed sharing. Maternal smoking during pregnancy has been found to be the most important preventable risk factor for SIDS [42], based on morphological and functional alterations of brainstem centers, such as hypodevelopment of the arcuate nucleus, somatostatin positive hypoglossus nucleus, tyrosine hydroxylase negativity in the locus coeruleus, gliosis, and hypoplasia of the hypoglossus nucleus, in addition to the early atherosclerotic lesions of the coronary arteries and of the arteries of the cardiac conduction system.

G. Ottaviani, *Crib Death - Sudden Infant Death Syndrome (SIDS): Sudden Infant and Perinatal Unexplained Death: The Pathologist's Viewpoint*,
DOI 10.1007/978-3-319-08347-6_5

There is an association between SIDS and sleep, and this is combined with data indicating impaired autonomic function in infants who subsequently die of SIDS or suffer from ALTE events. SIDS victims generally are found dead in the crib without prodromal signs; if the infant is seen in the agonal phase, it could be eventually saved with cardio-respiratory resuscitations. Cardiac massage, on the other hand, can damage the cardiac conduction system [27, 30, 57, 73]. The pathology of SIDS is included in the extended domain of perinatal pathology, particularly if within the diagnosis of SIDS one wishes to include so-called "borderline" SIDS not definitely separable from the unifying concept of the syndrome [19, 20, 56, 58, 59, 66].

Sudden intrauterine unexplained death (SIUD) is the late fetal death before the complete expulsion or removal of the fetus from the mother ≥22 weeks of gestation or ≥500 gm body mass which is unexpected by history and is unexplained after a thorough pathological exam of the fetus and the fetal adnexa [3, 5, 6, 61]. Advances in maternal and fetal care have produced a significant reduction in perinatal mortality, but have not significantly changed the prevalence of SIUD which represents about one-half of perinatal mortalities. In developed countries, one in 100–200 pregnancies ends in stillbirth [18], which has a six- to eightfold greater incidence than that of the SIDS and remains completely unexpected in 40–80% of cases, occurring in pregnancies that had seemed problem-free, and unexplained even after the performance of a routine postmortem examination [71, 80].

Sudden neonatal unexplained death (SNUD) and SIUD are both collected as sudden perinatal unexplained death (SPUD) which in turn should be regarded as part of the SIDS-SPUD complex because common developmental abnormalities have been detected in both SIDS and SPUD. The observation of frequent anomalies, mostly congenital, of the autonomic nervous system structures in SIDS-SPUD victims [9, 26, 28, 31] indicates a continuity between these two deadly forms of death.

Over the years, first at the Institute of Pathology and then, after its foundation, at the "Lino Rossi" Research Center, University of Milan, many cases of sudden infant and fetal death have been analyzed, since these institutions have been the referral center for SIDS and late unexplained fetal death of the Lombardy Region, according to the DGR n° 11693 of 06-20-2002. The Italian Law n° 31 of 02-02-2006 "Regulations for diagnostic *post mortem* investigation in victims of sudden infant death syndrome (SIDS) and unexpected fetal death" [2, 33] designates the Institute of Pathology and now the "Lino Rossi" research center of the University of Milan as the national referral center, being a recognized institution competent in this issue.

From even larger series, a total of 120 SIDS victims, 37 infant controls, 63 unexplained stillbirths, 16 unexplained neonatal death victims, and 19 perinatal controls were selected for this work. For each analyzed case, the cardiac conduction system is removed in two blocks for paraffin embedding: block one including the sinoatrial node, and block two including the atrioventricular system. Serial sections of the two blocks are stained alternately with H&E and Trichromic Heidenhain (Azan). The brainstem is divided into four blocks to analyze the brainstem nuclei, in particular, the arcuate nucleus and parabrachial/Kölliker-Fuse complex, using serial sections stained alternately with H&E and Klüver-Barrera stains. The neuronal cell body areas, neuronal density, transverse section areas and volume are evaluated. The carotid bifurcations, cardiac plexus ganglia and paraganglia are embedded separately and serially sectioned. In selected cases, immunohistochemistry studies are performed on sections of the cardiac conduction system, brainstem, and coronary arteries.

Overall, the SIDS-SPUD victims do not show any abnormality of the ordinary myocardium, while the core of the heart, where cardiac rhythm arises and spreads, showed pathological findings in almost all cases, such as impaired resorptive degeneration (in 97% of SIDS, 55% of SPUD cases), AVN/HB dispersion/septation (in 40% of SIDS, 64.5% of SPUD cases), persistent fetal dispersion (in 25% of SIDS and 73% of SPUD cases), accessory pathways, mainly Mahaim fibers (in 29% of SIDS and 20% of SPUD), cartilaginous meta/hyperplasia of the central fibrous body (in 6% of SIDS, 20% of SPUD cases), and dualism of the atrio-ventricular junction (in 3% of SIDS and SPUD cases). Under particular conditions and autonomic neuronal stimulation, the anomalies of the conduction represent the morphological substrates for potentially deadly arrhythmias, generally due to junctional reentry [21, 47–55, 61]. Despite the emphasis given to the association of QT prolongation with SIDS and stillbirth, no conclusions can be reached whenever the postmortem examination does not included an in-depth study of the cardiac conduction system and the brainstem.

The brainstem developmental abnormalities of SIDS-SPUD include long dendritic spines, markers of neuronal immaturity, and hypoplasia of the brainstem nuclei [7–14, 16, 17]. Mono- or bilateral hypoplasia or even agenesis of the ARCn occurs in at least 50% of cases, is pathognomonic and is frequently associated with pulmonary hypoplasia [28, 64]. Hyperplasia of the aorticopulmonary paraganglia was detected in 25% of the victims. Inflammatory foci in the right stellate ganglions were also observed [68–70].

Pre-/early atherosclerosis of the coronary and cardiac conduction arteries has been observed in 50–60% of SIDS-SPUD cases [15, 29, 32, 34, 36, 40, 45, 67] and fibromuscular hyperplasia of the pulmonary arteries has been detected in 7% of SIDS-SPUD cases [60, 63].

The observation of frequent anomalies, mostly congenital, of the autonomic nervous system and cardiac conduction structures, both in SIDS and in SPUD victims, indicates a continuity between these two common forms of death.

The herein presented research upholds a new approach to SIDS which involves the recognition of its analogical link with SPUD. The acronym SIDS-SPUD complex underlines the common morphological substrates and should be routinely adopted. Knowledge of the ante- and *post mortem* aspects of SIDS and SPUD is of international public concern, since its prevention would save a great number of potentially productive individuals.

From the pathologist's viewpoint, different findings have been detected as possible anatomo-pathological substrates: brainstem and cardiac conduction system developmental defects, immaturity of the lungs, and hyper- or hypoplasia of paraganglia and the carotid bodies [21–26, 37, 39, 64, 65]. Overall, the abnormalities detected represent a plausible morphological basis for a reflexogenic SIDS [37, 74–79]. Dive, feigned death, auditory, oculo-cardiac, trigemino-cardiac, vagal cardio-respiratory, Ondine's curse reflexes, if pathological, could lead to SIDS. Indeed, early SIDS may well depend on a postnatal block of respiratory reflexes for fetal survival, involving the parabrachial/Kölliker-Fuse complex, or upon impaired development of central circuitry for respiratory reflexogenesis. Hypoplasia with neuronal immaturity or agenesis of the parabrachial/Kölliker–Fuse has been observed in 35% of perinatal unexplained deaths, particularly intra-partum deaths [12, 13, 46].

The classification criteria for the SIDS-SPUD complex, the criteria for study and the methods of *post mortem* examination are still too multifaceted and little defined as internationally recognized guidelines. Nevertheless, in recent years, further progress in the diagnostic and scientific–instrumental procedures in SIDS-SPUD, "the last diagnosis", have opened to the anatomic and forensic pathologist important new avenues for research in this area.

In order to obtain a correct epicritic diagnosis, anatomic and forensic pathologists are required to analyze, in as complete a way as possible, all morphological aspects of each SIDS-SPUD suspected or diagnosed case. It is necessary that the pathologist applies new tools and methodologies of investigation to each case and acquires a deepening knowledge in order to be able to interpret those signs that may be considered significant.

The cardiac conduction findings in SIDS-SPUD, in association with altered neurovegetative stimuli [54], underlie potentially malignant arrhythmias, providing morphological support for the sudden cardiac death. In fact, the coincidence of other events, such as fever, vomiting or diarrhea and electrolytic imbalance, and active cell death in the conduction system seems to be crucial in causing crib death, whereas cell death and otherwise innocuous events are harmless if they occur separately. It is therefore important to recognize and act upon as many of these contributing causes, including sleeping position, as possible.

Respiratory derangements in infants appear to be predominantly neurogenic in nature since our observations indicate that such derangements can mainly be ascribed to prenatal and/or congenital developmental abnormalities compromising the reflexogenic neuroreceptors, whether central or peripheral. Their anatomical location and their particular functional effects are likely to interfere with the rhythmic and biochemical modulation of breathing and heartbeat. But what makes the problem more complicated is the dichotomous difference in reflexogenic physiology that may even become life-threatening during the pre- and postpartum periods. This may account for the fact that the problem of SIDS is still a perplexing and incompletely understood dilemma, and this has motivated coordinated investigations into the SIDS infant side by side with the SPUD or newborns, such deaths being intimately related to the pathological, anatomical or physiological problem of vital oxygen supply before and after birth [28, 41, 42, 72]. As the exact mechanism of cardiopulmonary failure in SIDS-SPUD is still unknown, all autonomic related central nervous system regions and neurotransmitters are open to further investigation, while much emphasis has been given to the genetic bases of SIDS.

At least five categories of genes are involved in the pathogenesis of SIDS: (1) genes for ion channel proteins involved in cardiac channelopathies; (2) genes for serotonin transporter based on decreased serotonergic receptor binding in brainstems; (3) genes pertinent to the autonomic nervous system (ANS) development; (4) genes regulating inflammation and infections; (5) genes regulating energy production, hypoglycemia, and thermal regulation. It should be stressed – and it could never be stressed enough – that no conclusions on inherited primary arrhythmia syndromes can ever be drawn without an accurate *post mortem* investigation of the cardiac conduction system carried out by an expert cardiovascular pathologist.

The pathologist might not be called to draw conclusions about the clinical conduct and prevention of SIDS, might also be involved too late to avoid the tragedy, yet has to carry out and underline the need for a thorough *post mortem* examination of every SIDS-SPUD victim.

Before submitting a case to molecular autopsy, the necessary cardiac and neuropathological studies must be performed seeking to identify the morphological substrates in sudden unexpected infant and perinatal death. The *post mortem* investigation requires homogeneous and standardized criteria and guidelines. In particular, a complete examination of the cardiac conduction and brainstem in serial sections allows an objective dimensional and architectural evaluation of all the inherent pertinent anatomic areas [31, 38, 44, 54]. This requires many sections and the systematic application of appropriate histological techniques (e.g. H&E, Klüver-Barrera, and trichromic Heidenhain stains), histochemical techniques (e.g. Glees-Marsland for neurons and neurofibrils, Bielschowsky for axons and dendrites, Mallory's PTAH for glia), and immunohistochemical techniques (to study apoptosis, various neuroreceptor structures, the expression of specific genes, etc.), and genetic techniques (e.g. Polymerase Chain Reaction – PCR, DNA Sequencing, etc.).

Such a complete *post mortem* examination system requires the availability of properly trained pathologists and histotechnicians. Furthermore, this study requires numerous histopthological sections, taking a histotechnician approximately one month of full-time work for a cost up to 2,500 Euros for each case. Government institutional funding and research grants have been covering most of these expenses.

A complete examination on serial sections allows an objective dimensional and architectural evaluation of all the pertinent anatomic structures. In fact, due to the architectural variability of the conduction system and brainstem, wrong indications on the involved structures and extension can result from the examination of single and casually chosen sections [31, 54]. It should be underlined that the autopsy protocol for SIDS victims, as already reported [35, 38, 43, 44, 62], should always include examination of the cardiac conduction and central, peripheral and autonomic nervous systems according to standardized guidelines, though this seldom occurs.

The parents or caregivers' neuropsychiatric disorders which may cause an apparently unexplained sudden infant and perinatal death have deliberately not been herein described in details, as the highly specialized medicolegal implications are beyond the pathologist's viewpoint. But it should be always kept in mind that any case of unexpected sudden infant and perinatal death should be considered as a murder until proven otherwise. In particular, the Munchausen syndrome by proxy, in which a psychopathic mother or other caregiver deliberately inflicts child's injuries, causing apnoeic attacks and suffocation [4], might try to involve the pediatrician and subsequently the pathologist in the false diagnostics of apnea-asphyxia-induced SIDS.

The pathological findings and arguments presented herein provide a brief report that wishes to open, rather than conclude, a far-reaching topic and to motivate pathologists, coroners, neonatologists, pediatricians, researchers and all the readers toward a more in-depth postmortem examination and study of the complex scenario sudden infant and perinatal death unexplained death.

In conclusion, it must be stressed that the morphologic examination of the cardiac conduction system and the brainstem on serial sections should be carried out as a gold standard procedure in any unexpected infant and perinatal death to elicit essential findings which are still lamentably lost in routine postmortem investigations, and even in molecular autopsies. In case such an investigation would not be feasible in the local facility, the anatomic specimens should be submitted to the referral specialized anatomo-pathological or medical-forensic centers.

The research will be continued for a better understanding of what is abnormal in the infant and perinatal cardiac conduction and nervous systems and the pathological findings presented herein seem to contribute to the literature for crib death as well as for unexplained perinatal death. To supplement the clinico-physio-pathological findings in infants and term fetuses dying suddenly and unexpectedly, a deeper insight is needed from pathological and molecular genetic research, the extreme specialization of which requires centers with the necessary expertise.

5.1 Review Questions

This test, composed of 10 multiple-choice questions, is designed to measure knowledge about the contents of this chapter on Concluding Remarks on Sudden Infant and Perinatal Unexplained Death. Questions have only one correct answer and cover the major content areas of this chapter. Check the correct responses and score your test using the answer keys on pages 190–191.

51. What is sudden intrauterine unexplained death (SIUD)?
    - □ A. Sudden intrauterine unexpected death (SIUD) is the fetal death before the complete expulsion or removal of the fetus from the mother at any gestational week.
    - □ B. Sudden intrauterine unexpected death (SIUD) is defined as the sudden unexpected death of a fetus from the 22nd gw or of a newborn since birth to the completion of the 1st month of postnatal life that remains unexplained after a thorough investigation of the case, including the review of the clinical history and the performance of a complete *post mortem* examination.
    - □ C. Sudden intrauterine unexplained death (SIUD) is the late fetal death before the complete expulsion or removal of the fetus from the mother

≥22 weeks of gestation or ≥500 gm body mass which is unexpected by history and is unexplained after a thorough pathological exam of the fetus and the fetal adnexa.

□ D. Sudden intrauterine unexplained death (SIUD) is defined as the sudden unexpected death of a term fetus from the 22nd gw or of a newborn since birth to the completion of the 1st month of postnatal life.

□ E. Sudden intrauterine unexplained death (SIUD) is defined as the sudden unexpected death of a term fetus from the 22nd gw or of an infant under one year of age that remains unexplained after a thorough investigation of the case, including the review of the clinical history and the performance of a complete *post mortem* examination.

52. Which of the following statements support the concept of continuity between sudden infant death syndrome (SIDS) and sudden perinatal unexplained death (SPUD)?

□ A. Observation of frequent anomalies of the autonomic nervous and cardiac conduction systems, both in SIDS and in SPUD victims, indicates a continuity between these two common forms of death.

□ B. This research data supports a new approach to SIDS which involves the recognition of its analogical link with SPUD, though the brainstem anomalies have been detected significantly more frequently in SIDS than SPUD.

□ C. There are no pathological findings supporting the SIDS-SPUD complex.

□ D. Observation of frequent anomalies of the autonomic nervous and cardiac conduction systems, both in SIDS and in SPUD victims, indicates a continuity between these two uncommon forms of death.

□ E. This research data supports a new approach to SIDS which involves the recognition of its analogical link with SPUD, though the cardiac conduction anomalies have been detected significantly more frequently in SIDS than SPUD.

53. Which of the following statements on risk factors for SIDS is correct?

□ A. Prone position in the crib has been found to be the most important preventable risk factor for SIDS, based on morphological and functional alterations of brainstem centers.

□ B. Maternal smoking during pregnancy has been found to be the most important preventable risk factor for SIDS, based on morphological and functional alterations of brainstem centers.

□ C. Only few risk factors are considered to be related to SIDS; they can be arbitrarily subdivided into non-amenable to prevention, such as gender, ethnicity, age or amenable to prevention, such as parental cigarette smoking, prone position in the crib, and bed sharing.

□ D. Many risk factors are considered to be related to SIDS; they are all amenable to prevention, such as parental cigarette smoking, prone position in the crib, and bed sharing.

□ E. Many risk factors are considered to be related to SIDS; they are all non-amenable to prevention, such as gender, ethnicity, and age.

54. What is the role of the Parabrachial/Kölliker-Fuse Complex in SIDS-SPUD?
    - □ A. The parabrachial/Kölliker-Fuse complex is a well-understood reflex-blocking center, exerting in the fetus the life-preserving excitatory action upon respiration.
    - □ B. Hypoplasia of the parabrachial/Kölliker–Fuse has been observed in 80% of SIDS-SPUD victims.
    - □ C. Hyperplasia of the parabrachial/Kölliker–Fuse has been observed in 35% of perinatal unexplained deaths, particularly intra-partum deaths.
    - □ D. The parabrachial/Kölliker–Fuse does not have any particular role in the pathology of SIDS-SPUD.
    - □ E. Hypoplasia with neuronal immaturity or agenesis of the parabrachial/Kölliker–Fuse has been observed in 35% of perinatal unexplained deaths, particularly intra-partum deaths.
55. How many categories of genes are involved in the pathogenesis of SIDS?
    - □ A. Five categories: genes for ion channel proteins involved in cardiac channelopathies; genes for serotonin transporter based on decreased serotonergic receptor binding in brainstems; genes pertinent to the autonomic nervous system (ANS) development; genes regulating inflammation and infections; genes regulating energy production, hypoglycemia, and thermal regulation.
    - □ B. Four categories: genes for ion channel proteins involved in cardiac channelopathies; genes for serotonin transporter based on decreased serotonergic receptor binding in brainstems; genes pertinent to autonomic nervous system (ANS) development; genes regulating inflammation and infections.
    - □ C. Three categories: genes for ion channel proteins involved in cardiac channelopathies; genes for serotonin transporter based on decreased serotonergic receptor binding in brainstems; genes pertinent to the autonomic nervous system (ANS) development.
    - □ D. Two categories: genes for ion channel proteins involved in cardiac channelopathies; genes for serotonin transporter based on decreased serotonergic receptor binding in brainstems.
    - □ E. One category: genes for ion channel proteins involved in cardiac channelopathies.
56. Which of the following statements on reflexogenic SIDS are correct?
    - □ A. SIDS is not reflexogenic in nature.
    - □ B. Dive, feigned death, auditory, oculo-cardiac, trigemino-cardiac, vagal cardio-respiratory, Ondine's curse reflexes are all pathognomonic for SIDS.
    - □ C. Dive, feigned death, auditory, oculo-cardiac, trigemino-cardiac, vagal cardio-respiratory, Ondine's curse reflexes could not lead to SIDS.
    - □ D. Abnormalities of the autonomic nervous and cardiac conduction systems, such as hypoplasia of the arcuate nucleus and Mahaim fibers, represent a plausible basis for a SIDS of reflexogenic nature. Dive, feigned death,

auditory, oculo-cardiac, trigemino-cardiac, vagal cardio-respiratory, Ondine's curse reflexes, if pathological, could lead to SIDS.

□ E. Dive is the only reflex that, if pathological, could lead to SIDS.

57. How is a case of SIDS analyzed?

□ A. The cardiac conduction system is removed in one block for paraffin embedding and the brainstem is divided into two blocks. Serial sections are stained alternately with H&E and Klüver-Barrera stains.

□ B. The cardiac conduction system is removed in two blocks for paraffin embedding: block one including the sinoatrial node, and block two including the atrioventricular system. Serial sections of the two blocks are stained alternately with H&E and Trichromic Heidenhain (Azan) stains. The brainstem is divided into four blocks to analyze the brainstem nuclei, in particular, the arcuate nucleus and parabrachial/Kölliker-Fuse complex, using serial sections stained alternately with H&E and Klüver-Barrera stains.

□ C. The cardiac conduction system is not analyzed The brainstem is divided into four blocks to analyze the brainstem nuclei, in particular, the arcuate nucleus and parabrachial/Kölliker-Fuse complex, using serial sections stained alternately with H&E and Klüver-Barrera stains.

□ D. The cardiac conduction system and the brainstem are removed in two blocks for paraffin embedding. Serial sections of the two blocks are stained alternately with H&E and Trichromic Heidenhain (Azan) stains.

□ E. The cardiac conduction system is removed in two blocks for paraffin embedding: block one including the sinoatrial node, and block two including the atrioventricular system. Serial sections of the two blocks are stained alternately with H&E and Trichromic Heidenhain (Azan) stains. The brainstem is not analyzed.

58. Which of the following statements regarding the SIDS-SPUD victims is correct?

□ A. Pre-/early atherosclerosis of the coronary and cardiac conduction arteries and fibromuscular hyperplasia of the pulmonary arteries have not been detected in SIDS-SPUD cases.

□ B. Pre-/early atherosclerosis of the coronary and cardiac conduction arteries and fibromuscular hyperplasia of the pulmonary arteries have been detected in almost all SIDS-SPUD cases.

□ C. Pre-/early atherosclerosis of the coronary and cardiac conduction arteries and fibromuscular hyperplasia of the pulmonary arteries have been detected respectively in 50–60% and 7% of SIDS-SPUD cases.

□ D. Pre-/early atherosclerosis of the coronary and cardiac conduction arteries and fibromuscular hyperplasia of the pulmonary arteries have been detected respectively in 7% and 50–60% of SIDS-SPUD cases.

□ E. Pre-/early atherosclerosis of the coronary and cardiac conduction arteries have been detected in 50–60% of SIDS-SPUD cases. No other artery abnormalities have been observed.

59. In the *post mortem* investigation of SIDS-SPUD which of the following statements is correct?
    - □ A. The morphologic examinations of the cardiac conduction system and the brainstem on serial sections should be carried out as a gold standard procedure.
    - □ B. The investigations should be focused on genetic molecular analyses as gold standard procedures.
    - □ C. The morphologic examination of the cardiac conduction system and the brainstem on serial sections and the genetic anases should both be carried out as gold standard procedures.
    - □ D. The clinical ECG findings of long QT syndrome is diagnostic itself and the clinical findings represent the gold standard in the SIDS-SPUD diagnostics.
    - □ E. The clinical ECG, the pathological and genetic analyses are, all together, the gold standard procedures in the SIDS-SPUD diagnostics.
60. Which of the following statements concerning the Munchausen syndrome by proxy is correct?
    - □ A. The Munchausen syndrome by proxy is a psychiatric disorder which is not a concern to SIDS diagnostics.
    - □ B. In Munchausen syndrome by proxy, a psychopathic mother, prone to self-feigned illness or to self-inflicted injuries, and might try to involve the pediatrician and subsequently the pathologist in false diagnostics, further suggesting the existence of apnea-asphyxia-induced SIDS.
    - □ C. The Munchausen syndrome by proxy is a psychiatric disorder of a psychopathic mother who deliberately self-inflicts injuries, causing apnoeic attacks and suffocation.
    - □ D. In the Munchausen syndrome by proxy a psychopathic mother or other caregiver deliberately inflicts child's injuries, causing apnoeic attacks and suffocation, might try to involve the pediatrician and subsequently the pathologist in false diagnostics, further suggesting the false existence of apnea-asphyxia-induced SIDS.
    - □ E. In the Munchausen syndrome by proxy a psychopathic mother self-inflicts injuries, involving the pathologist in false diagnostics.

5.2 Answer Keys

Block 5 (Questions 51–60)

51. C
52. A
53. B
54. E
55. A
56. D

57. B
58. C
59. A
60. D

References

1. Centers for Disease Control and Prevention (CDC) (2014) Linked birth/infant death records, 2007–2010 results. http://wonder.cdc.gov/lbd-current.html. Accessed July 26, 2014.
2. Constitution of the Italian Republic, February 2, 2006, Law n° 31 (2006) Regulations for diagnostic post mortem investigation in victims of sudden infant death syndrome and unexpected fetal death. Official Gazette of the Italian Republic General Series 34:4. http://users.unimi.it/giuliaottaviani/pdf/legge.pdf. Accessed July 26, 2014.
3. Cotzias CS, Paterson-Brown S, Fisk NM (1999) Prospective risk of unexplained stillbirth in singleton pregnancies at term: population based analysis. BMJ 319:287–288.
4. Craft AW, Hall DM (2004) Munchausen syndrome by proxy and sudden infant death. BMJ 328:1309–1312.
5. Frøen JF, Arnestad M, Vege A, Irgens LM, Rognum TO, Saugstad OD, Stray-Pedersen B (2002) Comparative epidemiology of sudden infant death syndrome and sudden intrauterine unexplained death. Arch Dis Child Fetal Neonatal Ed 87:F118–F121.
6. Kalousek DK, Gilbert-Barness E (1997) Causes of stillbirth and neonatal death. In: Potter's pathology of the fetus and infant. Mosby-Year book, New York, pp 128–162.
7. Lavezzi AM, Ottaviani G, Matturri L (2003) Identification of neurons responding to hypoxia in sudden infant death syndrome (SIDS). Pathol Int 53:769–774.
8. Lavezzi AM, Ottaviani G, Ballabio G, Rossi L, Matturri L (2004) Preliminary study on the cytoarchitecture of the human parabrachial/Kölliker-Fuse complex, with reference to sudden infant death syndrome and sudden intrauterine unexplained death. Pediatr Dev Pathol 7:171–179.
9. Lavezzi AM, Ottaviani G, Mauri M, Matturri L (2004) Hypoplasia of the arcuate nucleus and maternal smoking during pregnancy, in perinatal and infant sudden unexpected death. Neuropathology 24:284–289.
10. Lavezzi AM, Ottaviani G, Matturri L (2004) Involvement of somatostatin in breathing control before and after birth, and in perinatal and infant sudden unexplained death. Folia Neuropathol 42:59–65.
11. Lavezzi AM, Ottaviani G, Matturri L (2004) Role of somatostatin and apoptosis in breathing control in sudden perinatal and infant unexplained death. Clin Neuropathol 23:304–310.
12. Lavezzi AM, Ottaviani G, Rossi L, Matturri L (2004) Cytoarchitectural organization of the Parabrachial/Kölliker-Fuse complex in man. Brain Dev 26:316–320.
13. Lavezzi AM, Ottaviani G, Rossi L, Matturri L (2004) Hypoplasia of the parabrachial/Kölliker-Fuse complex in perinatal death. Biol Neonate 86:92–97.
14. Lavezzi AM, Ottaviani G, Matturri L (2005) Adverse effects of prenatal tobacco smoke exposure on biological parameters of the developing brainstem. Neurobiol Dis 20:601–607.
15. Lavezzi AM, Ottaviani G, Matturri L (2005) Biology of the smooth muscle cells in human atherosclerosis. APMIS 113:112–121.
16. Lavezzi AM, Ottaviani G, Mauri M, Terni L, Matturri L (2005) Involvement of the EN-2 gene in normal and abnormal development of the human arcuate nucleus. Int J Exp Pathol 86: 25–31.
17. Lavezzi AM, Ottaviani G, Mingrone R, Matturri L (2005) Analysis of the human locus coeruleus in perinatal and infant sudden unexplained deaths. Possible role of the cigarette smoking in the development of this nucleus. Brain Res Dev Brain Res 154:71–80.

18. MacDorman MF, Kirmeyer SE, Wilson EC (2012) Fetal and perinatal mortality, United States, 2006. Natl Vital Stat Rep 60:1–23. www.cdc.gov/nchs/data/nvsr/nvsr60/nvsr60_08.pdf. Accessed July 26, 2014.
19. Matturri L, Ottaviani G, Biondo B, Ramos SG, Rossi L (1998) Discrete T-lymphocytic leptomeningitis of the ventral medullary surface in a case of sudden unexpected infant death. Adv Clin Path 2:313–316.
20. Matturri L, Ottaviani G, Rossi L (1999) Sudden and unexpected infant death due to an hemangioendothelioma located in the medulla oblongata. Adv Clin Path 3:29–33.
21. Matturri L, Ottaviani G, Ramos SG, Rossi L (2000) Sudden infant death syndrome (SIDS). A study of cardiac conduction system. Cardiovasc Pathol 9:137–145.
22. Matturri L, Ottaviani G, Lavezzi AM, Turconi P, Cazzullo A, Rossi L (2001) Expression of apoptosis and proliferating cell nuclear antigen (PCNA) in the cardiac conduction system of crib death (SIDS). Adv Clin Path 5:79–86.
23. Matturri L, Lavezzi AM, Ottaviani G, Alfonsi G, Crippa M, Rossi L (2002) Anatomopathological techniques for the study of brainstem in sudden infant death syndrome (SIDS) and unexpected late fetal stillbirth. In: Proceedings of the 7th SIDS International Conference, Florence, pp 131–132.
24. Matturri L, Lavezzi AM, Ottaviani G, Rossi L (2002) Anatomia patologica della sindrome della morte improvvisa del lattante (SIDS) e della morte inaspettata del feto. In: Proceedings of the National Symposium "Sudden Infant Death Syndrome (SIDS) and Sudden Unexplained Intrauterine Death", Milan, pp 13–23.
25. Matturri L, Lavezzi AM, Rossi L (2002) Proposal to modify the definition of SIDS, with regard to the post-mortem exam. In: Proceedings of the 7th International Conference on SIDS, Florence, p 103.
26. Matturri L, Minoli I, Lavezzi AM, Cappellini A, Ramos S, Rossi L (2002) Hypoplasia of medullary arcuate nucleus in unexpected late fetal death (stillborn infants): a pathological study. Pediatrics 109:E43.
27. Matturri L, Ottaviani G, Rossi L (2002) Should overdone external cardiac massage in infants dying of SIDS be discouraged? In: Proceedings of the 7th International Conference on SIDS, Florence, p 136.
28. Matturri L, Lavezzi AM, Minoli I, Ottaviani G, Cappellini A, Rubino B, Rossi L (2003) Association between pulmonary hypoplasia and hypoplasia of arcuate nucleus in stillbirth. J Perinatol 23:328–332.
29. Matturri L, Lavezzi AM, Ottaviani G, Rossi L (2003) Intimal preatherosclerotic thickening of the coronary arteries in human fetuses of smoker mothers. J Thromb Haemost 1: 2234–2238.
30. Matturri L, Ottaviani G, Rossi L (2003) External cardiac massage in infants. Intensive Care Med 29:1199–1200.
31. Matturri L, Ottaviani G, Alfonsi G, Crippa M, Rossi L, Lavezzi AM (2004) Study of the brainstem, particularly the arcuate nucleus, in sudden infant death syndrome (SIDS) and sudden intrauterine unexplained death (SIUD). Am J Forensic Med Pathol 25:44–48.
32. Matturri L, Ottaviani G, Corti G, Lavezzi AM (2004) Pathogenesis of early atherosclerotic lesions in infants. Pathol Res Pract 200:403–410.
33. Matturri L, Ottaviani G, Lavezzi AM (2004) Autoptic examination in sudden infant death syndrome and sudden intrauterine unexpected death: proposal of a national law. J Matern Fetal Neonatal Med 16(Suppl 2):43–45.
34. Matturri L, Ottaviani G, Lavezzi AM, Rossi L (2004) Early atherosclerotic lesions of the cardiac conduction system arteries in infants. Cardiovasc Pathol 13:276–281.
35. Matturri L, Ottaviani G, Benedetti G, Agosta E, Lavezzi AM (2005) Unexpected perinatal death and sudden infant death syndrome (SIDS): anatomopathologic and legal aspects. Am J Forensic Med Pathol 26:155–160.
36. Matturri L, Ottaviani G, Lavezzi AM (2005) Early atherosclerotic lesions in infancy: role of parental cigarette smoking. Virchows Arch 447:74–80.
37. Matturri L, Ottaviani G, Lavezzi AM (2005) Sudden infant death triggered by dive reflex. J Clin Pathol 58:77–80.

38. Matturri L, Ottaviani G, Lavezzi AM (2005) Techniques and criteria in pathologic and forensic-medical diagnostics in sudden unexpected infant and perinatal death. Am J Clin Pathol 124:259–268.
39. Matturri L, Ottaviani G, Lavezzi AM (2005) Unexpected sudden death related to medullary brain lesions. Acta Neuropathol (Berl) 109:554–555.
40. Matturri L, Ottaviani G, Lavezzi AM, Grana D, Milei J (2005) Madres fumadoras y atherosclerosis prenatal. Rev Argent Cardiol 73:366–369.
41. Matturri L, Ottaviani G, Lavezzi AM, Ramos SG (2005) Peripheral chemoreceptors and sudden infant death syndrome: a wide open problem. Curr Cardiol Rev 1:65–70.
42. Matturri L, Ottaviani G, Lavezzi AM (2006) Maternal smoking and sudden infant death syndrome: epidemiological study related to pathology. Virchows Arch 449:697–706.
43. Matturri L, Giuliani P, Lavezzi AM, Ottaviani G, Minoli I, Colombi R, Nespoli L, Agosti M, Bulgheroni C, Cannatelli G, Farneti A, Lodi F, Cappellini A, Cattoretti G, Vergani P, Tagliabue P, Mosca F, Boffi R, Malaguti E, Merlino L, Lucchina C (2007) Protocollo diagnostico. Indagine anatomo-patologica e medico legale sulle vittime della sindrome della morte improvvisa del lattante (SIDS) e della morte inaspettata del feto. Regione Lombardia Sanità, Milan.
44. Matturri L, Ottaviani G, Lavezzi AM (2008) Guidelines for neuropathologic diagnostics of perinatal unexpected loss and sudden infant death syndrome (SIDS) – a technical protocol. Virchows Arch 452:19–25.
45. Milei J, Ottaviani G, Lavezzi AM, Grana DR, Stella I, Matturri L (2008) Perinatal and infant early atherosclerotic coronary lesions. Can J Cardiol 24:137–141.
46. Morpurgo CV, Lavezzi AM, Ottaviani G, Rossi L (2004) Bulbo-spinal pathology and sudden respiratory infant death syndrome. Eur J Anaesthesiol 21:589–593.
47. Ottaviani G, Ramos SG, Matturri L (1997) Defective "resorptive degeneration" of the heart's conduction system and sudden infant death syndrome. Ann Españ Pediatr 92(Suppl):53.
48. Ottaviani G, Goisis M, Ramos SG, Matturri L (1998) Dispersione del tessuto giunzionale e sue conseguenze in un caso di morte improvvisa del lattante. Cardiologia 43:737–739.
49. Ottaviani G, Matturri L, Ramos SG, Rossi L (1998) Resorptive degeneration of the heart's conduction system and sudden infant death syndrome: preliminary results. In: Proceedings of the 5th SIDS International Conference, Rouen, p 156.
50. Ottaviani G, Rossi L, Bondurri A, Ramos SG, Matturri L (1998) Morte improvvisa del lattante: un caso di sdoppiamento del nodo atrio-ventricolare. Riv Ital Pediatr 24:1165–1167.
51. Ottaviani G, James TN, Rossi L, Matturri L (2002) Significance of Mahaim fibers in crib death. In: Proceedings of the 7th SIDS International Conference, Florence, p 136.
52. Ottaviani G, Matturri L, Lavezzi AM, Rossi L, James TN (2002) Postnatal apoptosis of the cardiac conduction system in crib death: preliminary results. In: Proceedings of the 7th SIDS International Conference, Florence, p 132.
53. Ottaviani G, Matturri L, Rossi L, James TN (2002) Crib death: further support for the concept of fatal cardiac electrical instability as the final common pathway. In: Proceedings of the 7th SIDS International Conference, Florence, p 66.
54. Ottaviani G, Matturri L, Rossi L, James TN (2003) Crib death: further support for the concept of fatal cardiac electrical instability as the final common pathway. Int J Cardiol 92:17–26.
55. Ottaviani G, Lavezzi AM, Rossi L, Matturri L (2004) Sudden unexpected death of a term fetus in a anticardiolipin positive mother. Am J Perinatol 21:31–35.
56. Ottaviani G, Matturri L, Bruni B, Lavezzi AM (2005) Sudden infant death syndrome "gray zone" disclosed only by a study of the brain stem on serial sections. J Perinat Med 33:165–169.
57. Ottaviani G, Rossi L, Matturri L (2005) Myocardial injury attributable to external cardiac massage in infants. Cardiology 1:25–29.
58. Ottaviani G, Lavezzi AM, Matturri L (2006) Sudden infant death syndrome (SIDS) shortly after hexavalent vaccination: another pathology in suspected SIDS? Virchows Arch 448:100–104.
59. Ottaviani G, Matturri L, Mingrone R, Lavezzi AM (2006) Hypoplasia and neuronal immaturity of the hypoglossal nucleus in sudden infant death. J Clin Pathol 59:497–500.
60. Ottaviani G, Matturri L (2007) Fibromuscular hyperplasia of the pulmonary artery in sudden infant and perinatal unexpected death. 8th World Congress of Perinatal Medicine. Florence, Italy. J Perinat Med 35(Suppl):229.

61. Ottaviani G, Matturri L (2008) Histopathology of the cardiac conduction system in sudden intrauterine unexplained death. Cardiovasc Pathol 17:146–155.
62. Ottaviani G (2008) Sudden infant death syndrome (SIDS) – Standardised investigations and classification: Recommendations. JMSR 1:11–12.
63. Ottaviani G, Lavezzi AM, Matturri L (2009) Fibromuscular hyperplasia of the pulmonary artery in sudden infant and perinatal unexpected death. Cardiovasc Pathol 18:223–230.
64. Ottaviani G, Mingrone R, Lavezzi AM, Matturri L (2009) Infant and perinatal pulmonary hypoplasia frequently associated with brainstem hypodevelopment. Virchows Arch 454:451–456.
65. Ottaviani G (2010) In utero exposure to smoking and peripheral chemoreceptor function. Pediatrics [E-letter]. http://pediatrics.aappublications.org/content/125/3/e592/reply. Accessed July 26, 2014.
66. Ottaviani G (2011) Sudden infant and perinatal unexplained death: are we moving forward yet? Cardiovasc Pathol 10:302–306.
67. Ottaviani G (2012) Sudden death and coronary intimal thickening. Cardiovasc Pathol 21:e31–e32.
68. Ramos SG, Matturri L, Biondo B, Ottaviani G, Rossi L (1998) Hyperplasia of the aorticopulmonary paraganglia: a new insight into the pathogenesis of sudden infant death syndrome? Cardiologia 43:953–958.
69. Ramos SG, Matturri L, Ottaviani G, Rossi L (1998) Maternal smoking and aorticopulmonary paraganglia in sudden infant death syndrome. In: Proceedings of the 5th SIDS International Conference, Rouen, p 169.
70. Ramos SG, Ottaviani G, Biondo B, Rossi L, Matturri L (1999) Hyperplasia of the aorticopulmonary paraganglia in infants dying of SIDS: further supports for the cardio-respiratory hypothesis. In: Proceedings of the International Symposium on SIDS and Lombardy Region project for the reduction of the risk for sudden infant death and unexplained intrauterine death, Milan, pp 117–128.
71. Roberts D (2003) Histopathologic correlates of intrauterine fetal death. In: Proceed. Gynecologic and Obstetric Pathology Conference, Harvard Medical School, Boston.
72. Rossi L (1999) Bulbo-spinal pathology in neurocardiac sudden death of adults: a prognostic approach to a neglected problem. Int J Legal Med 112:83–90.
73. Rossi L, Matturri L (1988) His bundle haematoma and external cardiac massage: histopathological findings. Br Heart J 59:586–587.
74. Rossi L, Matturri L (1990) Clinicopathological approach to cardiac arrhythmias. A color atlas. Centro Scientifico Torinese, Turin.
75. Rossi L, Matturri L (1991) Anatomohistological features of sudden infant death. New Trends Arrhyt 6:135–142.
76. Rossi L, Matturri L (1995) Anatomo-histological features of the heart's conduction system and innervation in SIDS. In: Rognum TO (ed) Sudden infant death syndrome: new trends in the nineties. Scandinavian University Press, Oslo, pp 207–212.
77. Rossi L, Matturri L (1995) Cardiac conduction and nervous system in health disease and sudden death: an anatomoclinical overview. Osp Maggiore 89:239–257.
78. Schaller B, Cornelius JF, Prabhakar H, Koerbel A, Gnanalingham K, Sandu N, Ottaviani G, Filis A, Buchfelder M, Trigemino-Cardiac Reflex Examination Group (TCREG) (2009) The trigemino-cardiac reflex: an update of the current knowledge. J Neurosurg Anesthesiol 21:187–195.
79. Schaller B, Cornelius JF, Sandu N, Ottaviani G, Perez-Pinzon MA (2009) Oxygen-conserving reflexes of the brain: the current molecular knowledge. J Cell Mol Med 13:644–647.
80. Stillbirth Collaborative Research Network Writing Group (2011) Causes of death among stillbirths. JAMA 306:2459–2468.
81. Willinger M, James LS, Catz C (1991) Defining the sudden infant death syndrome (SIDS): deliberations of an expert panel convened by the National Institute of Child Health Development. Pediatr Pathol 11:677–684.

Acronyms and Abbreviations

AAP	American Academy of Pediatrics
ALTE	Apparent life-threatening event
ARCn	Arcuate nucleus
AV	Atrio-ventricular
AVJ	Atrio-ventricular junction
AVN	Atrio-ventricular node
Azan	Azocarmine aniline blue stain of Heidenhain (stain)
CCS	Cardiac conduction system
CDC	Centers for Disease Control and Prevention
cm	centimeter
ECG	Electrocardiogram
gm	gram
gw	gestational week
h	hour
HB	His bundle
H&E	Hematoxylin and eosin (stain)
LBB	Left bundle branch
lPB	Lateral parabrachial (nucleus)
LQT	Long QT (syndrome)
LW/BW	Lung weight/Body weight (ratio)
min	minute
mm	millimeter
mPB	Medial parabrachial (nucleus)
ms	millisecond
N/A	Not applicable
NICHD	National Institute of Child Health and Human Development
NICU	Neonatal intensive care unit
P	Pacemaker (cells)
PB/KF	Parabracial/Kölliker-Fuse (complex)
RAC	Radial alveolar count
RBB	Right bundle branch

G. Ottaviani, *Crib Death - Sudden Infant Death Syndrome (SIDS): Sudden Infant and Perinatal Unexplained Death: The Pathologist's Viewpoint*,
DOI 10.1007/978-3-319-08347-6

SAN	Sinoatrial node
SCP	Superior cerebellar peduncles
SEM	Standard error of the mean
SIDS	Sudden infant death syndrome
SIUD	Sudden intrauterine unexplained death
SNUD	Sudden neonatal unexplained death
SPUD	Sudden perinatal unexplained death
TCR	Trigemino-cardiac reflex
WPW	Wolff-Parkinson-White (syndrome)

Index

G. Ottaviani, *Crib Death - Sudden Infant Death Syndrome (SIDS): Sudden Infant and Perinatal Unexplained Death: The Pathologist's Viewpoint*,
DOI 10.1007/978-3-319-08347-6

GPSR Compliance

The European Union's (EU) General Product Safety Regulation (GPSR) is a set of rules that requires consumer products to be safe and our obligations to ensure this.

If you have any concerns about our products, you can contact us on ProductSafety@springernature.com

In case Publisher is established outside the EU, the EU authorized representative is:

Springer Nature Customer Service Center GmbH
Europaplatz 3
69115 Heidelberg, Germany

Batch number: 10837161

Printed by Printforce, the Netherlands